Understanding Perioperative Nursing

Edited by

Kate Nightingale BA, RGN, RMN, RNT

Nurse Educator and former Editor of the British Journal of Theatre Nursing

A member of the Hodder Headline Group
LONDON • SYDNEY • AUCKLAND

First published in Great Britain in 1999 by
Arnold, a member of the Hodder Headline Group,
338 Euston Road, London NW1 3BH

http://www.arnoldpublishers.com

© 1999 Arnold

British Library Cataloguing in Publication Data
A catalogue record for this book is available from the British Library

ISBN 0 340 70573 6

1 2 3 4 5 6 7 8 9 10

Commissioning Editor: Cathy Peck
Production Editor: Rada Radojicic
Production Controller: Priya Gohil
Project Editor: Paula O'Connell
Cover Design: Terry Griffiths

Typeset in 10/12pt Palatino by Saxon Graphics Ltd, Derby
Printed and bound in Great Britain by JW Arrowsmith Ltd, Bristol

What do you think about this book? Or any other Arnold title?
Please send your comments to feedback.arnold@hodder.co.uk

Understanding
Perioperative Nursing

Contents

Contributors

Bernadette Brennan RN, RNFA, Dip App Sc, FRCNA
Nurse Consultant, Bernadette Brennan Nurse Consultants and Healthcare Planners, Victoria, Australia

Margaret Brett SRN, FETC, Dip N(Lon), Dip N Ed(Lon), RNT, MA
Nursing Senior Lecturer, Perioperative Nursing, South Bank University, London, UK and Past President of AORNA

Libby Campbell OBE, MSc, RGN, RM
Director of Nursing and Quality, West Lothian NHS Trust, St John's Hospital, Livingston, West Lothian, UK and Past National Chairman of NATN

Ann-Carol Carrington RGN, DPSN
Theatre Staff Nurse (Nurse Bank), Day Procedure Unit, Solihull Hospital, Solihull, West Midlands, UK

Jennifer Cunningham RN, COTN, BN (Syd), MCN(NSW)
Nurse Educator, Perioperative Nursing Courses, The New South Wales College of Nursing, Sydney, New South Wales, Australia

Menna Davies RN, CM, COTN, BHSc(N), MHSc(N), FCN(NSW)
Nurse Educator, Perioperative Nursing Courses, The New South Wales College of Nursing, Sydney, New South Wales, Australia

Suzanne Fullbrook LLB (Hons), MPhil, RGN
Barrister and Independent Lecturer. Contact: Margaret Brett, Nursing Senior Lecturer, South Bank University, London, UK

Barbara J Gruendemann RN, MS, CNOR, FAAN
Educator, G4 Productions, Dallas, Texas, USA

Gitta Hutt BA, BSc (Hons), RGN, Dip OHN
Occupational Health Adviser, Metropolitan Police Service, London, UK and former Deputy Editor of the *British Journal of Theatre Nursing*

Doreen Kalideen MA BEd (Hons), RGN, Dip N(Lon), RCNT, Cert Ed(FE)
Primary Lecturer in Nursing, Nightingale Institute, King's College, London, UK

Inger Lönroth
Perioperative Nurse, Operating Department, Sahlgrenska University Hospital, Göteborg, Sweden

Kate Nightingale BA, RGN, RMN, RNT
Nurse Educator and former Editor of the *British Journal of Theatre Nursing*, UK

Colin Rees BSc, MSc, PGCE(FE)
Lecturer, School of Nursing Studies, University of Wales College of Medicine, St Cadoc's Hospital, Caerleon, Gwent, UK

Jane Rothrock DNSc, RN, CNOR
Professor of Perioperative Nursing and Past President of AORN, Delaware County Community College, Delaware, USA

Nicole Nightingale Sinclair
Formerly Territory Manager for Ethicon Endo Surgery (NE Scotland) and Olympus Keymed Ltd (Scotland), UK

Marilyn Williams RGN, Dip N, BSc (Hons), PGDE
Senior Lecturer, University of Wolverhampton, School of Nursing and Midwifery, UK

Foreword

The book you are holding has been developed by a nursing leader known to perioperative nurses in many parts of the world. Kate Nightingale, past editor of the *British Journal of Theatre Nursing*, has always brought her expertise to whatever project she is involved in and this book is no different. She has drawn together subjects of importance to perioperative nurses who are studying for a degree, but the book goes well beyond such a singular intent. Indeed, all of us are trying to meet the increasing demands of teaching and learning in an environment characterised by rapid change, enormous amounts of information and less time. The subject matter of this book is relevant to our learning, but more importantly, it encourages us to think. Whether you are a student or practising nurse, this book is a wonderful reference manual. You will find an extensive list of references to substantiate the validity of the information presented and which serves to simultaneously encourage your additional investigation.

Organisation of the book

The organising principles of this book permit you to look at the past, our current environment and to speculate about the future. Chapter 1 sets the stage by exploring the development of this speciality since the 1970s as we have moved from the initiation of education and training programmes, working diligently to stay abreast of the current changes in our field, only to find ourselves faced with new and more challenging issues in the 1990s. Subsequent chapters review these challenges, delving into topics such as planning patient care, advanced practice, education for perioperative nursing, research, minimally invasive surgery and infection control. The reader is presented with the essential principles that we must all embrace as we manage risk and maintain quality, become leaders, learn to manage change and acquaint ourselves with important concepts of the legal and ethical premises governing our practice and provoking dilemmas in everyday patient care. Finally, we are provided with the development of perioperative nursing within Europe, a review of political influences that have shaped our history and will shape our future, and then reminded of the value of education in charting that future.

Unifying principle

If there is one thing that we could point to as we describe what we are all about, the reason we are who we are and do what we do, it is the principle of caring. Caring is an elusive concept, individualised to each encounter and yet is at the same time paradoxically universal to us all. It brings together the things we do each day with our heads (as we think through what is needed for this patient); our hands (as we get all the things ready for this patient); and our hearts (as we attend to the special needs, fears and worries that this patient comes with). Thus, we are a thinking, doing, caring group of professional nurses who have a specialised body of knowledge based on the basic sciences, research and humanism. Our importance to a patient during a critical life event such as surgery requires us to blend our scientific use of knowledge with the therapeutic use of self in an act of caring, supporting, teaching and bonding.

Let us look at each of these a little more closely. In the operating department, we 'do' many things. In fact, to the untrained observer, it may appear that we are just doing things, but it is in the 'doing' of those things that we demonstrate care and caring. Doing more is what we do every time we do things that go beyond what is just required for the surgery to get accomplished. When you do more, you reach out to the patient, get closer to them and take more time than might usually be required. Despite everything else that is going on in that operating room, you focus on the patient, acknowledging their concerns and needs, so you can provide care that meets those needs. You make eye contact, offer emotional support and use a soft, concerned tone of voice. You comfort and connect with that patient.

'Doing for' is when you primarily respond to a patient's request. You are pleasant and considerate as you give assistance. This 'doing for' is characterised by the little things you do each and every time, with each and every patient. 'Doing with' is when you have something to do and you involve the patient in it. You seek the patient's feelings and perceptions. 'How does this feel? Are you cold? I'll get you a warm blanket. Do you need a pillow under your back so you are more comfortable?'

In all of these things that we do, we use touch. We use caring touch when we want to soothe, quiet, reassure or encourage our patient. This kind of touch demonstrates your caring and concern every time you use it. We also use protective touch in many of the things we do: moving the patient, positioning, applying devices and equipment so the patient is not injured.

Concluding remarks

One of the things that is special and unique about perioperative nurses around the world is the care we provide every day to our patients. Caring for and about patients has been described as the central focus of nursing's body of knowledge and our practice as nurses. People who are sick, in need, or undergoing a frightening life event like surgery need caring from their perioperative nurse. This book, in its many facets, is a celebration of that caring. All over the world perioperative nurses are working to define and redefine themselves in the midst of constant new scientific advances and the changing needs of society. As we engage in this transition, we need to find our own voice and speak of our contributions and accomplishments. We are coming of age as a caring profession and this is where we were destined to be. Our caring practices are grounded in ancient and timeless traditions. In order to get where we need to be, we have to see anew the art and science of human caring in our nursing practice, to shed light where there has been darkness. This book, in no small measure, reflects the spirit of the Nightingales – Kate and Florence – in allowing us to experience and feel the warm rays of light and energy that shine forth from the spirit of caring.

Jane C Rothrock DNSc, RN, CNOR

Preface

As I have edited this book it has become increasingly clear to me that the term perioperative nurse or perioperative nursing must be adopted and finally accepted by those who have resisted its introduction. I hope I have edited out all terms such as 'theatre nurse' or 'operating room nurse' and replaced them by 'perioperative nursing', though old habits die hard.

Some nursing organisations have already changed their names to include the word 'perioperative' and I know others are thinking about it. Some of those organisations have well-loved titles and snappy acronyms by which they are well known, so it is quite a wrench to think of changing. APN, NAPN, ACPN or EPNA do not have quite the familiar ring of AORN, NATN, ACORN or EORNA. Perhaps we can keep the acronyms but change the names?

Why do I feel that 'perioperative nurse' is a good description? Firstly, it describes a specific area of nursing practice that has now been defined and agreed globally. It is not just stating where a nurse works, or with whom she works. It is nurse and patient-focused, and can be applied in different situations. I know some groups have tried to hijack the use of the term, but I think that this book will show clearly what perioperative nurses mean when they use the term.

This book has not been written as a textbook. I make no apologies to those who feel that there are aspects of perioperative practice which may be missing from the book. The authors were invited to contribute and given a free hand on how they addressed their brief. Nearly all of them are senior nurses who have regarded themselves throughout their professional lives as primarily perioperative nurses. Many of them have moved on to other areas during their career. Most of them have other qualifications and it is this second qualification which has added a new depth to their writing. This further education in management, education, research, the law, occupational health and experience in industry, higher education or higher levels of management has given a new perspective to the discussions.

I regard each chapter as a contribution to the debate on perioperative nursing which I believe needs to be carried out as publicly as possible. National and international groups, conferences, seminars and masterclasses are wonderful and contribute largely to the body of knowledge. They also inspire those who attend, but too often we preach to the converted. By inviting some of those inspirational speakers to contribute to this book I hope to bring some of their wisdom to a wider audience, an audience which includes both nurses and others.

I know that one of the criticisms levelled at a book like this will be that it ignores the existence of those non-nursing members of the staff of operating departments. Perioperative nurses share their working days, not only with surgeons, anaesthetists and other health professionals, but with non-registered technicians and operating department practitioners who share many of their skills and, in some instances, add their own special skills to the work of the operating team. Sometimes there can be conflict, more often there is mutual respect and joint efforts to achieve high standards of practice and quality patient care. This book is about perioperative nurses and is about nursing issues which is why it concentrates primarily on nursing.

Kate Nightingale BA, RGN, RMN, RNT

Acknowledgements

I would like to express my gratitude to all those who have contributed to this book and whose names appear in the book. Their contributions to perioperative nursing have been much greater than mine.

I would like to dedicate the book to past and present members of the Editorial Board of the *British Journal of Theatre Nursing*, in particular to Isobel Curry who edited the journal for 15 years and inspired many of us to put pen to paper.

PART ONE

The development of perioperative nursing

The past as prologue to the future

Kate Nightingale

This chapter is concerned with perioperative nursing as an element in the development of professional nursing. It looks back at events during the last hundred years to link developments in health care systems with developments in nursing, more especially with those nursing activities carried out before, during and after surgery.

Local initiatives as well as broader ideas have affected the process by which perioperative nursing became a separate and specialist branch of nursing. An eclectic selection of extracts from nursing literature has been used alongside the main text to illustrate contemporary attitudes and values of the branch of the profession we now know as perioperative nursing. The argument advanced in this chapter is that perioperative practice has not been entirely isolated behind the closed doors of the operating department, elitist and behind the mask, but that the social and political context of the times and professional changes have had an unavoidable effect on the perioperative nurse.

Nursing as an occupation began to grow towards professionalism in a world which did not yet hold the belief that the state had an obligation to ensure the health and wellbeing of all its citizens, including those who worked for little financial reward. The medical profession was powerful and paternalistic; nursing, then a strictly female occupation apart from mental nursing, had only begun to move along the road leading to slow recognition as a profession.

The nursing profession itself has not always been ready to recognise the particular competences of those members we now call perioperative nurses, possibly because, initially, all nurses were expected to have some training to assist in the operating department. Working in a variety of capacities before, during and after surgery and anaesthesia, perioperative nurses are aware that they must preach not only to the converted but must access other nurses and non-nurses to demonstrate their contribution to the care of all surgical patients. They also have specialised knowledge and skills to contribute to the education and training of other nurses who are now being increasingly called upon to assist in day and outpatient surgery.

Most of the comments in the chapter are based on changes in the UK. However, despite variations in the health systems and operating departments of different countries, the ideological bases from which health systems grew are common throughout the Western world. At the end of the 20th century, perioperative nurses across the globe face many of the same issues, share the same ideas and are learning from each other to make innovations in practice.

Nursing is defined by the society in which it is practised. It is sometimes hard for nurses to realise this as the legal and professional limitations of their role and function are mediated through the statutory body which controls the profession. In recent years the changing philosophies and policies underpinning health care have brought this fact home to all nurses. Only rarely have nurses worked as independently accountable practitioners in the past. Only recently has the nursing literature broadened to include issues beyond the practical skills of patient care or sharp reminders on appropriate and deferential behaviour on duty. The expectations of those for whom and with whom they have worked have also influenced the content of nurses' work. This is true as much for perioperative nurses as it is for any other nurse.

Before considering the political changes which have affected health care during the reforms of the last 20 years, a brief review of some significant social changes attempts to throw light on the attitudes and relationships within operating department teams. Nursing, as a recognised occupation, has been growing for little more than 100 years and, as a profession, for much less time than that. The society which saw the birth of nurse training after 1860 was very different from the society of today and there have been many social and political changes during that time.

Ideology and the health services

During the 19th century, hospitals were developing and dedicated operating theatres were being built to provide a dedicated area for surgery. The relationship between the medical staff using the hospitals and the staff preparing the theatre and assisting the surgeon was different from that in the public hospitals of today. Surgeons had honorary appointments to the hospital, often their own teaching hospital. They had their own male assistants, box carriers,

Collectivism

The reforming governments of the early years of the 20th century introduced a number of welfare initiatives including the first old age pensions and a non-contributory national insurance scheme in response to information from a number of private and public investigations into poverty. Recruitment for the Boer War had also shown up the poor health and physique of a high proportion of young men and led to an investigation into physical deterioration and the development of the concept of 'national efficiency'. Politicians began to realise that government had a responsibility to ensure that the population remained healthy and able to contribute to the common weal. This was the beginning of the 'collectivist' approach to health and welfare (Peden, 1995, pp.15–32).

The first major change of view expressed by an official body was the Minority Report of the Royal Commission on the Poor Laws and the Relief of Distress. This (minority) report was written by the Fabians, Beatrice and Sidney Webb, and signed by several other members of the Commission including the London socialist, George Lansbury, and a future Bishop of Birmingham. The minority report was concerned that the Poor Law approach was a policing exercise, concerned with keeping down costs of relief rather than providing state support intended to make it easier for individuals to help themselves. Suggestions included transfer of responsibilities from the Poor Law Guardians to the new local authorities with specialist departments responsible for education, asylums and health and the creation of a national authority with responsibility to oversee local authorities in areas such as unemployment relief (Clarke *et al.*, 1992, pp.50–51). This is a shift in position which would be pursued for the future of the welfare state. Doctors were, as usual, politically involved but we do not hear too much of the political opinions of nurses of the time.

Medical attitudes

An interesting light is cast on the attitudes of doctors at the beginning of this century by the British Medical Association (BMA) response to national health insurance. The government realised that they needed the cooperation of the medical profession and had the awful example of a medical strike in Leipzig in 1904 to demonstrate what could happen without the doctors. The BMA wanted a state medical service, but on their terms, to give them a safe and substantial income. Competition between doctors for the friendly societies' work had forced fees down at a time when voluntary hospital funds were low. To ensure secure incomes doctors wanted to restrict national insurance to those with an annual income under £100, leaving other workers to be treated as before, as private patients. Lloyd George, however, insisted on £160 minimum income but did not succeed in forcing this through until 1912 (Peden, 1995, p.29).

> **1914**
> **War Office. *Royal Army Medical Corps Training*. 1911**
> **reprinted 1914. London, HMSO. (Price ninepence)**
>
> This textbook is for doctors in the RAMC who are involved in training orderlies. Sisters of Queen Alexandra's Imperial Nursing Service are occasionally mentioned.
>
> The chapter on surgical nursing concentrates on two principles: cleanliness and rest.
>
> ### Sterilisation and cleaning of instruments
>
> Instruments except knives are sterilised by boiling. They are put into boiling water to which one per cent of bicarbonate of soda has been added, and are boiled for 10 minutes. Knives should not be boiled as it blunts their edges. They may be sterilised by being wiped with pure carbolic on a sterilised swab, then placed in ether for ten minutes, or be sterilised in other ways according to the instruction of the surgeon ...
>
> After boiling or sterilising, instruments are placed in trays containing carbolic lotion 1 in 60 by means of a pair of sterile forceps; on no account must they be touched with the hands. Should an instrument be dropped or touch anything while being conveyed to the tray, it must be resterilised immediately. After use instruments are washed in tepid water, scrubbed with soap and water and bicarbonate, rinsed in water and dipped into methylated spirit.

Changing attitudes

This century has seen a realisation that people are not out of work and poor because they are feckless but, rather, that mass unemployment is the result of the changes in society following industrialisation and technological advances. Keynesian economic theories have shown politicians that labour and capital do not always balance out in response to market forces. A healthy economy could exist with large scale unemployment. We have seen a further resurgence of unemployment in our own times and renewed condemnatory attitudes to those out of work among those in work and paying taxes.

Keynesian economics

Following the labour disputes of the 1920s, Maynard Keynes grasped that managing the market did not necessarily lead to full employment and that governments must manage the demands on the economy, considering five factors:

- national income
- consumption

- private investment
- government expenditure
- exports and imports.

Before Keynes, taxation was raised to balance the budget. With the advent of Keynesian economics it was possible to work with a budget deficit to allow government intervention to reduce unemployment. Keynes died in 1946, but his theories of budget management published in 1936 have continued to be used by government and reinterpreted by other economists until 1976, when it was replaced by monetarist economic policies. These focus on control of the money supply (Johnson, 1994, pp.192–3).

1935
Rutherford Darling, H.C. 1935 *Surgical nursing and after treatment. A handbook for nurses and others*, 5th edition. London, J.A. Churchill

The chapter on ligatures and sutures includes detailed instructions on the preparation and sterilisation of catgut, silk, linen, not to mention kangaroo tendon. The description of saline solutions indicates that the importance of different concentrations are being recognised:

Strong salt solution (a solution consisting of 5% and 2% sodium chloride) has recently been used in the treatment of wounds ... although inducing a copious flow of serum from a wound ... (it) has a repellent action against the migration of leucocytes ...

A whole chapter is devoted to the operating theatre which has some familiar features, a Plenum ventilation system, scialytic lighting, for instance:

Electricity is best for the artificial lighting ...

The diagram of the places of the scrubbed team around the table is familiar (Figure 1.2).

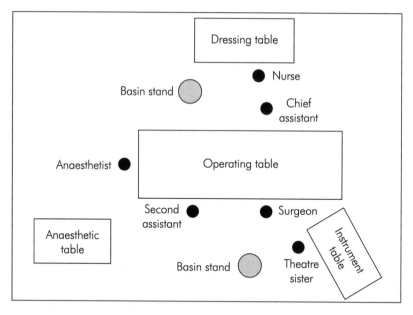

Figure 1.2 An interesting diagram of a recommended theatre layout from 1935. Note the position of the scrub nurse and theatre sister. Also recommended were an oxygen cylinder and an emergency table to make up saline infusions. From: Rutherford Darling, H.C. 1935 *Surgical nursing and after treatment,* p. 186.

Water is sterilised by the use of boiled water tanks which were in use in many modern operating theatres until the early 1970s. A room is provided for scrubbing used mackintoshes before they are re-sterilised and high pressure steam sterilisers have now appeared.

Surgery may still be carried out at home. Phenol, or carbolic, is still recommended for use on floors and walls. The operating table may be a portable affair brought by the surgeon or one selected in the patient's own house:

> Care should be taken to select a table with firm strong legs as the operator and his assistant may lean on it and this, combined with the weight of the patient, would be liable to break off the legs if they were rickety or weak.

Improvisation is the order of the day.

Surgical Instruments
Instruments for what we would call a 'general set' are as follows:

- 2 scalpels
- 2 dissecting forceps
- 12 artery forceps (Spencer Wells)
- 2 probes (large and small)
- 1 director
- 3 scissors (straight, curved and angular)
- 2 retractors

- 2 aneurism (sic) needles
- 6 suture needles (straight, three-eighths and half circle)
- 2 needle holders
- 6 towel holding forceps.

For incising abscess or opening sinus:

- 1 Volkman's spoon
- 1 sinus forceps (Lister's).

There is not much on general anaesthesia except in relation to preparing the theatre and postoperative care but spinal anaesthesia and the use of avertin as a rectal anaesthesia are included.

This information came from the textbook quoted above (Rutherford Darling, 1935), written by an Australian surgeon and dedicated to the Australian Trained Nurses' Association, but published in London. The aspects which were regarded as essential for training nurses in the operating department were already related to the technical aspects of assisting the surgeon and anaesthetist. More general aspects of patient care were assumed to be part of the nurse's general training. Notice that it is still largely surgeons who write the textbooks but there is some consultation and recognition across boundaries. Assumptions are made about the reliable qualities of the trained nurse but her duties are still of a very practical nature as instructed by the surgeon.

The welfare state

We find it difficult to think ourselves into the attitudes and concerns of the past including the belief that each person was solely responsible for their own well-being and should work to ensure the health and prosperity of self and family.

The term 'welfare state' is often associated with Archbishop Temple's famous wartime comparison between the 'power state' of Nazi Germany and the 'welfare state' to be achieved after the war. A welfare state was to be concerned with the individual welfare of all members of the state in contrast to protection of the wellbeing of the state as a whole which would be ensured in a power state (Pierson, 1991, p.102).

During the 1930s and 1940s, the growth of rational social planning, utilising experts like Beveridge and Keynes, made it feasible to envisage a state in which the whole population would be able to realise equality of opportunity, full employment and the end of poverty.

The Beveridge Report (1942) encapsulated the aims of the British welfare state:

New Britain should be free, as free as possible, of the five giant evils, of Want, of Disease, of Ignorance, of Squalor and of Idleness.

Beveridge (1943, p.81).

These were seen as ideals worth fighting for to ensure both preventive and therapeutic care for all. The shift in public opinion was carefully nurtured during the war and social reform was planned for when peace arrived.

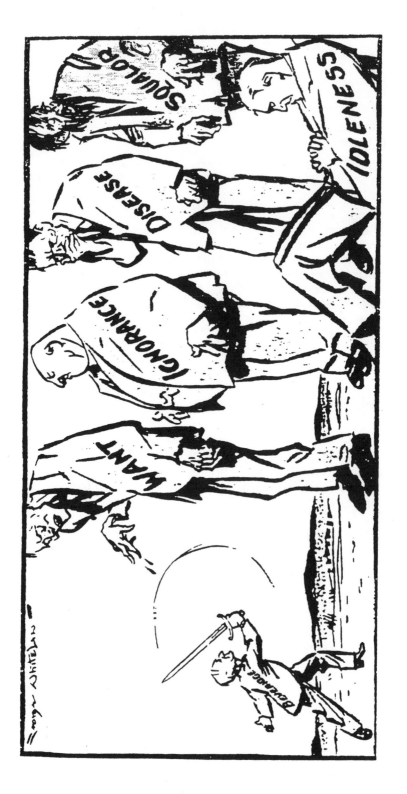

Figure 1.3 This cartoon appeared in the *Daily Herald* newspaper in 1942. Beveridge saw idleness as the greatest of these evils because he saw full employment as the most effective way to promote individual health and wellbeing. Reprinted from Johnson 1994.

Looking back from the uplands of 50 years' experience we can see that it was never going to be easy. Nor is it easy to remember the idealism and hope in the minds of those who saw the coming welfare state as an answer to the social evils that had become so obvious during the development of the industrial world and the recent World War. Most of us have practised throughout our professional lives in a health service built on these collectivist principles which have formed our attitudes to our patients and to our working practices.

1954
Gration, H.M. & Holland, D.L. 1954 *The practice of nursing*, 4th edition. London, Faber & Faber

This textbook is, at last, written by nurses for nurses. The care of the patient is dealt with in some detail in the body of the book whilst a section devoted to 'The Operating Theatre' is included later in the book. Patients are routinely admitted 2 days preoperatively to allow a thorough physical and psychological preparation.

> Five minutes before going to theatre the bladder must be emptied ... The patient must be sent to theatre comfortably warm but in hot weather it is important to see that she is not so warm as to perspire as a considerable amount of fluid can be lost by the skin in this manner ... Common sense should dictate how many blankets should be put over the patient.

The nurse who accompanies the patient to theatre expects to stay until the patient is anaesthetised:

> It gives the patient confidence if someone who knows her is present. She may like to grip the nurse's hand.

In the postoperative period, patient care focuses on keeping the patient comfortable and, in principle, is not so far from modern nursing care though not so technical. For instance, half a page is devoted to nursing actions to encourage the patient to pass urine if there is a degree of retention.

The chapter on the operating theatre is for those nurses who are assisting in theatre. It begins by evaluating aseptic and antiseptic techniques, emphasising that the aseptic method is now fully accepted, and details some of the disadvantages of using carbolic so widely. It goes on to describe the geography of theatres, clothes of the staff and daily routine, including the daily 'wet-dusting' routine and the use of 'recovered' spirit to polish glass and shiny surfaces.

> Unnecessary traffic in and out of theatres is avoided.

A sister or senior nurse selects instruments from the cupboard and wraps them in a towel and places them on a labelled tray for sterilisation. Drums of sterile towels are put out. Lifting forceps are ready to lift instruments. Sterilisers (boilers) are brought to the boil. Scrub sinks are provided with soap, scrubbing brush and a bowl of disinfectant. Drums of sterile gowns, masks and gloves are put out with several pairs of Cheatle (lifting) forceps in disinfectant.

The patient is positioned on the table by two nurses whilst the theatre sister is in charge of the whole procedure.

The nurse watches each step carefully and tries to anticipate the wants of the surgeon. To do this she must be intelligent and alert and listen carefully to his remarks as he goes along. With experience, the nurse assisting the surgeon learns the technique of the various operations and is able to save time by her efficiency. This time factor is important in the prevention of shock ...

Large swabs which have been introduced into a cavity are counted before the surgeon closes the cavity ... black tapes may be attached to these swabs so that they are readily recognisable.

Little is disposable and needles and sharp instruments are kept in trays of lysol after boiling for 20 minutes. Sharps are sterilised by 3 minutes soaking in pure lysol. Hot air ovens are now in use for syringes, glass and hypodermic needles.

This operating theatre would look familiar in general layout though there are no disposables and no electronic monitors as routine. Less storage space is needed but more changing and preparation areas as the department would wash, recycle and re-sterilise its own instruments, gowns and gloves as well as other equipment.

This brings us to within 50 years of the present and despite the fact that authors claim to write for their own clinical areas or their own hospital, it is already possible to see that there has been interchange of ideas over considerable areas. Surgeons are still dictating practice though some nurses have gained considerable recognition and respect. There is no mention in these textbooks of health policies, managers or costs. Excellence was the aim, not value for money. Patients are told what is best for them, not given any choices.

1962
Brigden, J.R. 1962 *Operating theatre technique.* Edinburgh, E & S Livingstone

This was an early textbook for specialist operating department nurses 'and others', written by a nurse who was familiar with and committed to the speciality. It was until very recently an essential item on the bookshelf of every operating department in the UK (see also Clarke & Jones, 1998).

The preface to the first edition is illuminating. It shows how technical patient care in the operating theatre had now become. For instance:

The chapters on electricity and static electricity have been included because it is felt that these subjects are of increasing importance to theatre staff. A better understanding of electrical apparatus and lighting will ensure a sensible approach to the use of such equipment in a modern operating theatre.

Emphasis has been placed upon a packet system of sterilisation and the use of heat rather than chemicals whenever possible.

Although nylon has been described as a wrapping material, it is accepted that many units are using paper or linen for this purpose.

This is, of course, a matter of individual preference.

The chapter on ligatures and suture materials has been made comprehensive in order that it may be used for reference.

The instruments described for various operations are those in common use and are arranged in sets. Substitution of instruments may be necessary according to a surgeon's individual preferences, but those shown should be adequate for the particular procedure.

The outline of procedures for each operation is not intended to replace the many excellent textbooks on operative procedure, but rather to act as a general guide and handy source of reference. The reader is referred to the appropriate surgery textbook if further details are required.

Imperfections and criticism

There have been paradoxical results from the development of a welfare state. The expected reduction of sickness with reduced demands on the health services has not occurred and better social policies have not banished poverty despite increasing economic progress. The increasing costs of health care and rising patient expectations about the affordability of health services have created problems in advanced countries, whether the health care system has been primarily based on a public health care system or whether it has been based on a system of personal health insurance. Attempts to resolve the economic problems, rising costs and scarce resources, have brought both systems closer together in recent years, ready to explore alternative ways to cost-effectiveness. By 1985 the welfare state was subject to criticism from both political wings. The consensus across the political spectrum which had supported the welfare state broke down. The Conservative government of the day, claiming that the health service was safe in their hands, launched a Green Paper which proposed a radical restructuring based once more on a narrow, *laissez-faire* 'market' ideology (DOH, 1989).

The market-oriented NHS

The 1948 welfare state was built on a fully-employed population who would easily pay enough contributions to support the unfortunate few who were ill or out of work. By the 1980s there was:

- rising unemployment
- deepening poverty of women
- deepening poverty of ethnic groups

- alienation of the young
- an economic recession.

The increased demands on the health services were, as a result, far greater than the reduced financial contributions from national insurance even when supported from taxation and by payment for some services at point of delivery.

Once again there was a resurgence of the idea of self-help with pressure to take steps to insure self and family before problems arose. The Thatcher government philosophy stated that individuals should take responsibility for the wellbeing of themselves and their family. This was a time of market-oriented satisfaction of personal needs, of conspicuous consumption. The reformed National Health Service went forward based on an internal market with the money following the patient. The general practitioners, the purchasers, controlled the money as they bought in services for their patients from service providers, mainly the hospitals.

The New Right

The New Right can be defined as a group of people who hold monetarist, market-oriented ideas. Its propositions are that:

1 Individualism and freedom are co-dependent, but they accept some collective protection is required against poverty in the way of old age pensions and sickness and unemployment pay.

2 Bureaucratic administration to meet needs of individuals will overload the system and lead to unequal distribution of resources. It is more efficient for people to pay for what they need.

3 Universal free services provided by the state benefit the middle classes more than the poor.

4 Free or subsidised welfare creates shortages which would be removed by the operation of market forces.

5 Welfare benefits encourage dependency on the state.

6 Welfare costs tend to rise, thereby increasing taxation and reducing enterprise (Peden, 1995, pp.216–18.)

The New Right Conservative government, under Margaret Thatcher and John Major, questioned both the efficiency and the objectives of the welfare system in general, and the health service in particular. They argued that only 'the market' had the ability to respond to changing needs and to satisfy them cost-effectively, hence the introduction of an 'internal market' with purchasers and providers across the health service. Health professionals were concerned at this perceived attack and the early 1990s saw concerns with professional roles and limits of professional responsibility.

1992

UKCC. 1992 *The scope of professional practice*. London, UKCC

In 1992 the UKCC document, *The scope of professional practice* clarified the move from task-oriented training by defining the principles for nursing practice. It recognised the need to meet patient or client needs, the need to maintain competence and to acknowledge limits to meeting patient needs. More importantly it pointed out the individual accountability of a nurse and the fact that enlarging the scope of professional practice must not interfere with the existing aspects of nursing practice and care. There was also a recognition of the need for collaboration within health care teams (UKCC, 1992, p.6). In considering the extension of nursing practice the section concludes:

> The reality is that the practice of nursing, and education for that practice, will continue to be shaped by developments in care and treatment, and by other events which influence it ...

> In order to bring into proper focus the professional responsibility and consequent accountability of individual practitioners it is the Council's principles for practice rather than certificates for tasks which should form the basis for adjustments to the scope of practice (p.8).

The New Right, as evinced in the nearly 20-year span of Conservative rule from 1979, were also concerned with the monopoly position of the medical profession. The government was not able to give the health consumers the financial power they would have liked because of the public feelings for the Health Service. Neither privatisation nor the use of 'health vouchers' was an option (Johnson, 1994, pp.369–70).[1]

Purchasers or patients

The transformation of the NHS from 'service' to 'market' saw the patients changed into customers, consumers who were offered choices whilst the purchasers, on their behalf, expected quality. Hence, we saw the emergence of consumer and management practices which were often copied from those already introduced in the growing private health care sector. Quality assurance, risk assessment, clinical and financial audits and resource management became the management tools of the time (Lowe, 1993, pp.320–22).

The first reactions of the professions to new policies implemented by newly powerful managers was resistance and resentment at interference with their clinical standards and a threat to their professional power (Hugman, 1991). It is not easy to ignore the way in which such profound social and political changes have impinged on our roles and practice. It was even less easy for apolitical nurses to be aware of the changing ideology which resulted in the changes. An understanding of the way in which political and economic pressures, past, present and future, have directly and indirectly influenced nursing practice can help perioperative nurses to make decisions about the way forward as health policies change and, in turn, cause changes in the way nurses are expected to work.

Minimal access therapy as a catalyst

ORGANISATIONAL

The coincidental growth of minimal access therapy (MAS) gave politicians and managers an opportunity to meet changed patient expectations by offering day surgery units and 'ambulatory' surgery. The early rapid development of day surgery was patient-driven and took place, in large part, in the private sector. Patients saw day surgery as a convenient way of controlling the time and place of their operation with a minimal time in hospital before and after the procedure. All of this was true, but put pressure on surgeons and institutions to move forward rapidly. Managers and politicians, however, saw this clinical development as a new means to achieve economies in the health services. Late admission and early discharge can be seen as a way to reduce the cost of a single operative episode, but it also increases the number of operations which can be completed in a given time. In the private sector, where costs are passed on directly to the patient, this increases income. In a public health service where the day surgery is funded by a fixed budget, it increases the costs over a given time. In a market-oriented service, the day surgery service will be funded by the demands of the purchaser and limited by the resources of the purchasers.

CLINICAL

Minimal invasive therapy became a catalyst for many other changes of the 1990s – development of day-care units, team working, multiskilling and skill mix changes. Professional organisations, manufacturers and individuals have cooperated to set up training courses. Doctors cooperated with nurses to enable nurses to take over preassessment of patients and with Trusts to allow advanced nurse practitioners to run day surgery units. By allowing a nurse manager to run the unit, prepare and provide the services and follow up patients with pain control services and other postoperative care, managers and doctors found that efficiency, as measured by non-show rates, for example, and by patient satisfaction, was improved (Neasham, 1996).

In addition to the financial management lessons, nurses gained new insights into aspects of perioperative nursing care in the day surgery units which were built in response to the growth of minimal access interventions. Isolated from confusion with the care given by other nurses it was now possible to see the full scope of perioperative nursing care. It was also possible to see how perioperative nurses could extend their practice preoperatively and postoperatively in new ways. One possible aspect for the future is the increased development of outreach into the community by perioperative nurses, especially in the control of pain and distress following surgery.

Professional advances

Demographic effects

Demographic changes have continued to be unpredictable but influential. The rise in the birth rate affected unemployment in the 1920s; declining birth rates before 1941 reduced family size and, thereby, poverty in the 1940s; by 1950 the population was visibly ageing and the 1960s, despite the advent of the contraceptive pill, saw a 'baby boom' (after Feinstein in Johnson, 1994, pp.94–6). The predicted 'demographic time-bomb' of the 1980s which was to have such a devastating effect on nursing recruitment did not materialise as expected, though a major reorganisation of nursing and nurse education did go ahead. Instead, we have seen a reduction of qualified nursing posts, a change in the role and function of many nurses and an increase in the use of unregistered staff in hospitals.

The role and function of the nurse

The concern of professional nurses over the blurring of roles and overlap of duties has led to a number of initiatives to define professional nursing practice much of which has been included in UKCC publications and other professional strategy documents (UKCC, 1992); (Scottish NNMCC, 1992). This has not occurred too early for perioperative nurses as it has helped them to define their nursing role and function, and their perioperative nursing role, despite what has been added to or taken away from the jobs which they were currently filling (NATN, 1996).

1992
Scottish National Nursing and Midwifery Consultative Committee. 1992 *The role and function of the professional nurse*. Edinburgh, Scottish Office

In 1991 the Scottish National Nursing and Midwifery Consultative Committee (NNMCC) examined and defined the future role of the nurse, midwife and health visitor and their interface with support workers. They defined the key aspects of the role and function of the professional nurse as follows:

- The planning of nursing required for each individual patient.
- The delivery of direct care.
- Identifying when it is appropriate for the nursing care to be undertaken by those without a professional nursing qualification.
- Preparing and supporting those who do not have a professional nursing qualification to undertake such activities as are delegated to them by the professional nurse.

- The effective and efficient management and organisation of the resources of personnel, equipment and services directly controlled or requisitioned by the professional nurse.
- Standard setting, nursing audit and clinical audit.

Such documents, backed up by publications from perioperative nursing associations, have been of considerable use to perioperative nurses as they develop new roles, work in teams and become involved in skills sharing.

More recently, as nurse preparation moves from training into higher education, nurses worldwide felt the need to define themselves and their practice and to develop a knowledge base for nursing practice that is patient-centred, uses a problem solving approach, and identifies and meets the holistic needs of the patient (WHO, 1977).

Following the emphasis laid by the World Health Organization on the role of the nurse in promoting health across the world, the profession, worldwide, has redefined nursing to focus on assisting patients to maintain or regain health or to compensate for deficiencies in the ability to do that (WHO, 1985).

1977

World Health Organization. 1977 *The nursing process. Report on the first meeting of a technical advisory group*. Geneva, WHO

From the 1970s nursing went through a major change from a purely skills based vocational activity to a practical profession basing activities on a sound theoretical basis, though not without criticism. The nursing process was defined by the WHO as a 'system of characteristic nursing interventions':

In detail it involves the use of scientific methods for identifying the health needs of the patient ... and for using these to select those which can most effectively be met by nursing care; it also includes planning to meet these needs, provide the care and evaluate the results. The nurse in collaboration with other members of the health care team and the individual ... being served, defines objectives, sets priorities, identifies care to be given and mobilises resources. He/she then provides the nursing services either directly or indirectly. Subsequently he/she evaluates the outcome ... In this way, nursing becomes a dynamic process lending itself to adaptation and improvement.

Nursing was starting to be seen as capable of creative decision made as the result of applying sound theory and expertise to care situations.

Specialist nurse practitioners

As the first nurses to specialise and become involved in the more technical aspects of surgery, perioperative nurses have experienced some difficulties in justifying their inclusion as specialist nurses within the new limits of the profession (Casey, 1993). Perioperative nurses, worldwide, have always believed that the need for nursing care does not cease purely because the patient is unconscious or out of the ward and would wish to point out that the addition of technological aspects to their role does not obviate their ability to practice the nursing skills needed to meet the sometimes urgent needs of a patient at a particularly stressful time. The American Association of Operating Room Nurses (AORN) was the first perioperative nursing body to define the responsibility of the professional nurse caring for the patient during the perioperative period as:

> The identification of the physiological, psychological and sociological needs of patients, and the implementation of an individual program of nursing care that co-ordinates the nursing actions based on a knowledge of the natural behavioural sciences, in order to restore or maintain the health and welfare of the patient before, during and after surgical intervention.
>
> AORN (1969).

Nursing and anaesthetic practice

As perioperative nursing roles increase, an important issue is the changing relationships between nursing, surgical and anaesthetic practitioners in the operating department. It would be impossible to address the proliferation of perioperative nursing roles without mention of the relationship between nurses and anaesthetists. In the USA, operating room nurses were joined in the department by nurse anaesthetists. Some European countries followed the American example. Even though nurse anaesthetists have worked there, the UK, Canada and Australia have been slow to adopt this second anaesthetic professional, preferring to opt for anaesthetic nurses.

Anaesthetic and recovery nurses have sometimes seen themselves as separate from theatre nurses, perhaps because many of them came into the operating department from a ward or critical care background and had not worked with the surgical team during an operation. This is one area where local solutions to skill mixes have created anomalies. However, the difference between a nurse anaesthetist and anaesthetic nurse is more than one of semantics. It defines whether the person concerned practices as a nurse or as an anaesthetist and defines his or her accountability. By 1997, the UK and Australia remain as the countries whose anaesthetists resist the addition of nurse anaesthetists to the anaesthetic team. Whether different initiatives in other countries or politico-economic pressures on the health services will result in a re-thinking of this approach is yet to be seen.

The issue highlights the fact that there is a variety of ways in which the role of the specialist perioperative nurse can be advanced. Some of these are explored in this book. There are many other opportunities – in research, in education, managerially in a variety of routes and, now, clinically as assistant to the surgeon.[2]

Perioperative practitioners

The period from 1970 saw the development of theatre technicians, orderlies and porters into non-professionalised but respected and well-trained members of the operating department team. The development of such initiatives as vocational training in the UK and the role of non-licensed assistants in the USA caused this group of theatre workers, also, to consider ways of enhancing their status and job satisfaction. The gradations and duties of operating department staff became bafflingly complex even across a single health authority as so many different practitioners became integrated into theatre teams. Despite seeing many similar political and professional changes on a worldwide basis, operating departments have always been subject to local change to meet the organisational and clinical needs in individual centres. It is these initiatives to meet the demands on the theatre teams which have resulted in the varied job demarcations in operating departments.

Medical and nursing professionals, with traditional values rooted in their belief in the pre-eminence of their own hospital and the limits of the accountability and knowledge base of their own profession, have been defining their own practice at local level for many years. Surgeons dominated their own operating room, working for the benefit of their own patients, their own hospital and their own practise and success. In the 20 years from 1960, perioperative nurses made great professional strides, sharing conferences and learning from each other across national boundaries, setting clinical standards, defining curricula and finding solutions to common problems. Indeed, perioperative nurses are now well known as one of the groups of nurses who have a strong and meaningful international voice.

By the mid-1980s, expectations of citizens, who are, by definition, potential patients, were greater and the ability to meet those expectations was increasing all the time (DOH, 1991). However, the means to investigate and treat patients, especially by surgery, was ever more expensive. Governments realised that a crisis in welfare and health care was upon them and required major reform. This had enormous and unexpected repercussions for all health care professions, not least for perioperative nurses. The advances, led until then by perioperative nursing associations, had now to come into line with wider changes in the nursing profession and have had to adapt to the repercussions of the health care reforms.

New initiatives

Salvage (1988) has criticised nursing in the UK for being too concerned with a professionalisation which is not in step with the reality of nursing work. She felt that there should have been a model of 'occupational authority' rather than a

covert bid for professionalism. Perioperative nurses have pursued the occupational authority model for some considerable time and found themselves in a
position where they were open to the criticism of neglecting real nursing work.

Globalisation

It was the need for peer support which led to national and international
networking. In the early days much of the work was related to sharing experience of working conditions, considering working practices and setting standards for practice and training. The Association of Operating Room Nurses
(AORN) took the lead in establishing international links, planning and organising the biennial World Conference of Operating Room Nurses (WCORN) and
establishing overseas chapters of their association whilst nurses from many
countries attend the AORN Congress as well as other national conferences,
including the National Association of Theatre Nurses (NATN) Congress in the
UK. The European Operating Room Nurses Association (EORNA) developed
from informal links in the early 1980s, well supported by those countries, such as
the UK, whose associations had already forged ahead with perioperative
education and standard setting. EORNA was originally intended to include only
those countries belonging to the European Union but now has representatives
from an increasing number of European perioperative nursing associations.

An early priority was seen to be a European Common Core Curriculum
for operating department nurses (Brett, 1997) which was published in 1997
to coincide with the first European (EORNA) conference held in Brussels.
Canada and Australia, also leading centres of perioperative nurse
education, have responded to the particular needs of their widespread and
sparsely populated countries by developing distance learning theatre
courses, initiatives which have been taken up across the Pacific (NSW
College of Nursing, 1993).[3]

1997
Brett, M.(ed). 1997 European common core curriculum for operating department nursing. Edinburgh, EORNA

As the European Union developed, operating nurses became one of the first groups
of nurses to develop networks. An early aim was to work towards standardisation
of operating room practice across Europe. This led to the development of a
common core curriculum flexible enough to be interpreted within the standards of
the nursing body of each member country.

Philosophy

- Individuals undergoing anaesthetic and/or invasive surgical procedures have the
  right to be cared for by appropriately qualified staff in a safe supportive
  environment whilst in the preoperative department.

- Those qualified and experienced staff working within the multidisciplinary team should be expected to perform in a competent manner, displaying an awareness of current developments in research and knowledge relating to the operating department and perioperative care.
- A systematic approach to holistic care should maintain the identity and dignity of each individual patient without prejudice to health status, their nationality, creed or other beliefs.
- Both the patient, the relatives and any significant others are entitled to receive the necessary information and physical and emotional support needed to help them through the stages of perioperative care.

The contents of the curriculum have moved far beyond the basic skills training of the earlier part of the century and include understanding of the history and development of nursing in general and perioperative nursing in particular. The knowledge base required also includes attitudes towards health, society and individual patients and personal and professional development.

Post-registration specialisation, such as perioperative nursing, is now seen as requiring education to first degree level, at least, and ultimately to master level. There has been considerable discussion on how one should define 'degree level practice'. How does such advanced practice differ from the lower level practice of the recently qualified nurse practitioner?

The work done by perioperative nursing associations has been important in ensuring that both nursing and technical aspects of perioperative practice remain a part of the postgraduate education and training of perioperative nurses whilst bearing in mind the educationalists' work on the elements of advanced practice. The positive result has been inclusion once more in the broad mainstream of nursing.

Localisation

Witz (in Gabe *et al.*, 1994, pp.23–41) points out that nursing eventually validated itself by the standardisation and control of nurse education. She also points out that nursing interests have only succeeded when they coincide with the interests of more powerful groups.

As power was decentralised in the health service, local needs began to influence training and educational needs once more. The variety of new roles and moves to meet service needs compounded the confusion. The shortage of doctors has influenced decisions by politicians and managers to promote the enhancement of nursing roles in new ways. Only nurses were in a position to take over some of the functions carried out by doctors. It is also more cost-effective to employ a nurse than a doctor. The presence of more highly educated and autonomous nursing practitioners fitted well with both managerial needs to replace junior doctors after the health reforms and the aspirations of nurses. In operating departments unlicensed practitioners and assistants took over many routine jobs whilst specialist nurses developed advanced roles. These processes continue whilst strategy and consultative groups refine their recommendations.

As postgraduate nurse education moved into the universities, individual centres were able to approve curricula to meet local needs. Medical and nursing roles have begun to overlap in a number of new ways – surgeons' assistants posts have been created and filled by nurses in a variety of ways, preassessment of patients for day surgery is increasingly carried out by nurses, nurse practitioners are surgical unit managers. Much soul-searching to explain how a nurse, a doctor and a non-registered operating department assistant can all have the same jobs as part of their practice has been needed to clarify some of the confusion. Concepts such as multiskilling, team care and collaborative care and the broadening and clarification of the scope of nursing practice (UKCC, 1992) and deeper understanding of the true nature of accountability have resulted as the professions seek to resolve some of the issues.

1996: NATN Position Statement
NATN, 1996 *The scope of perioperative practice, British Journal of Theatre Nursing* **6 (5), 49**

By this time specialist nursing organisations such as NATN, were publishing guidelines for their own specialist practitioners. This position statement drew attention to already published documents and defined the following principles to be followed when developing new perioperative nursing roles:

- Parameters of the role
- Training and education required
- Professional implications
- Ethical and legal considerations
- Managerial issues.

Such documents and strategic initiatives have become a necessary support for nurses when roles are being extended or changed.

Flexible working practices

The NHS Management Executive in their review of skill mix in operating departments (Dyson & Naylor 1992) identify the restrictive practices which account for such skill mix variations as:

- Professional rules: right of professions to withdraw training approval.
- Custom and practice: medical preferences and formal protocols.
- Labour supply: recruiting and retaining staff.
- Budgetary constraints: need to retain an essential but expensive service.

The paper goes on to outline ways in which the theatre manager or director can introduce flexibility into the operating department. It concentrates particularly on the use of multiskilling, the sharing of skills between professionals within a team, and the effective use of well-supervised support workers. It is this road which has been followed in many centres. A particularly interesting aspect of this paper was the recognition given by a government department to decisions reached by surgeons and perioperative nurses themselves, perhaps not always implemented in the way in which the professionals had envisaged (Bevan 1989; NATN, 1990).[3]

Perioperative nurses have always worked as team members. Flexibility within that team, rather than being disapproved of, is now an accepted part of life in health care. Now that employers clearly define what they allow their staff to do and what they are insured to do, practitioners themselves are less rigid about the limits of their practice but more aware of their accountability. Nurses have found that the acquisition of new skills and the development of responsible and interesting roles which fit in with the new health care ideologies and with modern philosophies of nursing need not erode nursing practice and autonomy. They have also discovered that 'flexibility' can be a double-edged tool when used to reduce staff numbers and keep within budget limits.

1990
Rothrock, J.C. 1990 *Perioperative nursing care planning.* St Louis, Mosby

Rothrock makes a significant remark in the preface to *Perioperative nurse care planning*:

> You must make the patient care you deliver evident.
> We cannot afford to keep this our secret.

Activities dictated by the policy of the institution or as part of the medical regime can be completed without awareness of individual needs. Management of the patient's environment can be achieved in a standardised way without considering the unique needs of each patient. The perioperative nurse meets needs of the individual by a preoperative nursing assessment to plan the care to be delivered before, during and after surgery. Taking over the junior doctor's role in completing medical preassessment or in achieving pain control combines well with the nursing priority to meet the needs of individual patients.

Conclusion

Despite the reorganisation by the 'New Right' governments, health services are still facing economic problems. Many surgical procedures drain enormous resources in preoperative diagnoses and workups as well as in the cost of effective operations with prolonged after care. The increase in life expectancy means that many who live longer also make greater demands on surgical services. Not only do patients have greater expectations but, as 'knowledgeable consumers' they find themselves more ready to criticise if all is not well.

There has been a swing away from punitive right wing governments to social democratic regimes, but there can be no return to the bright morning of the early collectivist welfare state now we know that no juggling of public medicine can treat an increasingly dependent population at low cost whether funding is found from the public purse or supplemented from private resources. We have recently lived though a crisis in welfare provisions which was painful for some, involving as it did major reorganisations, restrictions and demoralisation. The welfare state remains a dominant institution in modern states but it will change. We no longer live in a world which accepts state obligation to fill the gap completely when people cannot meet their own health needs. New Left governments appear to be reaching a new consensus with the New Right on a market-oriented approach to funding the welfare state. Pierson (1991) proposes two methods to do this. One is what he calls 'enhancement of citizenship'. This could mean an increase in the voluntary sector of health care, setting a minimum level of rights only. The other is an increase in investment, an increased commitment to collective ownership of the economy, perhaps as compulsory state insurance.

> For many, the crisis was real enough, but is now passing ... Questions about the relationship between economic and social policy, between employment and income, between political decision making, between state and market, between this and subsequent generations, will have to be addressed anew. When they are, the consensus presently formed around the market may look no stronger than the consensus which once seemed to cocoon the welfare state.
>
> Pierson (1991).

Will Hutton, editor of the *Observer* believes that we should not worry about the rise of public expenditure and higher taxes as they are necessary to public services such as health and that such a 'stake holder' economy opens the way to a better democracy. He also points out that we, the people, have the final responsibility for the way forward as it is we who vote in the government (Hutton, 1997). Nurses have a further responsibility. The health services remain technocratic and centralised. Managers and consultants still have their hands on the levers of power. As Rothrock (1990) said, we cannot afford to keep our contributions or our views a secret. They must be made public for the sake of both perioperative nurses and their patients.

Reflective activities

This chapter has been presented in a style which has reviewed the political and economic developments alongside developments in the nursing profession which have particularly affected perioperative nurses. Perioperative nurses, as represented by their professional organisations, have never lost sight of their accountability as nurses whilst being aware of the importance of the technical aspects of their work. At first these specialist nursing organisations were concerned with setting standards for practice but during recent years these same organisations have cooperated with educators and used their journals to integrate the caring and technical aspects of perioperative nursing practice.

Use the selected excerpts from perioperative nursing literature quoted in this chapter to consider how nursing during the perioperative period has developed (pp.7–10 and 21–8).

1 Identify principles of operating department practice which were already recognised as part of the role of the nurse during the first part of the century. Reflect on the reasons for nursing in the operating department being seen as an essential part of a nurse's experience at the time whilst, nowadays, some nursing schools no longer regard this as essential. Can this be a mistake in this time of rapid change?

2 How did new nursing theories and philosophies help perioperative nurses to identify and develop their unique role?

3 Using your own experience and refering to this chapter, consider both politico-economic and organisational factors which have contributed to making the perioperative nurse of today very different from her or his predecessor in 1900.

Endnotes

1 For further information on the New Right criticism of state welfare and comparison with Victorian *laissez-faire* ideas see:
Frederick von Hayeck's *Road to Serfdom* (1944) Routledge and Keegan Paul.

2 Bernadette Brennan explores new advanced perioperative roles in Chapter 3 and compares developments across the world.

3 See Menna Davies' and Jennifer Cunningham's interesting chapter on the development of distance learning for perioperative nurses in Australia (Chapter 4, pp.79–99).

References

AORN Statement Committee. 1969 Definition and objectives for clinical practice of professional operating room nursing. *American Operating Room Journal* **10** (5), 43–8.

Bevan Report. 1989 *Management and utilisation of operating departments.* London, NHSME, HMSO.

Beveridge, W. 1942 *Social insurance and allied services.* Cmnd. 6404. London, HMSO.

Beveridge, W. 1943 *The pillars of security* and other wartime essays and addresses. London, George Allen & Unwin.

Brett, M. (ed.) 1997 *European Common Core Curriculum for Operating Department Nursing.* Edinburgh, EORNA.

Brigden, J.R. 1962 *Operating theatre technique.* Edinburgh, E & S Livingstone.

Cameron, H.C. 1954 *Mr Guy's Hospital. 1726–1948.* London, Longman's, Green & Co.

Casey, N. 1993 Editorial. *Nursing Standard* April, **7** (31), 3.

Clarke, J., Cochrane, A. & Smart, C. 1992 Ideologies of welfare. *From dreams to disillusion.* London, Routledge.

Clarke, P. & Jones, J. 1998 *Brigden's Operating Department Practice.* Edinburgh, Churchill Livingstone.

DOH. 1989 *Working for patients.* Cmd. 555. London, HMSO.

DOH. 1991 *The Patient's Charter.* London, HMSO.

Dyson, R. & Naylor, A. 1992 *Skill mix issues and choices in hospital theatres.* (For the Personnel Development Unit, DOH.) London, HMSO.

Feinstein, C.H. 1972 *Statistical tables of national income, expenditure and output of the United Kingdom, 1855–1965.* Cambridge, T120–21.

Gabe, J., Keller, D. & Williams, G. (eds.) 1994 *Challenging medicine.* London & New York, Routledge.

Gration, H.M. & Holland, D.L. 1954 *The practice of nursing,* 4th edition. London, Faber & Faber.

Hugman, R. 1991 *Power in caring professions.* London, Macmillan.

Hutton, W. 1997 *The state to come.* (From extracts published in the *Observer.*) London, Vintage.

Johnson, P. (ed.) 1994 *Twentieth century Britain: economic, social and cultural change.* London & New York, Longman.

Lowe, R. 1993 *The welfare state in Britain since 1945.* London, Macmillan.

NATN. 1990 *Operating department: Identifying non-medical staff skills-mix.* Harrogate, NATN.

NATN. 1996 Position statement. The scope of perioperative practice. *British Journal of Theatre Nursing* August, **6** (5), 49.

Neasham, J. 1996 Nurse led pre-assessment clinics. *British Journal of Theatre Nursing* November, **6** (8), 5–10.

New South Wales College of Nursing. 1993 *Perioperative nursing course curriculum,* 3rd edition. Sydney, NSW College.

Nightingale, F. 1860 *Notes on nursing.* London, Harrison, bookseller to the Queen.

Oxford, M.N. 1900 *A handbook of nursing.* London, Methuen & Co.

Peden, G.C. 1995 *British Economic and Social Policy Lloyd George to Margaret Thatcher,* 2nd edition. Oxford, Phillip Allen.

Pierson, C. 1991 *Beyond the welfare state.* Oxford, Polity Press.

Rothrock, J.C. 1990 *Perioperative nursing care planning.* St. Louis, Mosby.

Rutherford Darling, H.C. 1935 *Surgical nursing and after treatment. A handbook for nurses and others,* 5th edition. London, J.A. Churchill.

Salvage, J. 1988 *The politics of nursing.* Oxford, Heinemann.

Scottish National Nursing and Midwifery Consultative Committee. 1992 *The role and function of the professional nurse.* Edinburgh, Scottish Office.

UKCC. 1992 *The scope of professional practice.* London, UKCC.

War Office. 1911 reprinted 1914 *Royal Army Medical Corps Training.* London, HMSO. (Price ninepence.)

Witz, A. 1994 The challenge of nursing. In: Gabe, Keller & Williams (eds.) *Challenging medicine.* London & New York, Routledge.

World Health Organization. 1977 *The nursing process.* Report on the first meeting of a technical advisory group. Geneva, WHO.

World Health Organization. 1985 *Health for all by the year 2000.* Copenhagen, WHO.

2 Delivering planned perioperative care

Doreen Kalideen

Doreen Kalideen led one of the earliest approved postgraduate courses to be set up in the UK. At the time when the nursing profession was moving towards the 'nursing process' and 'theatre' nurses were becoming aware of the American concept of perioperative nursing, she pioneered the first English National Board (ENB) 183 course. This 15 month course provided education for nurses to work in anaesthetics, the operating theatre and recovery room – perioperative nursing, in fact. Her experience fits her to discuss the process by which perioperative nursing has been developed in recent times.

This chapter will be particularly valuable for those nurses who have come into perioperative nursing since the changes introduced during the last 20 years and will help them to understand some of the anomalies in practice and the misunderstandings which have grown up among those who are not perioperative nurses. The chapter comes right up to date in discussing the aspirations of the specialist practitioners as innovators and change agents, and the part many perioperative nurses will have to play in that particular team approach to care known as planned collaborative care.

The chapter reviews the previous organisation of work in the operating department, which utilised task allocation. It describes how the operating department nurses of the time integrated the technical aspects of their job with a patient-centred approach to patient care during the perioperative period, despite the difficulties many found in changing their attitudes. For some, it was a threat to their pride in a well-organised theatre team to unpick the team structure and rebuild it on different principles. Yet, nurses who worked in the operating department never stopped regarding themselves as nurses who use their nursing skills to care for patients throughout the perioperative period and many were ready to integrate the 'nursing process' into their work.

The term 'theatre nurse' has been retained in this chapter, where it is appropriate, to indicate an earlier attitude to those nurses who work in operating departments in the UK. The authors are aware that it is still used but is now rather imprecise. The term 'perioperative nurse' can be taken to cover all nurses who care for the patient before, during and immediately after surgery whatever their role may be.

When I started my theatre nursing career, the concept of planned, individualised care in the operating theatre was of little consideration. This is not to imply that, as a nurse, I was not concerned with giving the best possible care to my patients. However, the culture of nursing and expectations of society at that time gave little attention to the notion of planned nursing care or consideration of the holistic elements of individualised care. Why should this be? In spite of the fact that theatre nursing is regarded as one of the first areas in which nurses began to specialise (Fennell, 1989), the need to acquire those specialist skills led to a concentration on the technical nature of the work, with a focus on developing the necessary skills to provide assistance for the anaesthetist or surgeon.

The past

The 1960s was a decade of rapid progress, with, for example, pioneering cardiovascular surgery and the beginnings of the transplant programme. The nurse's role was to ensure patients' safety during surgery by providing skilled assistance to the surgical team. With the surgeon as 'captain of the ship', it was easy to see how 'keeping the surgeon happy' during long and complex procedures led to a concentration on the preparation and maintenance of the safe physical environment in terms of ensuring that the correct instruments and equipment were available, safe and immediately to hand throughout. This was achieved by delegating elements of care to different team members; in effect working within a framework of 'task allocation.'

Table 2.1   Task-centred v. patient-centred nursing.

	Task-centred mode	Nursing process mode
Assessment	Verbal information only Stereotyped reports No direct accountability of individual nurse	Full nursing history documented Personalised reports Individual accountability demonstrated
Planning work	Sister delegates workload No involvement of patient in planning Individual nurse has little control Tasks recorded in workbook Nurse satisfies Sister Limited definition of nursing	Nurses plan own work schedule Patients involved Individual nurse in control Individual care documented. Nurse satisfies patient Wider definition of nursing

Table 2.1   continued

	Task-centred mode	Nursing process mode
Implementing care	Task allocation	Patient allocation
	Task hierarchy	Total patient care
	Transient patient contact	Extended patient contact
	Limited interaction	Greater interaction
	Fixed work schedules	Flexible work schedules
Evaluation	Patient and family passive recipients	Patients and family involved
	Social and culture element not important	Social and cultural elements important
	Relationships with patient undesirable	Relationship with patient necessary
	Explicit hierarchy	Implicit hierarchy
	Rank important	Rank unimportant
	Sister is manager/accountable	Sister is colleague/professional nurse
	Medicine dominates	Medical dominates
	Nursing theory not explicit	Nursing theory explicit
	Taught through practice	Formally taught

Source: Adapted from Webb (1982).

Organisation of nursing work

Task allocation was generally seen as an effective way to get nursing work done and, according to Menzies (1970), reduced the stress of nursing which resulted from intense personal interactions with patients. However, it provided little opportunity to examine the theory underpinning practice which became ritualistic and hierarchical. There was little involvement of the patient or the family in decision making and limited personal accountability for nursing actions taken. This, it should be remembered, applied equally to ward nursing at the time.

In the operating department, detachment from the patient was assisted by environmental factors which separated the operating theatres from the main-stream of the hospital in purpose built units. Physical barriers, erected as a means of controlling infection, also banned 'unauthorised persons' from entry. This included family members and any significant others who were important for the patients' psychological wellbeing at this stressful time. Patients and those who were permitted to enter were required to change into theatre clothing and observe strict protocols related to entry and exit, a policy which created more psychological barriers between patient and carers whilst being seen as an important element of infection control.

Thus, the nurses working in the operating department became 'lost behind the theatre mask', maintaining little contact with ward nursing colleagues, a factor identified by Rait (1975) who noted the increasing isolation of the 'theatre nurse' with detrimental effects for the patient. The ward nurses became responsible for the preoperative preparation of the patient, who was delivered to the theatre door, often as 'the next cholecystectomy' with no previous contact with those who would be caring for him or her during the perioperative period. This gave little chance for the theatre nurse to establish any meaningful relationship with a stressed and anxious patient who assumed a passive role as the recipient of technical care. The nurse was also largely dependent on information passed on by the surgeons for information necessary to plan the care to be given during surgery, often dictated purely by surgical strategies and needs rather than patient needs.

As surgical and anaesthetic techniques advanced, care within the operating department became further fragmented with the need for specialist assistance in the anaesthetic room, the need for increasing technical knowledge and the development of postanaesthetic recovery rooms. Perioperative nurses in the UK were lured into this technological 'roller-coaster' by the advent of the Joint Board of Clinical Nursing Studies (JBCNS), as a result of the exponential developments in medical technology. This required a coordinated postregistration training approach to provide and prepare skilled nursing assistance, not only in operating departments but also intensive care units and renal units. Thus, as Barnett (1975) wrote:

> The age of technology has affected hospitals as any other area of our daily life ... a new breed of nurse has arisen to meet this new need – the technical specialist – able to carry out procedures and even institute treatment without close supervision.
>
> Barnett (1975, p.59).

Whilst emphasising the fact that medicine had moved from the patient's well-being to a 'scientific result', she also warned that the technicalisation of nursing and empathetic care must not become mutually exclusive.

Many nurses regarded the acquisition of a post basic qualification in these highly technical areas of nursing as a symbol of their advanced knowledge and skills. With openings for perceived 'high status' work opportunities, both in the UK and abroad, such courses were in high demand. However, both renal and intensive care nursing offered the opportunity for intensive personal interaction between nurse, patient and family members which is less obvious in the operating theatre. The challenge for the theatre nurse was in balancing the demands of increasingly sophisticated anaesthetic and surgical techniques with an individual, patient-centred approach.

To balance individual patient needs with the technical demands of the surgeon and the anaesthetist required cooperation and collaboration between ward and theatre staff. However, care remained fragmented. The nursing assessment, conducted by the ward nurses on the patient's admission, was often unavailable to theatre staff. Thus, there was no way of knowing whether or not a patient had a particular anxiety or psychological need, nor indeed whether the patient was 'at risk' of specific physiological threats, such as hypothermia or pressure sores during surgery.

Despite these limitations, skilled nurses became adept at intuitive assessment of need, responding quickly to physiological changes during surgery to ensure physical needs were met and postoperative risks were minimised. This ability to think on their feet was often seen as a challenge for perioperative nurses, who gained great satisfaction from knowing they were part of a team committed to an individual patient with a specific work outcome (Kalideen,1994). However, this intuitive approach did not help in defining what perioperative nursing was or, indeed, in demonstrating effective outcomes.

In common with many other areas of nursing practice, defining the unique function of the perioperative nurse proved elusive. It was equally difficult to provide evidence of the perioperative nurse's contribution to care. Apart from the official theatre register which documented information about the surgery and anaesthetic, with space to record those involved in the surgical procedure, including nurses, the only documented evidence of care provided by the nurse related to the swab count and, perhaps, to information concerning pathology specimens. There were no nursing records in which information was recorded about patient positioning, strategies used to prevent injury through positioning or on maintaining homeostasis related to body temperature or prevention of infection. This is not to imply that these strategies were not employed but without documented evidence it was impossible to examine outcomes or to evaluate the standard of care provided during the intraoperative period. Whilst theatre nurses were coming to terms with the exponential increase in technology, nursing outside the theatre doors was moving forward.

Towards a new way of nursing

The advent of patient-centred nursing during the early 1970s was one result of the growing dissatisfaction with the task allocation approach to nursing work which was highlighted by the Briggs Committee (1972). Concerned with the high attrition rates from nursing it was an attempt to introduce a system which could unite the study of nursing with nursing practice in an attempt to overcome some of the 'reality shock' to student nurses (Kramer, 1974) and introduce a more patient orientated approach to nursing care (Heath, 1995).

Originating from a business management system, the 'process' approach to nursing provided a systematic approach to problem solving in a nursing context which was accepted by the General Nursing Council (GNC, 1977)[1] as the unifying thread between theory and practice. Like much of early nursing theory, the nursing process had its roots in the United States, where it was hailed as a means of achieving professional status through enhanced patient care. It was adapted for use in the UK to accommodate the British health care settings and became embodied in the 1983 Nurses, Midwives and Health Visitors' Act which requires all first level nurses to:

> Assess, plan, implement and evaluate nursing care (Rule 18, Nurses, Midwives and Health Visitors' Act, 1983).

In practice, the introduction of the nursing process caused much furore, particularly from the medical profession, who saw it as a paper exercise, removing the nurse from direct patient care, and as a means of 'empire building' for nursing rather than any real attempt to improve the quality of care given (Burn, 1984; Michell, 1984). It may be that the underlying medical concern was

Despite a plethora of literature from nurses in the UK to support these views, for example, Wicker (1980); Kalideen (1991) and many others, all supporting a more holistic role for the theatre nurse, there was, at first, little real evidence that perioperative nurses were embracing a perioperative perspective.

Changing priorities

To some extent, the apparent low enthusiasm could be attributed to a lack of management commitment. Ongoing recruitment and staffing problems in operating departments put pressures on both managers and practitioners to cover surgical lists and emergency surgery. This left little time for preoperative visiting. Perioperative nurses were also threatened by the implications of the Bevan enquiry (1989)[2] which recommended more flexible working practices within the operating theatre and the development of a new grade of staff, the operating department practitioner (ODP).

The inability of perioperative nurses to shape their role development created a negative cycle in which nurses became so embroiled in the technical nature of the work that there was little opportunity to demonstrate the caring aspect of perioperative nursing. In such a situation perioperative nurses were perceived as little more than technicians but more costly to train and recruit. This became a salient issue in the new National Health Service committed to efficiency, effectiveness and value for money! The new ethos of 'business management' stimulated by the Griffith enquiry (1983) challenged health authorities to examine skill mix in health care as a way of controlling unit labour costs. Since nursing salaries were estimated to cost the health service between 40 and 60% of the total NHS budget (DOH, 1993), one can see the economic attraction for managers in replacing highly qualified nursing staff by less qualified alternatives. The advent of the ODP and health care assistant (HCA) was seen as a cost-effective means to provide a service which drew from a range of grades, each with a specific job description centred on the surgical process. This further fragmented the notion of holistic care and created a dilemma for the theatre nurse who was now faced with the choice of promoting innovation and change through skill mix review and role re-definition or acceptance of professional nursing values responsive to individual patient care needs.

Yet, ironically, the NHS reforms which challenged the power and autonomy of the medical profession may have proved the final catalyst for the acceptance of nurse's professionalisation.

The 1990 NHS and Community Care Act, with its introduction of the internal health care market, can be seen as an attempt to shift the balance of power in British health care from doctors to managers. This is set in the context of an improvement in the efficient use of resources. Competition within the internal market to provide health care renewed an interest in quality and value for money. As major users of NHS resources operating departments had already come under scrutiny from the Bevan working party and were to suffer considerable changes in the future as managers attempted to act on the Bevan recommendations.

At the same time there was a focus on consumerism in health care. Individual health authorities and Trusts were charged with meeting Patient Charter Standards (DOH, 1992a; 1995), which aimed to put the patient first, recognise local and national needs and standards and recognise the views of consumers. By 1999 the Patient's Charter had almost been forgotten by the majority of patients. Many claimed never to have seen such a document, despite the fact that every household received a pristine copy of the Patient's Charter through the letter-box. On its publication, the National Association of Theatre Nurses (NATN 1992) had noted the contents and had produced its own 'Patient's Charter for the Operating Department' (1995) which was presented as a poster for the department and individual cards for patients.

Charter Standards explicitly stated that:

> You can expect a qualified nurse, midwife or Health Visitor to be responsible for your nursing or midwifery care. You will be told their name.
>
> Patient's Charter (1995, p.14).

Such a statement was seen as placing the onus on all nurses, in whatever setting, to examine how nursing care could be organised to meet this standard which required the named nurse to be accountable for the delivery of care, and to be accessible and visible to the patient. The National Association of Theatre Nurses (NATN) advocated that, in the operating department:

> each patient ... shall receive individual care planned to meet his or her special needs throughout the perioperative period.
>
> NATN (1992, p.3).

Furthermore, the NATN Strategy for Nursing (1991) had emphasised the need for a planned, systematic problem solving approach to care planning which reflects:

> an holistic concept, respects human values and maintains the identity and dignity of each patient.
>
> NATN (1991, p.4).

Clearly, these objectives were only to be achieved by active involvement in the preoperative assessment when the named nurse had an opportunity to meet the patient, gather information to enable the planning of perioperative care and to provide physical and psychological support to enable the patient to cope with the stresses of the surgical experience. In this way, the named nurse would become the team leader, documenting individual care needs, communicating and collaborating with other members of the health care team and negotiating care strategies to ensure identified outcomes were achieved and evaluated. In this way, also, core standards were to be defined and monitored through quality audit, thereby meeting many of the Charter standards.

At time of writing, the Patient's Charter has been discredited by its lack of effectiveness. Whether this is because of consumer unawareness or because the lack of nursing staff has made its standards unachievable, or because there have been so many changes during the last decade, remains to be seen.

Meanwhile, the Department of Health raised important issues for the future of nursing. In May 1993 the Chief Nurses of the four countries of the UK invited a group of nursing leaders and other professional colleagues to a seminar at Heathrow. They believed that there were important technological, demographic and organisational matters which would influence future health care and which should be discussed as a matter of urgency. The report on the 'Heathrow Debate' is well worth re-reading to assess how far change is affecting the profession and to recognise how diverse the profession has become. One significant comment states that:

> the role of the nurse vis-à-vis other professions and non-professional groups, will depend on how well they all defend or develop their own image and status.
>
> The Heathrow Debate (1993).

Towards the new millennium

As we reach the new millennium, there is no doubt that the public will expect an effective National Health Service which combines all the best of their past experience with the innovations and expectations of modern health care. However, providers and commissioners of health care will be looking to maximise their returns from finite resources. As a result, nurses, in whatever setting, will need to prove they can offer quality and effectiveness. This will require a rigorous analysis of the skills required to provide such quality nursing care. It is also predicted that by 2002, 60% of all surgery will be on a day-care basis and 80% of surgical interventions will be by minimal access (DOH, 1993). This will affect the role of the nurse in the operating department. One major driver towards cost-effective care will be the search for a less costly substitute for the registered perioperative nurse or a search to use such registered nurses in different roles.

If it can be shown that theatre nursing skills are relatively more expensive than the alternatives, they may be threatened. The real strength of nursing should be in its focus on people, how they live and feel, recognising the link between health and wholeness, physical, psychological, social and spiritual. In this way, care becomes a process of human interaction, not just mechanistic repair.

Perioperative nurses are at a crossroad in their future career pathway. New management structures will continue to challenge traditional ways of working, blurring the boundaries of established practice. Skill mix review, restructuring and re-engineering can be seen as a challenge or a threat to professional nursing values. We have the choice of redefining our roles in becoming 'technical assistants' to the surgeon or anaesthetist, or accepting the challenge of the Scope of Professional Practice (UKCC, 1992a and b; UKCC 1996a and b; UKCC, 1998) in identifying new and innovative roles which enhance nursing values.

Although the two pathways are not mutually exclusive, the key features of expanding nursing roles within the Scope of Practice are that they:

- should be patient-focused
- benefit existing services

- involve collaborative working
- provide appropriate delegation and show recognition of limitations.

The nurse is personally accountable for her own expanded practice to new levels whilst ensuring that existing aspects of his or her practice are not compromised. The necessary skills, knowledge and competencies are to be formally developed and practice is well-documented to provide evidence that the nurse has honoured her duty of care (UKCC, 1992a; 1996b; 1998).

However, as Read (1995) writes:

> The introduction of innovative nursing roles is not easy, nor cheap, and requires good management support and real enthusiasm for success.
>
> Read (1995, p.1).

Examples of expanded roles include nurses within the day surgery unit who have taken on the responsibility for the preoperative assessment of patients for day surgery. Others include case managers who coordinate care for patients undergoing surgery or day surgery liaison nurses, who liaise between patients, carers and community services to ensure those patients who have surgery on a day-care basis have the appropriate after care and support. All these roles provide opportunities for perioperative nurses to demonstrate their nursing expertise in:

> psychological assessment and intervention, patient teaching, health maintenance and caring and comforting.
>
> Dressier (1994), cited in Gee (1995, p.639).

This ensures that patients do receive care which is planned to meet their holistic perioperative needs.

Why plan perioperative care?

Firstly, patients deserve and expect a coordinated approach to their care. A more articulate and informed society is willing to challenge the standard of care they receive, hence the increase in patient complaints and litigation. The changing nature of surgery, with increasing numbers of patients being treated on a day-care basis has important implications for how their surgical experience is managed. If the government is to achieve its target for surgery to be carried out on a day-care basis by 2002, the key to success is in effective planning; selecting only those patients, or clients, who meet the physical, psychological and social criteria. Care must be planned to minimise the risk of adverse effects or complications and effective discharge planning will be necessary to ensure that clients and their families can cope with the consequences and make a rapid recovery. Those who will continue to require inpatient surgery will be the most vulnerable; those at the extremes of the age range, either the elderly or the very young and those requiring major surgery or surgery for trauma. All will demand a planned and coordinated approach to perioperative care to ensure that the best possible outcomes are achieved.

Secondly, if nurses are to continue to play a role in perioperative care, they need to be able to demonstrate what this role is and why it has value. In seeking to determine their collective beliefs and values in philosophy statements they can explore a model of care for perioperative practice. McGee (1991), suggests that the nature of nursing in the operating theatre has four dimensions. These are:

- Infection control
- Safety
- Management
- Performance of a specialist role.

In exploring the knowledge base underpinning these dimensions, a theory of perioperative practice will begin to emerge. This could be used to develop a care plan relevant to theatre practitioners which demonstrates that individual patient needs are assessed, identified nursing actions are planned and goals evaluated. The result will also provide a documented record of interventions which can be used to ensure both continuity of care and as the basis for quality audit. Evidence is crucial in determining which interventions are effective and establishing the cost/benefit ratio of alternative options. In planning to meet the patient's perioperative needs, we can establish what resources are needed and ensure these are used efficiently.

Risk management is a big issue for most NHS trusts. This has been defined as:

> The reduction of harm to an organisation by identifying and, as far as possible, eliminating risk.
>
> Clements (1995).

One aspect of risk management is the reduction or elimination of harm to patients and commitment to dealing promptly with any untoward incidents which may give rise to litigation. Perioperative nurses have always been conscious of safety issues related to intraoperative care, in applying 'blanket' safety measures, when checking identity and consent, in ensuring electrosurgical safety and in applying stringent infection control measures[3] and by ensuring that swabs, needles and instruments are accounted for. These risks can be classed as 'normative', as in general, they apply to any patient undergoing surgery. However, normative care planning will not identify the patient with a specific risk factor: the elderly, malnourished patient at risk of hypothermia or pressure area damage or the highly anxious, vulnerable patient who may be at risk of poor pain management, postoperative nausea and possible prolonged recovery. Besides causing unnecessary pain and suffering, such incidents have heavy financial penalties in terms of increased hospitalisation costs and the potential for litigation. Planned perioperative care should identify those patients with specific risk factors so that resources can be targeted, to ensure appropriate, effective and efficient use.

How can we plan perioperative care effectively?

The ideals of the specialist practitioner provide one of the best opportunities for promoting planned individualised patient care by encouraging the development of innovative nursing roles involving interdisciplinary coordination and collaboration.[4] Specialist practitioners should be able to act as change agents, challenging established practices and supporting individuals and teams in providing 'seamless care'. This means no overlaps, no gaps, no omissions but care that is *planned* to meet specific outcomes. These roles will be for the few. The rest of us will have to find ways of communicating our desire for information related to the patient's needs and collaborate with colleagues to ensure these needs are met. This can be achieved through collaborative care planning, where all parties, including medical staff, therapists and nurses are involved in determining critical pathways and care protocols. Various terms have been used to describe this approach to care, including case management, managed care, patient-focused care. In essence, all profess to provide a model of care which integrates patient and provider satisfaction within an economic framework. The qualities of a managed care approach are that they can optimise patients' self care abilities, decrease fragmentation of care and provide quality care across a continuum (Girard, 1994). Case management through managed care protocols can offer the opportunity to provide cost-effective care whilst also reconciling the holistic needs of individual patients. It lends itself well to perioperative care, both on a day-care or inpatient basis, because of the clearly defined clinical progression of surgery with its preoperative preparation, the intraoperative care and the postoperative and rehabilitative needs. Collaborative care plans which promote health and wellbeing, reflect the holistic nature of nursing and involve significant others, can then become a reality. The perioperative nurse must contribute to the development of appropriate care protocols if the environment of care during the perioperative period is to be properly considered.

Conclusion

Many changes have taken place since I first started working as a perioperative nurse. Fortunately, many of the rituals are now gone. Instead, these activities have been replaced by more technical acts, such as the time consuming preparation for minimum access surgery or the ordering of expensive aids to surgery. The perioperative nurse is expected to be practitioner, manager, teacher and budget holder. Somehow we always seem to have filled the gaps, but is this in the patient's best interest?

Despite a continually expanding body of research-based knowledge related to perioperative care, can we honestly say that it is influencing our practices? Have we changed enough to fulfil our role within the UKCC Scope of Practice in exercising a duty of care based on a holistic assessment of our patients ' needs? For theatre nurses to become true perioperative nurses they will need to participate in new care delivery modes, they must continue to develop a professional knowledge base which provides the framework for standards of care in the perioperative setting. They need to be proactive in determining what information they require to plan effective interventions which meet the patient's physical, psychological, spiritual and social wellbeing. This requires a critical appraisal of perioperative practices which are efficient, effective and appropriate, in demonstrating positive nursing outcomes.

Greater liaison with ward nursing colleagues will ensure that the rituals of the past are not perpetuated in, for example, prolonged fasting times for patients awaiting surgery or the indignity of patients being deprived of their dentures or hearing aids for prolonged periods of time. Collaboration in care will ensure that postoperative pain is effectively managed, that those patients at risk of pressure area damage or hypothermia are identified and expensive resources are used appropriately to minimise risks. Better communication between health care workers should ensure that patients receive accurate, relevant and appropriate information about their surgery and the postoperative sequalae. In sharing knowledge and experience all parties will benefit.

As minimal access surgery advances, the technological element of care will escalate, while patients will become increasingly vulnerable. The nurse's role should be to protect that vulnerability through a coordinating role. In collaborating and communicating with other health care workers as well as with their patients, an agreed philosophy of care can be negotiated which will ensure a comprehensive assessment and appropriate protocols for delivering planned care. Not only will this help clarify the perioperative nurses' own role, but it will contribute to their professional autonomy and accountability, translating visions and dreams into reality.

Reflective activities

In this chapter we have explored the development of perioperative nursing from the earlier task orientated medical model when nurses in the operating department were in danger of being overtaken by the technical aspects of their work. The chapter has discussed how the introduction of new approaches in nursing gave perioperative nurses the impetus needed for them to focus their work on patient needs and has finally come to consider the new roles and expanded practice which are now in the process of being developed.

It would be possible to criticise the chapter because it refers largely to nursing theory developed between the mid-1970s and 1992. This is because this was the period during which perioperative nursing moved from a task-centred to a patient-centred approach. Once this change had been effected and accepted as the basis of nursing practice the discussions in the professional press focused on other issues and other aspects of patient care which are discussed elsewhere in this book, most particularly in this first section and in the final chapter of the book.

1 Consider your own perioperative practice. How far is your nursing practice truly patient-centred? How far do the technical aspects of your role interfere with the time you can spend on patient care? Does the need to support the surgeon or anaesthetist get first priority? Are there specialist nurse practitioners or registered nurse surgeons assistants/ RNFAs?

2 All these aspects of work in the operating department are important. Has the work in your department been divided so that the right person(s) with the right expertise is concentrating on:

- care of instruments and equipment
- support for the surgeon and anaesthetist
- delivering planned patient care throughout the perioperative period.

If not, what changes could be made?

3 Day surgery (ambulatory surgery) units have given perioperative nurses new opportunities to practice perioperative nursing. Try to find the opportunity to visit a 'stand alone' day surgery unit to see how new nursing roles, relationships and responsibilities in new areas have been developed.

In the UK, nurses from other areas who are not perioperatively qualified have often come into new surgical units, such as day units. There are also many non-nursing personnel in operating departments. In your experience are perioperative nurses working to establish good team relationships and to develop understanding of perioperative patient care?

Endnotes

1 The General Nursing Council (GNC) was the statutory body responsible for nursing in the United Kingdom until replaced after 1983 by the present United Kingdom Central Council for Nursing, Midwifery and Health Visiting (UKCC).

2 The Bevan report is discussed in some detail in Chapter 15.

3 Risk management is explored further in Chapter 11, pp.247–67.

4 Chapter 3 focuses on expanded roles of perioperative nurses and is based on research carried out by the author.

References

Barnett, D. 1975 Standards of nursing care – why are they falling? *Nursing Mirror* June 26, 58–60.

Benner, P. 1984 *From novice to expert: excellence and power in clinical nursing practice.* California, Addison-Wesley.

Bevan, P. 1989 *The management and utilisation of operating departments.* Report. National Health Service Management Executive. London, HMSO.

Boore, J. 1978 *A prescription for recovery.* London, Royal College of Nursing.

Briggs, A. 1972 *Report of the Committee on Nursing.* London, HMSO.

Burn, J. 1984 Letter. *British Medical Journal* **288**, 528.

Clements, R. 1995 Essentials of clinical risk management. *Quality in Health Care* **4**, 129–34.

DOH. 1992a *The Patient's Charter.* London, HMSO.

DOH. 1992b *The health of the nation: a strategy for health in England.* London, HMSO.

DOH. 1993 *The challenge for nursing and midwifery in the 21st century.* Heathrow Debate. London, HMSO.

DOH. 1995 *The Patient's Charter and you.* London, HMSO.

Emden, C. 1983 Operating suite nurses – can we face a challenge to professional practice? *Gown and Glove* Suppl., Winter, 1–11.

Fennell, L. 1989 But is it nursing? *British Journal of Theatre Nursing* February, **26** (2), 13–17.

Gee, K. 1995 Competency through being: the enemy within? *British Journal of Nursing* **4** (11), 637–40.

General Nursing Council. 1977 *A statement for educational policy.* Circular 77/19/A GNC. London.

Girard, N. 1994 The case management model of patient care delivery. *AORN Journal* **60** (3), 403–15.

Griffith, R. 1983 *The NHS management enquiry.* Report. London, DHSS.

Hayward, J. 1975 *Information: a prescription against pain.* London, Royal College of Nursing.

Heath, H. 1995 (ed.) *Potter and Perry's foundations in nursing theory and practice.* New York, Mosby.

Jackson, M. 1986 On maps and models. *Senior Nurse* **5** (4), 24–6.

Kalideen, D. 1991 The case for preoperative visiting. *British Journal of Theatre Nursing,* August, **1** (5), 19–21.

Kalideen, D. 1994 Why nurses choose theatre nursing. *British Journal of Theatre Nursing.* **3** (10), 16–25

Kramer, M. 1974 *Reality shock: why nurses leave nursing.* St Louis, Mosby.

Kratz, C. 1976 Talking point: Roles and reality. *Nursing Times* June 17th, **92**, 3.

Kneedler, J. 1979 Perioperative role in three dimension. *AORN Journal* November 859–74.

McGee, P. 1991 Perioperative nursing: a review of the literature. *British Journal of Theatre Nursing* October **1** (7), 12–17.

Menzies, L. 1970 *The functioning of social systems as a defence against anxiety.* Pamphlet No. 5. London, Tavistock.

Meerabeau, L. 1992 Tacit nursing knowledge: An untapped resource or a methodological headache? *Journal of Advanced Nursing* **17**, 108–112.

Michell, J. 1984 Is nursing any business of doctors? A simple guide to the nursing process. *British Medical Journal* **288**, 216–19.

Miller, A. 1985 Are you using the nursing process? *Nursing Times* **11**, 36–9.

NATN. 1991 *A strategy for nursing in the operating department.* Harrogate, NATN.

NATN. 1992 *The named nurse in the operating department.* Harrogate, NATN.

Nurses Midwives and Health Visitors' Act. (1983) London, HMSO.

Orem, D. 1991 *Nursing: Concepts of practice.* New York, McGraw-Hill.

Pearson, A. & Vaughan, B. 1986 *Nursing models for practice.* London, Heinemann.

Rait, A. 1975 Introduction to the pre- and post-operative visit concept. *Nursing Times* October, Suppl., iv.

Read, S. 1995 *Catching the tide: new voyages in nursing?* Occasional Paper 1. Sheffield, Sheffield Centre for Health and Related Research.

Robinson, K. 1990 Nursing models – the hidden costs. *Surgical Nurse* **3** (1), 11–14.

Roper, N., Logan, W., Tierney, A. 1980 *The elements of nursing.* Edinburgh, Churchill Livingstone.

Roy, C. 1980 *Conceptual models for practice.* New York, Appleton-Century-Croft.

Salvage, J. 1990 *The theory and practice of the new nursing.* Occasional Paper. *Nursing Times* **86** (4), 42–5.

Shaw, H. 1976 The nursing process – the operating theatre and the patient. *NAT News* November, 20–22.

UKCC. 1992a *Code of professional conduct.* London, UKCC.

UKCC. 1992b *Scope of professional practice.* London, UKCC.

UKCC. 1996a *Scope in practice.* London, UKCC.

UKCC. 1996b *Guidelines for professional practice.* London, UKCC.

UKCC. 1998 *Guidelines for records and record keeping.* London, UKCC.

Webb, C. 1982 A comparison of task centred and patient centred nursing. *Journal of Advanced Nursing* **6**, 369–76.

Wicker, P. 1980 A reassuring presence. *Nursing Times* **86** (29), 59–61.

Yura, H. & Walsh, M. 1978 *The nursing process: assessing, planning, implementing and evaluating,* 4th edition. Norwalk, Appleton Century.

The challenge of tomorrow

Bernadette Brennan

Bernadette Brennan is particularly fitted to write this chapter on extending and expanding perioperative nursing practice. She is an Australian perioperative nurse of many years' experience. She has researched her topic in considerable detail and, in this chapter, pulls together much of the information and discussions from many countries. She discusses and compares extended and expanded roles in perioperative practice, most particularly in relation to nurses acting as first assistants to the surgeon. She also discusses the differing roles played by nurses when working with the anaesthetist. The issue of nurses and operating department practitioners who are not qualified nurses but who may be required to carry out similar roles and duties is also explored. This chapter is extremely well-referenced, but the detailed discussion on the topic of advanced perioperative practice will not only give perioperative nurses pause for thought, but offers others involved in the operating department a closer insight into the views of perioperative nurses worldwide. It may help to give politicians and health care managers a deeper understanding of the issues which are being raised by their need to implement a cost-effective service.

Jane Rothrock, who has worked with Bernadette Brennan on this issue has pointed out that the role of Registered Nurse First Assistant (RNFA) is not, in itself, regarded as an advanced role in the USA, though it is an expansion of perioperative nursing practice. After reading this chapter you will see that Australian nurses are working to develop this first assistant role as an element of advanced perioperative practice. The UK differentiates between first assistant as part of the role of perioperative nursing and the more advanced role of surgeon's assistant. In countries such as the UK, with a more developed training for non-nursing perioperative practitioners we also see them undertaking these new roles. It is important to remember that the role of surgeon's assistant is still an evolving role which may be integrated into practice in a variety of ways.

Introduction

The challenges we face today, in a global sense, provide opportunities for tomorrow, in the third millennium. Perioperative nursing practice is in a phase of evolution. There is a need to explore developing roles as perioperative nurses walk into the future and accept the challenge of providing cost-effective perioperative nursing care which will result in quality outcomes for patients. Consideration must be given to advanced perioperative practice, the expansion and extension of perioperative nursing roles. Rothrock (1997) states that:

> the potential for professional growth in perioperative nursing is vast; however, if we are not prepared or only perceive change as an obstacle to our success, we will never see all of the potential nurturing options for our future as perioperative nurses.

Porter-O'Grady (1996) believes that the new health care delivery, particularly the focus on the continuum of care, will drive the need for nursing to develop new approaches to the service it delivers. He expounds the theory that the emerging practice of nursing will require integration, coordination, insight, energy and commitment to enable it to meet the needs of patients and the community. Advanced practice will mean the end of task-based intervention and the introduction of partnerships and collaboration with other members of the health care team. However, in order to introduce changes in perioperative nursing practice, it is essential to begin to understand the new and emerging reality of advanced practice.

Mitchinson & Goodlad (1996) discuss the changing of the traditional boundaries of nursing and the necessity to explore the implications of the evolution of advanced practice as it affects the nursing workload, the quality of patient care and the level of extension which the increased responsibility will generate. It is suggested by Mitchinson & Goodlad (1996 p.734) that although opportunities will be created by the development of nursing roles, professional concerns must be considered. The perceived advantages of a fuller, more stimulating and autonomous role would appear to place the nursing profession where it should be as the 21st century approaches and not where it has been, in its traditional 'handmaiden' role. Bowey & Caballero (1996) argue that nursing is undergoing a struggle in its attempt to find a definition, a future direction, including the development of goals and professional standards. This future direction is surely that of advanced practice.

The shift of surgical care from inpatient to outpatient settings will inevitably alter perioperative nursing as we know it today. The development of advanced practice roles in perioperative nursing is gaining momentum. Advanced practice implies leadership, research and professional pioneering. It is not product driven but process driven. Advanced practice provides the skills to effect change to care modalities as patient need and service provision change.

Hamilton (1998) believes that the roles, practice environments, titles and scope of responsibilities for nursing practice are 'very broad and diverse.' She states that 'nurses could be forgiven for being even more confused about this burgeoning dimension of advanced nursing practice.' Definitions lack both accuracy and clarity. It is necessary to explore developing roles in an endeavour to provide a lucid and distinct description of the roles.

The terms 'nurse practitioner' and 'advanced nursing practice' have different connotations dependent on the country where the practice is occurring. In the USA and the UK, the role of nurse practitioner has been clearly defined but, in other countries, the role continues to be perceived as ambiguous and confusing (Hamilton, 1998, p.5). It is believed that the title 'nurse practitioner' is not sufficiently defined and therefore does not provide a differentiation from other levels of nursing practice. There are many titles for nurses undertaking developing roles which constitute what is described as advanced practice. Our medical colleagues perceive the word 'practitioner' when it describes a nursing role as a threat. But do they have an embargo on the word 'practitioner'? We nurses must convince our medical colleagues that we practice at all times within a nursing framework: our practice is to provide nursing care to the patient at all times. The fact that we are capable of providing interventional care which until now has been traditionally regarded as the domain of the medical fraternity, by the medical fraternity, appears to cause some angst in medical circles.

Advanced practice

What is advanced practice? Who practices in an advanced role? A condensed definition is a registered nurse who employs advanced skills including the evaluation, diagnosis and treatment of patients with diseases and adverse health conditions. Advanced practice nurses ensure continuity of care, manage use of resources and coordinate patient services which will result in cost savings. These nurses provide access to quality health care across the continuum by improving continuity of care.

In the perioperative role, the continuity of care spans the pre-, intra- and postoperative phases of the patient's surgical experience. This includes preoperative history taking and testing, expanding the teaching of the patient and family undertaken by the surgeon, identifying intraoperative needs and planning and implementing the care during the procedure. During the intraoperative phase the advanced practice nurse assists the surgeon during the surgical procedure. Evaluation of the care given follows postoperatively and the discharge planning process is commenced.

Extension and expansion of nursing roles have been discussed in the literature, at conferences and in other public forums. The terms 'extension' and 'expansion' of roles are often used inconsistently and interchangeably. They do have quite different meetings which should be clarified before going further. How do we prepare for an 'extended' or 'expanded' role? Any registered nurse who practices in an expanded role should have completed an accredited college or university graduate programme and acquired the knowledge and practice skills in order to function effectively.

An extended role

An extended role has been defined as involving 'tasks' borrowed from other professions; these tasks are executed by the nurse at the discretion and convenience of others. The role includes training, and supervision by other professionals. *The Scope of Professional Practice* published in 1992 by the United Kingdom Central Council for Nursing, Midwifery and Health Visiting (UKCC) refers to the scope and extended practice of nursing. This document states that the terms 'extended' or 'extending' which have been associated with the traditional base or system upon which the practice of nursing has existed until now are no longer suitable since they limit, rather than extend, the parameters of practice. As a result, many practitioners have been prevented from fulfilling their potential for the benefit of patients. It is also believed that a concentration on 'activities' or 'tasks' can detract from the importance of integrated nursing care. Extension occurs when we add on narrow fields of advanced practice – we develop different skills like 'teaching a monkey new tricks' but little reference is made to issues of accountability or additional knowledge to support it – we just add skills on to an existing repertoire.

Mitchinson & Goodlad (1996, p.734) believe that the adoption of the extended role, that is, taking on a series of tasks passed from one profession to another can result in the nurse operating in a narrow field delegated to and supervised by another profession. The interdependent and collaborative relationship is not present. The role has been described in the literature as augmenting the role of technical assistant to the doctor while increasing the nursing workload.

An expanded role

An expanded role, on the other hand, involves a higher level of nursing practice within the existing boundaries of nursing. This is the result of the development of knowledge from research, experience and continuing education which allows the nurse to incorporate new skills from this knowledge base. This role is described as a collaborative role which promotes continuity between the professions and a resultant higher standard of interprofessional care. Bowey & Caballero (1996, p.30) describe the expansion of the scope of professional practice as including:

- The result of a considered judgement by the professional.
- A continuous process involving far more than a technical expertise or focus.
- Responsibilities and skills which will intensify the curative and recuperative components of a practitioner role and the provision of the continuum of care.

Henderson (1969) identified two components of the expanded role:

- The first component is a unique nursing role, divided into clinical, management and teaching, the province of the nurse and from which the expanded role arises.
- Secondly, the collaborative role, which is shared with other health professionals.

The expanded role promotes continuity between the professions and a resultant higher standard of interprofessional care, although some nurses have difficulty in understanding the parameters of this role and how it will revolutionise their practice.

The expanded role should be integrated into nursing education at postgraduate level.[1] The apparent advantages in the expanded role benefit the patient in the quality of care given, the education, the provision of information and improved continuity of care. In perioperative practice, the surgeon can be relieved from pressure of work; there is less necessity to undertake the day-to-day assignments which are repetitive. These assignments can be undertaken by the registered nurse, in collaboration with the surgeon, which will result in increased efficiency in perioperative practice. The health care facility can perceive improved cost-effectiveness. It is a well-documented fact that nurses are a more economical option.

Peter Lovett, educational officer for the UKCC, speaking at the National Association of Theatre Nurses (NATN) Conference in Harrogate in 1996 outlined the expansion of the nurse's role. In part, he said:

> … When a nurse takes on the skills traditionally belonging to another professional group, and incorporates them into her own repertoire, they become part of her programme of care delivery. So it is not an issue about taking on someone else's cast-offs, it's about widening and enriching the contribution the nurse can make. And the value added is not in that she carries out another skill for the patient, but that she can do it immediately because she's there, she can do it with reference to everything else she does for a patient and she can do it with reference to good communication, good interpersonal relationships, health education, all the things that nurses do and know about.

A pithy description of what perioperative nurses are beginning to achieve within their practice currently and what can be aspired to and achieved in the future!

The expanded role is flexible – it can be developed according to the local need and the health care facility should be setting the parameters of each individual role, as needs dictate.

An exemplar of a comprehensive model of perioperative nursing

To illustrate how the expanded role may be developed for perioperative nursing, let us consider a comprehensive model of perioperative practice being proposed in the USA.

The Association of Operating Room Nurses (AORN) is currently developing a comprehensive model for perioperative nursing practice. A working document was published in the *AORN Journal,* January, 1998, for discussion at the AORN Congress in Orlando, Florida, in the House of Delegates on 30 March 1998. The development of this model followed a redefinition and reconceptualisation of perioperative nursing by AORN, in an effort to position American perioperative nurses for the future. This model has been designed to meet the needs of patients within various practice settings. AORN believes that perioperative nursing must have flexible boundaries that are responsive to the needs of the patient and the environment where care is delivered. This includes the increased use of ambulatory surgery and surgery in the community. These new boundaries require an expanding knowledge base. Therefore perioperative nursing is perceived as being provided at three levels. Within each level of practice, individual nurses demonstrate competence along the continuum of novice to expert (Benner, 1984, p.56). Additionally, within each role, perioperative nurses can choose to develop expertise in specific surgical specialties.

The definition of these models provides direction for clinical nurses, educators, administrators. The three conceptual roles are:

- perioperative clinician
- perioperative care coordinator
- perioperative advanced practitioner.

A perioperative clinician is defined as a perioperative nurse responsible for the care of the patient during the preoperative, intraoperative and postoperative period. The core activities encompass the current anaesthetic, instrument, circulating and postanaesthetic roles.

The perioperative care coordinator functions in an expanded role, responsible and accountable for optimising the available resources and independently and collaboratively assessing, planning, implementing and evaluating the care of the patient. Critical thinking, communication and leadership skills are required together with data-assisted decision making and the provision of formal and informal education to patients, other members of the health care team, family, community, industry, insurers and regulatory bodies. This role includes amongst others, the Registered Nurse First Assistant (RNFA).

The perioperative advanced practitioner is a master-prepared nurse who is competent to manage patient health/illness status, disease prevention and health promotion in a broad context. Comprehensive health assessments in collaborative and collegial relationships with other health professionals is part of this role together with clinical decision making, diagnosing and prescribing treatment modalities. The advanced practitioner integrates clinical practice, education, research, management, leadership and consultation into a single role.

This model is interesting and in several countries, including Australia, there are moves to undertake much of the work in perioperative nursing outlined in this model, although it has not been defined or articulated. It is necessary to reflect on and begin to accept that, as the new millennium approaches, the traditional or discrete perioperative roles, that is anaesthetic, instrument, circulating and postanaesthetic roles, will become blurred and the beginning of integrated or expanded roles will become emergent. Busen and Engleman (1996) suggest that there will be a realisation that perioperative nursing roles have flexible boundaries and that, dependent on the needs of patients, the differing places of health care delivery and the expansion of the perioperative knowledge base itself, there will be a need to respond to change as it manifests itself. There is a requirement to consider how to develop these expanded roles in perioperative nursing. The 'have to do more with less' philosophy coupled with the burgeoning of new complex technology forces an acknowledgement that change is necessary in order to provide cost-effective continuity of care for the patient.

Developments in advanced perioperative nursing

Canada appears to have limited documented evidence of nurses practising in advanced perioperative roles although Gruendemann & Fernsebner (1995), in describing global perioperative nursing, refer to future trends in Canada, including the registered nurse acting as first assistant to the surgeon and acting as assistant to the anaesthetist, which will be an expansion of the circulating role. Other anticipated areas of expansion include specialising in particular sub-specialties of surgery, providing strong patient advocacy and resources to surgeons and being involved in community teaching and case management in an outpatient setting. It appears that the evolution of the Registered Nurse First Assistant (RNFA) role has commenced: several programmes are being offered in different provinces. An article authored by Groetzsch (1997) and published in the *Canadian Operating Room Nursing Journal* highlights the uncoordinated approach to the preparation of the RNFA in Canada. The provincial operating room nursing associations are working towards the development of the Perioperative Nurse – Surgery (RNFA) role. However, the author's research identified the absence of a core curriculum and the need for the Operating Room Nurses Association of Canada (ORNAC) to promote and influence the implementation of the role.

In the Republic of South Africa, the perioperative nurse has a high profile, providing seamless care from admission to discharge although at this juncture, advanced roles within perioperative nursing do not appear to be highly developed.

Perioperative nursing in Chile is considered very specialised because of burgeoning technology and the complexity of surgical procedures. There appears to be little evolution of advanced roles.

In Australia there are concerted moves, caused by financial constraints, to erode the role of the perioperative registered nurse.[2] To prevent the continuation of this trend, the Australian Confederation of Operating Room Nurses (ACORN) has made a commitment to developing roles in the operating suite, whether in the acute hospital setting or ambulatory surgery. In 1990, ACORN was asked for direction on the increasing use of registered nurses as first assistants brought about by the tyranny of distance and the lack of registrars and interns in some public and private health care facilities. A policy statement was developed and included the criteria which should be set regarding the role, what limitations should be set, the necessity for the patient to be informed before giving consent, the nurse's right to refuse to fulfil the role, the issue of rostering extra registered nurses for this role, the requirement for specific education and experience, reimbursement and who completes the surgery in case the surgeon becomes ill during the procedure. Legal advice was obtained which covered several issues including duty of care, informed consent, negligence and vicarious liability. Other issues for consideration were professional conduct, accountability, reimbursement, professional indemnity and collaborative practice. A review of this information led to the development of an outcome standard which was published in May, 1995 and has recently been reviewed and rewritten.

There is a growing trend in Australia for perioperative nurses to undertake the role of first assistant. This trend has in part been influenced by the shortage of doctors in rural areas. The Australian Medical Workforce Data Review Committee's Annual Report in 1995 highlighted a downward trend in the number of doctors graduating from 1996 to 2000. It is expected that this projected decline will accelerate the development of the advanced nurse practitioner in the operating suite. The ACORN Council and the Australian Nursing Federation (ANF), the principal nursing union in Australia, have an agreed position that patient care must be undertaken by registered nurses in one of the most critical areas of the patient's hospital experience, i.e. the operating suite. It was jointly agreed that exploration of the development of the role of the RN as First Assistant be undertaken and that the development of a suitable post registration course in Australia to educate the registered nurse as first assistant be developed as an adjunct to this.

In 1996, the ACORN Council granted a Fellowship to research developing roles in perioperative nursing. Relevant information was needed for consideration to be given to new and expanded roles in other countries and their development. A study tour was undertaken in the USA and the UK where these roles are clearly defined and being practised in a variety of settings. An industry partnership with a university has been formed and the first distance education course commenced in February 1999.[3]

In the USA, advanced practice roles are well developed. In 1979 the Association of Operating Room Nurses (AORN, 1998) House of Delegates approved the following statement: '… in the absence of a qualified physician, the registered nurse who possesses appropriate knowledge and technical skills is the best qualified non-physician to serve as the first assistant.' In 1980 AORN developed guidelines for the registered nurse who functioned as the first assistant. Emphasis was placed on the necessity for the assigned duties to fall within the scope of the various State Nurse Practice Acts.

By 1983 the RN was permitted to act as first assistant in many States although there was an expressed concern that this role was not within the scope of the

Nurse Practice Acts. The majority of States considered this to be a delegated medical function or a function regulated by hospital policy. In 1983 AORN appointed a task force to study and clarify the role and qualifications of the RNFA. In 1989, at the AORN Congress in Anaheim, the House of Delegates approved a motion for the Board of Directors to charge a committee to develop a generic curriculum for the RNFA. The curriculum was developed and there are now 15 courses for the RNFA in America. There is existing legislation regarding the legality of nurses working as first assistants and the reimbursement offered for this work (Rothrock,1998).

In the UK a similar development has taken place following protracted deliberation and discussion by NATN. Several years ago two documents were produced by NATN on the two roles which were considered necessary – one was the Nurse as First Assistant to the Surgeon in the Operating Department, the second the Nurse as Surgeon's Assistant. The difference between the two roles was that the Surgeon's Assistant is able to undertake surgical interventions. These interventions were initially always performed under direct supervision of the surgeon, though some nurses are now taking clinical responsibility for surgical interventions under more indirect supervision by the surgeon (NATN, 1993a and b).

The first external course was developed for the Nurse as First Assistant to the Surgeon by Shropshire and Staffordshire College of Nursing and Midwifery. An inhouse course for the Nurse as Surgical Assistant to the Surgeon was introduced at Papworth Hospital, Cambridge in 1996 and other centres have followed these leads. Many innovative roles have been developed in the UK. Examples are of a laparoscopic nurse practitioner who undertakes a complete role from assessment of the patient to discharge and follow-up. Wirral Hospitals Trust sanctioned the training of a perioperative nurse to undertake minor routine surgery following acceptance of a proposal and support by the consultant surgeons (Leifer, 1996). Vincent (1996) cited changes in surgical and anaesthetic practice as reasons for the development of expanded roles in perioperative nursing. Vincent gives examples of the movement of the domain of perioperative nursing from the conventional operating suite to areas such as ambulatory surgery units, medical imaging, cardiac catheter laboratories, radiology departments, endoscopy units and emergency departments. She discusses the proposal by Bevan (1989) that perioperative nurses and Operating Department Assistants/Operating Department Practitioners (ODAs/ODPs) 'become more interchangeable'. This recommendation raises the question of the need for registered nurses in the operating suite. Vincent discusses the view of NATN that these roles can, to an extent be complementary, but that they are both required. She provides a clear and concise overview of the registered nurse's role in delivering patient-focused care which embraces the 'totality of perioperative activity' and includes the utilisation of research-based knowledge. This multifaceted approach places the perioperative nurse in a 'unique position.' However, Vincent warns that the new roles which are emerging as a result of restructuring of areas and the reduction of junior doctors' hours may have been initiated without full consideration of the implications.

Nurse anaesthetists

The consideration of nurse anaesthetists inevitably causes some lively discussion amongst nurses and our medical colleagues. The use of nurse anaesthetists in the USA has an extensive history in the development of the role. America is the only English-speaking country purported to use nurse anaesthetists. The Guidelines and Standards of Practice for Nurse Anaesthesia Practice generated by the American Association of Nurse Anaesthetists (AANA, 1992) specifies their scope of practice, standards for nurses' anaesthesia practice, patient monitoring standards, guidelines for granting clinical privileges and a model of a position description. This document, in part, refers to the practice of anaesthesia as being a recognised specialty within the profession of nursing. Another document, published by the International Federation of Nurse Anaesthetists Committee on Education (1990) states in the preamble that nurse anaesthetists are prepared and utilised in many countries throughout the world. The writers of this statement could be forgiven for a slight exaggeration, as analysis of the situation seems to indicate that it is not as widespread as our American colleagues would have us believe.

In 1996, the President of the Association of Anaesthetists of Great Britain and Ireland Education and Research Trust circulated a letter to all UK and Republic of Ireland consultants and trainee members of the Association. In part, this letter referred to a working party of the Association set up in 1992 which considered the introduction of nurses administering anaesthesia in Great Britain and Ireland. The conclusion drawn was that there would be little advantage to be gained for patients, the specialty of anaesthesia or for anaesthetists. In 1994 a further working party was convened with the same result. It was felt by the Association that the impetus to look at the introduction of nurse anaesthetists was initiated by the nursing profession and management. A multidisciplinary 'Scoping Study' on Professional Roles in Anaesthetics was commissioned by the National Health Service (NHS) Executive in October, 1996. The brief for this study was to:

- identify current practices in the delivery of anaesthetics;
- set out a range of options for service provision;
- outline actual and potential skills and roles within anaesthetics;
- describe the key educational implications that need to be addressed if substantial changes in patterns of service are to be effected.

Several recommendations were made as a result of this study. These include the finding of 'no support' from any national medical or nursing body for the introduction of nurse anaesthetists. The Royal College of Anaesthetists, the Royal College of Surgeons and the Association of Anaesthetists were reported as strongly opposing any such moves. There was, however, considerable support for the definition and development of an anaesthetic assistant whether it be a registered nurse or an (ODA) as part of the anaesthetic team. The reasons given for the lack of support for nurse anaesthetists was the perceived 'animosity' between nurse anaesthetists and anaesthesiologists in the USA. It was reported in the 'Scoping Study' document that there is a steady decline in the number of nurses entering courses for the education of nurse anaesthetists. Information was presented which cited higher incidences of adverse outcomes in countries where nurses administer anaesthetics (Chopra *et al.*, 1990). The principal concern amongst all parties was that the quality of patient care is not compromised. Woodhead (1995) expresses concern for the lack of clarification and definition of extended roles and the ad hoc development which has resulted in confusion for the nursing profession.

In Scandinavia, it was reported that nurses administer anaesthesia to low-risk healthy patients (Baxter, 1993). In Denmark and Holland, the nurse anaesthetist maintains intraoperative anaesthesia while the anaesthetist undertakes the induction and recovery phases. In France, a 2-year programme resulting in a Diploma in Anaesthesia enables registered nurses and midwives to deliver anaesthesia (Brett, 1996).

In Australia, there has been some protracted discussion regarding the development of a nurse anaesthetist role. To date there has been no overall support for this development, although some educational institutions have been researching the possibility of developing such a course. ACORN has discussed this role within their Council meetings and do not support its development at this stage. The general opinion expressed, indicates that should registered nurses wish to expand their professional expertise in this direction, the course to be pursued would be a medical degree. (This argument is similar to the contention that if technicians wish to undertake nursing care of patients, they would need to undertake a nursing degree.) Registered nurses are not a substitute medical practitioner, but should be perceived as supplemental to the anaesthetist, providing a collaborative partnership.

Current trends in education in advanced practice

What are the current and future trends in education for advanced perioperative nursing practice? In order to briefly explore these trends in differing countries, cognisance must be made of the employment of technicians or assistive personnel, whether licensed or unlicensed, in these countries.

Brett (1996, p.5) in a paper published in the *British Journal of Theatre Nursing* discussed operating suite nurse education in Europe.[4] The European Health Committee Working Party on the Role and Education of Nurses declared in a document on the European Agreement on the Instruction and Education of Nurses that nursing was both an art and a science. Four attributes were cited: patient care, teaching, developing practice and acting as an expert in a multidisciplinary team. These attributes were all considered part of the role of the perioperative nurse.

In Spain, Portugal and Italy, education in the perioperative stream is difficult to access. It is necessary for these nurses, if they wish to undertake a course, to travel to neighbouring countries. Recognition of these courses is not always assured.

In Portugal, a 2-year course in anaesthetic nursing has been accepted providing the prospective student has completed a basic nursing course, and subsequently has 2 years' experience, one year of which is in perioperative nursing. As in other countries perioperative nurses are under threat from the employment of technicians in the operating suite, as always because of perceived cost-effectiveness.

The situation in Italy is similar, with a one year anaesthetic nursing course being recognised, but there are few opportunities to practice. Operating suite technicians are employed purely for technical support.

In the early part of the 1990s in Spain, there was little specialist education in perioperative nursing. A government study in 1991 recommended the implementation of specialist nursing courses which were developed.

In other parts of Europe, namely Germany, the Netherlands, Norway and Switzerland, postbasic nursing courses are highly developed in differing ways. Germany's course is of 5 years' duration – 3 years of basic education followed by an intensive 2-year postbasic course. The Netherlands, on the other hand, require their course to be undertaken in a continuous 5-year progression. Switzerland requires that one year of nursing is completed before a perioperative course can be undertaken. Norway mandates a one week update, every 2 years as continuing professional development. This is exclusively for registered nurses – second level nurses and technicians are not permitted to register for these courses. The employment of technicians in Germany and Switzerland is offered coupled with an education programme.

In Scandinavian countries, differing approaches to perioperative education are offered. There is no specific perioperative education in Denmark. However, advanced practice, for example nurse management of resources including the medical team is exercised in some of the clinics. Clinical practice is highly developed with a strong component of research contained in the courses offered in Scandinavia. There is a requirement to possess basic education plus experience before commencing work in the operating suite. Sweden commenced offering perioperative postbasic courses in the mid 1990s and demonstrates a strong commitment to the employment of registered nurses in the operating suite – they do not employ either technicians or assistants. These Scandinavian countries are advanced in their provision of nursing education with many college-based courses being offered.

In Belgium, the country has two divisions – in the French speaking areas in 1995, a diploma course was commenced. The Flemish area, at the time of publication of Brett's paper, was considering the future education of perioperative nurses and the Belgian national perioperative association was hoping that the European Operating Room Nurses' Association (EORNA) core curriculum would be accepted as suitable. A degree in nursing management is offered in Flemish Belgium, but is not available for perioperative nursing. It is apparent in this country that there is medical dominance in the education and practice of perioperative nurses. However, the positive side of this question is that legislation exists in Belgium which precludes the use of assistive personnel to undertake nursing practice.

France has been successful in ensuring that the education of nurses remains under the control of nurses. Additionally, a 2-year Diploma of Anaesthesia is offered which, when completed, allows registered nurses and midwives to administer anaesthetics. In Greece, the nursing courses offered are curtailed because of the lack of educators. The credibility of perioperative nurses differs from north to south, with those in the south being held in low esteem.

It is obvious when assessing the situation in Europe that advanced practice is in its infancy. Generally, differences in requirements for practice in each country makes portability difficult to achieve. Further education may need to be undertaken to allow practice in differing countries.

In Canada, by 2000, the requirement will be for registered nurses to have a baccalaureate degree in nursing in a 4-year university programme. In 1995 there were approximately ten postgraduate perioperative programs offered, of 3 to 6 months' duration. Several of the 3-month programmes are designed for home study and have limited attached clinical experience. In many health care facilities in Canada, registered nurses undertake 'on-the-job' training in the operating room (Gruendemann & Fernsebner, 1995, p.335).

In the USA, the development of perioperative nursing roles is well-advanced and has been undertaken because of the influence of major social, political and economic changes in health care. These roles include the RNFA, Perioperative Nurse Practitioner and Advanced Nurse Practitioner in the perioperative area.

South African registered nurses possess a diploma or degree in nursing from a recognised tertiary institution. If not in possession of either of these, proof of an acceptable qualification and/or experience must be presented to the South African Nursing Council. The scope of practice in South Africa allows the performance of any task or work for which a registered nurse has been educated and is capable of performing. Retention of accountability is an important part of the scope of practice responsibilities (Gruendemann & Fernsebner, 1995, p.342).

The education of perioperative nurses in Chile is somewhat haphazard with little consensus on educational requirements: each facility has its own criteria for selection of registered nurses and the educational courses undertaken. Examples of this are that the circulating nurse and the assistant to the anaesthetist are not necessarily registered nurses, but auxiliary nurses. The instrument nurse may be a medical assistant. Some institutions will employ registered nurses who have completed a college course, but generally these are only for working with complex technological equipment or complicated procedures (Gruendemann & Fernsebner, 1995, p.346).

In Australia, perioperative nursing education has moved from hospital based programmes to universities and colleges. Baccalaureate degrees and diplomas are required in the basic nursing courses with graduate diplomas being offered in perioperative nursing. There is a concerted move for registered nurses to continue their education by undertaking a Master's degree. The development of advanced practice is gaining momentum and several educational institutions are offering postgraduate courses in specialised advanced practice nursing.

There are varying opinions regarding the necessary education for expanded practice roles in the USA. Discussion with colleagues and educators elicited the belief by some that a Master's degree was not required for the RNFA role but that it was necessary for advanced practice nursing. It is believed that a Master's degree is required to provide the academic and practice preparation for clinical decision making and patient management in the perioperative setting. The advance practice role is effective in other specialty settings and can be readily developed in a variety of surgical settings.

The most important challenge for perioperative nurse practitioners is to embrace the expanded role and not perceive it as that of a 'physician extender'. Rather, it is a role that encompasses advanced decision making in complex acute care settings. Clinical competence and credibility together with collaborative and interdisciplinary practice must be achieved. The movement of nurse practitioners into specialty settings is still in its early stages in the USA, as elsewhere, but preliminary data suggest that this role is an effective response to the needs of patients in acute care settings.

Keane & Richmond (1993) express the opinion that advanced nursing practice has developed in the last 20 years into 'two related but distinct directions: the nurse practitioner and the clinical specialist.' It is suggested that this development has been in response to the demands society makes, that is, increased access to primary health care that is affordable, quality driven and that it is available to provide specialised nursing for the increasing complexity of conditions which patients manifest.

AORN has a position statement on the definition of Perioperative Advanced Practice (Box 3.1). This statement is contained in the AORN Standards, Recommended Practices and Guidelines (1998), and had been adopted by the House of Delegates in Atlanta, Georgia, in 1995. In this definition AORN believes that the Advanced Practice Nurse 'should possess a graduate degree in nursing that forms the foundation for an advanced practice role.'

Box 3.1 AORN Position Statement. Reprinted with permission from AORN *Standards, Recommended Practices, and Guidelines,* 1999, p.126. Copyright © AORN, Inc., 2170 South Parker Road, Suite 300, Denver, CO 80231.

Definition of perioperative advanced practice

The perioperative advanced practice nurse (APN) is a registered professional nurse who uses specialised knowledge and skills in the care of patients and families undergoing operative and other invasive procedures. The APN possesses a graduate degree in nursing that forms the foundation for an advanced practice role. The perioperative APN conducts comprehensive health assessments and demonstrates autonomy and skill in diagnosing and treating complex responses of clients (i.e. patient, family, community) to actual and potential health problems that are related to the prospect or performances of operative or other invasive procedures. The perioperative APN formulates clinical decisions to manage acute and chronic illness by assessing, diagnosing and prescribing treatment modalities, including pharmacological agents. The perioperative APN integrates clinical practice, education, research, management, leadership, and consultation into a single role. The perioperative APN functions in a collegial relationship with nurses, physicians and others who influence the health environment.

Suggested reading

Coalition of Nurse Practitioners. Agenda item 12.2.5. item presented at the Coalition of Nurse Practitioners Constituent Assembly, 2–3 December 1993.

Mirr, M.P. 'Advanced clinical practice: A reconceptualised role.' *AACN Clinical Issues in Critical Care Nursing* 4 November 1993, 600.

Submitted: 3/95
Adopted: 3/95
House of Delegates,
Atlanta, Georgia
Sunset review: 3/2000

Issues for exploration in the development of advanced perioperative practice

(a)   Legal issues

The nursing profession is very aware of the legal duty of care which must be provided for patients. Health care facilities have a duty of care also, defined by professional standards, government regulation and by various legislation. The nursing profession's responsibility to patients must be met, by ensuring that they have an acceptable standard of care, and to employers by upholding the policies of the facility. In acting in advanced practice roles, for example the RNFA, this duty of care must be upheld (AORN, 1998b). If an RN believes that this role cannot be practised safely, their obligation to both patient and employer is to communicate this fact.

Friend (1996) highlights the need for a 'new understanding of the changing role of nurses' and suggests that a process of filtration into the legal system will have to occur. Revision of the 'nurse as handmaiden' concept will need to be dealt with by legal practitioners, health care authorities and insurance funds.

All registered nurses are aware of the importance of informed consent and of ensuring that the patient is made fully aware of, and consents to, treatment. When a patient enters a health care facility, a contract is entered into with the administrators of the institution. If the patient is a private patient, he enters into a contract with his medical practitioner also. The registered nurse is perceived to be acting in the capacity of 'servant' or agent of the hospital. Outside this situation, as an independent or advanced practitioner, for example, the nurse enters into a direct contractual relationship with the patient. This is exemplified when the RN works as an independent practitioner, as a first assistant to the surgeon.

It is important to remember that 'every human being of adult years and sound mind has a right to determine what shall be done with his own body.' (Schloendorff v. Society of New York Hospital as cited in *Nursing and the Law,* Staunton & Whyburn, 1993.)

Legal opinions have indicated that just as a patient gives consent for a surgeon to operate or to treatment by a medical practitioner, consent should be obtained for an assistant to be utilised, be they a medical practitioner or a registered nurse. Friend, (1996, p.27) cites a research paper which determined that patients must be informed of the role and education of the health care workers involved in their care and this includes new clinical roles such a surgical or first assistant.

The question of negligence highlights the need for the nurse to act in a way that a 'reasonable nurse' with the same level of training and skill would act. Failure to do so would constitute negligence, if the breach of the duty of care caused damage to the patient. Competence in advanced practice roles will be a requirement and must be demonstrated.

Advanced practice roles such as the first assistant elicit the question of professional indemnity cover. It is considered in Australia that the surgeon is vicariously liable for medical indemnity covering all assistants. In addition, the employer is vicariously liable for the action of its employee. If an employee acts outside the scope of his or her employment and outside the authority of that employment, the employer will not be liable for damage arising out of the employee's actions. But the definition of employer is not easy to interpret. Is the employer the hospital or the surgeon, in this instance? In the USA, health care facilities employ registered nurses as first assistants. Will other countries follow suit as advanced perioperative practice develops? Will surgeons employ their own registered nurses as first assistants? Will health care facilities provide the first assistant from their perioperative nursing staff and charge the surgeon a fee? (Nurse Practitioner Project, 1995.)

An opinion offered by the Medical Defence Union in Australia states:

> A nurse is required to exercise a level of care and skill consistent with her qualifications and any special skills and qualifications she professes to have. Thus, a nurse who undertakes a role of first assistant, holds her or himself out as having the competence to perform that role and is required to exercise the care and skill which a person having that competence should exercise.

A further consideration is that the perioperative nurse acting as the first assistant is under the direct supervision of the surgeon and this, therefore, would relieve the RN from the responsibility in respect of any action or procedure undertaken by the proper direction of the surgeon. The lawyers considered that no liability could attach to a nurse who competently carried out such a direction. But they went on to make the point that the nurse would be required to exhibit the standard of care and skill consistent with that expected of a perioperative nurse who undertook the role of first assistant.

If, however, the RNFA was routinely rostered on the operating list as a first assistant and the RN performed first assisting duties on a regular basis, the surgeon may be entitled to rely on the skills and expertise of the nurse. Therefore, the nurse and/or health care facility may be held responsible for requiring the nurse to perform those duties.

The primary responsibility lies with the employer who presumably is aware that first assisting is routinely performed by registered nurses. It is deemed necessary that the employer provides necessary guidelines for this level of practice. It was generally agreed that the nurse undertaking this role:

- is an experienced perioperative nurse
- has completed an appropriate course
- has a demonstrated skill in performing the required duties.

(b)   Reimbursement

The question of reimbursement is complex and will differ from country to country. In Australia, questions which have been raised include:

- If the registered nurse acts as first assistant and is employed by a hospital or other facility, will this role become classified as part of a Nurses' Award?
- Will there be a classified payment by the hospital for this expanded role?
- Will surgeons employ RNs as first assistants, and will this be reimbursed by health insurance funds as is the current situation for medical practitioners ?

The versatility of the registered nurse in providing all phases of patient care will not only benefit the ever-diminishing hospital budget, but will provide an optimal and safe level of patient care in the operating suite and ambulatory surgery centres. Perioperative nurses will broaden their responsibility to encompass a multifaceted role, that is, they will undertake:

- preoperative assessment
- patient preparation and education
- intraoperative nursing practice including assisting the surgeon
- postoperative recovery
- evaluation of the surgical experience
- discharge planning and return to the community.

The cost benefits to be gained by initiating a multifaceted role will became an ever-increasing consideration for health care administrators. Although some health professionals espouse specialisation in perioperative nursing, in reality it is widely believed that this path will fragment the role of the registered nurse in the operating suite and affect staffing requirements in the budget. The role of the perioperative advanced nurse practitioner which incorporates that of the registered nurse as first assistant to the surgeon will have the potential ability to provide cost-effective nursing care and the versatility to undertake all roles in perioperative nursing. The ability to undertake other roles in the operating suite when not acting as first assistant has cost benefits to the facility. It provides a multiskilled approach which is reflected in a realistic staffing budget. The perceived benefits resultant from the development of this role include:

- improvement in the quality of patient care
- improved communication between care groups
- an increase in the continuity of patient care
- improvement in the standards of surgical teamwork
- provision of highly educated health professionals.

In Australia, continuing discussions between the Federal Minister for Health and the Federal Secretary of the Australian Nursing Federation have included a proposed reimbursement for nursing practice similar to Medicare.[5] However, there is still much work to be completed.

In the USA, reimbursement for nurse practitioners, clinical nurse specialists and certified midwives who are also RNFAs is set at 85% of the fee an assisting physician would receive. Prior to legislation passed in 1997, such reimbursement varied from state to state and practitioner to practitioner. Now, that reimbursement is unconstrained by geographic location or practice arrangement (see also AORN 1998b). Currently the question of Medicare reimbursement is being strongly lobbied for RNFAs in the US Congress.

(c)   Accountability

While the perioperative nurse works in collaboration with other health professionals to determine and meet patient needs, the nurse has primary responsibility and accountability for the nursing care of patients undergoing surgical intervention.

Accountability for practice by a registered nurse involves acting in such a manner as to enhance the general health and harmony of the community, justify public trust and confidence, and enhance the reputation of the profession and safeguard the interests of individual patients. Therefore, nurses must only carry out those clinical procedures for which they have been prepared. This preparation must include theory and supervised practice until competence has been assessed. Maintenance of knowledge and skills in performing clinical procedures is essential and measures must be in place to ensure regular review of competence. Nurses are at all times responsible for their own practice. They are expected to be aware of the limits of their abilities and to function within these limits. Nurses should be aware of the policies and procedures of their employing organisation. However, it should be noted that within a guideline or policy statement of an employer, any other organisation or professional group does not relieve the nurse of responsibility for his or her own actions and may not provide immunity in case of negligence. Accountability and responsibility coupled with the right of refusal to undertake any procedures for which preparation is inadequate are significant components of the role of the registered nurse as first assistant.

(d)   Professional practice

Most professions have established 'Standards of Practice' which provide a legal and professional framework for practice. They are defined in legislation by state or national authorities. The nursing profession is bound to comply with these standards of practice which are also defined by collegiate means through the statements such as the codes of conduct and practice issued by the professional nursing organisations.

(e)   Collaborative practice

Collaboration 'combines the activities of cooperation, or concern for another's interests, with assertiveness, or concern for one's own interests' (King et al., 1996). Its purpose is to enhance the quality of care and to improve patient outcomes. It is suggested that this could not be achieved when practised differently, for example, by separate and discrete medical and nursing models of care which would lack the communication which is part of collaborative practice.

Many health care facilities are introducing collaborative practice models which flow on from the introduction of shared governance (Porter-O'Grady, 1992). However, in the operating room the concept of collaborative practice has been part of the operating team approach for many years. Perioperative education provides the knowledge and expertise necessary to undertake such a role. The expanded role of the RNFA is perceived as a further development in collaboration. It is crucial that a registered nurse fulfils the perioperative role because first assisting in and of itself is not nursing but a medically supervised supportive service. This distinction has serious ramifications for collaborative relationships. Collaborative practice can be achieved only among groups with accountability, responsibility and authority for their own profession and practice. It is a complementary relationship, not a subordinate one.

As a perioperative nurse, the RNFA operates within the framework of nursing, although being supervised by the surgeon during the act of assisting. Registered nurses and doctors each offer areas of expertise making them interdependent in providing a total plan of care. This is a most significant development in health care. Neither medicine nor nursing alone can totally meet a patient's needs. Teamwork can only be achieved when doctors and nurses each decide that working together in the interest of the patient will bring them to their fullest professional potential.

Assistive personnel – a threat to perioperative nursing[6,7]

The health care needs of patients have become more complex as technology and science advance and change. The resultant treatment options have also increased in complexity. This necessitates that the provision of nursing care be undertaken by professionals who can demonstrate a substantial education in nursing and related sciences with a continuing commitment to accountable nursing practice.

In the current climate of economic constraint, management teams in health care facilities are seeking ways of saving money in high cost centres such as the operating suite. There is a concerted move by hospital administrators to employ technicians in nursing roles in the operating suite.

Concern has been expressed by several nursing bodies that standards of patient care are being, or will be, jeopardised by the employment of non-nursing personnel, that is, assistive personnel in the operating suite. In many areas, these workers are unlicensed. It is the responsibility of the nursing profession to endeavour to address this situation for the safety of patients.

Registered nurses undertake all roles in the operating suite, i.e. instrument, circulating, anaesthetic and postanaesthetic nurse in many countries. Only the registered nurse has the necessary theoretical knowledge, clinical expertise and the legal responsibility to practise perioperative nursing. The provision of complex nursing care which is part of the role of the perioperative nurse is considered the practice domain of the registered nurse. It is believed that the use of unlicensed assistive personnel to provide this level of nursing care is not based on consideration of who is the most suitably qualified but rather on economic considerations. The versatility of the registered nurse in providing all phases of perioperative care not only supports hospital budgets but also provides safe patient care.

Registered nurses have studied anatomy and the physiological alterations relating to disease, anaesthetics and surgery. They are aware of the consequences for the patients, the intraoperative risks, the potential for injuries and how to prevent them. They are also aware of the psychological implications of surgery and how to support the patient through the process. These qualifications work to ensure that patients have the highest quality of clinical and emotional care. There is a role for the technician in the operating suite and technicians are valuable members of the multidisciplinary team. However, they must provide specific technical support only and not undertake direct patient care.

In Australia, registered nurses and medical practitioners have responsibilities under state Drugs and Poisons Acts and Regulations which cannot be delegated to technicians. Legislation in individual states ascribes responsibility for the safe handling and administration of S4 and S8 drugs to the registered nurse. Any person described as a technician is not authorised to handle these drugs and if found in possession, notwithstanding the presence of an anaesthetist, is committing an offence under the various state acts and is liable to a penalty.

Nursing care of patients in all health care environments is and shall remain the responsibility of the profession of nursing. Medical practitioners and nurses must continue to work together as a collaborative team dedicated to and responsible for the provision of optimal patient care in all health care environments.

The Australian and New Zealand College of Anaesthetists (ANZCA) released their revised policy document on *The Assistant for the Anaesthetist* in February 1998. This document outlines the principles, the educational programme and the recommended content of the training courses. Nurses have some major concerns with the contents of this document such as the basic sciences to be taught, the invasive techniques which these assistants will undertake, e.g. insertion of intravenous, central venous and pulmonary artery catheters and arterial lines and their ongoing management. A further example is the administration of all drugs, fluids and other therapeutic substances during anaesthesia. An in-depth understanding as well as appropriate practical experience is to be obtained while providing assistance to the anaesthetists. Unfortunately, any person can undertake these courses provided they have a suitable educational standard. The duration of the course is 3 years' full-time employment for those without previous hospital experience, 2 years for an enrolled nurse and one year for a registered nurse. These personnel will be anaesthesia assistants. This situation was discussed at an open forum at the recent (1998) ACORN Triennial National Conference. A resolution was passed that ACORN and the ANF seek consultation with the peak nursing organisations in Australia to consider further action.

The situation in Canada is that surgical technicians are minimally employed and only undertake the instrument role (Gruendemann & Fernsebner, 1995, p.338).

In South Africa, all other personnel function only under the supervision of the registered nurse (Gruendemann & Fernsebner, 1995, p.343).

In Chile, technicians are utilised as required in surgical procedures, for example, as X-ray technologists and in cardiac surgery as perfusionists (Gruendemann & Fernsebner, 1995, p.348).

As discussed previously, in Portugal, perioperative nursing positions are under threat because of the perceived cost benefit of employing technicians in the operating suite.

There is a different situation in Italy where operating suite technicians are employed purely for technical support (Brett, 1996, p.5).

In Australia, the escalating use of technicians to undertake care of the patient which is deemed to be nursing has caused grave concern and is being urgently addressed. The use of enrolled nurses is perceived to be of limited use in the operating room because of the necessity to directly supervise these personnel when engaged in direct patient care. Assistants at surgery are either registrars, interns or registered nurses.

In the UK, because of staffing shortages, for many years health care facilities have been utilising Operating Department Assistants (ODAs). These personnel are not registered nurses. The introduction of paramedical personnel originated from cost containment and registered nurses staffing shortages, now allied with the need to provide specialist support as junior doctors hours are reduced. Traditionally, in the UK the ODA supported the anaesthetist. ODA training was introduced as a result of a shortage of 'theatre' nurses in 1973. In 1976, as part of the recommendations of the Lewin Report, training criteria and an examination were implemented for ODAs. The Bevan Report in 1989 recommended the development of a common training with defined levels of competence for anaesthetic and surgical support personnel. A 'theatre person' to be known as an Operating Department Practitioner (ODP) was expected to have the knowledge and ability to practise in all theatre situations and was expected to supersede and interchange with, but not replace, the traditional roles of, the registered nurse and the ODA. Bevan used ODP as a generic term 'referring to a theatre worker' but there could be some confusion between this level of worker and those designated as ODPs and certified by City and Guilds at a Practice Level 3 (Ince, 1995, p.80).

It is evident that these assistant roles were developed because the initial 'training' of Registered General Nurses and State Enrolled Nurses was undertaken on an ad hoc basis. The Lewin Report in its recommendation for specific training obviously intended to ensure that standards were maintained and that assistants had the skills to assist in the provision of safe medical practice. Unfortunately, this would appear to affect the utilisation of nurses in the operating suite and a resultant fragmentation of patient care. Ince described the introduction of Additional Accredited Units by the National Council for Vocational Qualifications (NCVQ) with significant medical input in their development. Assessment and certification were provided for each unit and, as understanding improved, it was believed that nurses and ODAs would feel 'less threatened'. Ince (1995, p.83), in his conclusion, referred to the reduction in hours of the junior doctors and the resultant need to have other personnel available to undertake the work. He believes that the tasks currently performed by doctors 'could be safely delegated to non-medical staff' but he also states that ODAs and ODPs 'must have a professional register and be fully accountable'. Registered nurses already possess a professional register and are fully accountable. It is postulated that registered nurses have permitted these and other similar situations to develop because of lack of care or motivation until it was already too late. The concern which is felt by the nursing profession is that assistants and other unlicensed personnel, although performing nursing roles, are not responsible to the nursing division within a health care facility. They may be controlled by the medical division or the allied health division. These personnel are utilised in many health care facilities. Some form of action must be taken by the nursing profession to retain the regulation of these personnel under the 'umbrella' of nursing which will ensure that the protection of patients' rights will be ensured.

The challenge for the future

We have a challenge as we move towards the third millennium. We must consider a new and dynamic approach, to adapt to new practice modalities. Challenges are demanding but they provide opportunities for enormous growth and development. To undertake such an approach requires courage and commitment. Dr Jane Rothrock who has been so involved in developing the RNFA role in the USA inspires us to find the courage to discover new ways to provide care for patients during their perioperative experience and entreats us to increase our knowledge base about how best to achieve this. We must set out on a journey into a future which is dazzling in its promise of advanced practice. Our journey of courage will require us to embrace change and travel across unfamiliar boundaries. As we travel, it is important to remember that the roles which are evolving are nursing roles, developed and practised within the framework of the profession of nursing.

At the National Association of Theatre Nurses Annual Conference in Harrogate in 1996, during the presentation of one of the papers defining the evolving roles in perioperative nursing, a significant statement was made:

> We (nurses) are not surrogate doctors, not technicians and certainly not power-crazy elitists but nurses with vision, self-respect and confidence in ourselves and our profession.

Let us accept the challenges, let us seize the opportunities, let us commence the journey, let us walk into the future with renewed vigour inspired with the clarity of our vision for perioperative nursing. Our allegiance to our profession will allow us to do no less.

Reflective activities

It should now be clear that a considerable amount of work has been carried out into new roles and relationships for perioperative nurses. In line with developments in other branches of nursing there is a move to replace highly paid nurses with non-registered (or unlicenced or assistive) staff who have been vocationally trained to acquire the practical skills needed in a specific area of practice.

The development of the advanced nursing practitioner, leading a team of lesser qualified assistants, is resulting in the development of a valuable, and cost-effective member of the operating department team who will be able to undertake a variety of roles. In addition to a clinical intraoperative role this nurse will liaise with wards and assess patients preoperatively, manage theatre suites intraoperatively and will be able to outreach to the community to give clinical and educational support to both patients and their carers.

1 Consider your own role in the operating department. How far are your moving towards advanced practice? Make sure that you are clear about your own professional role and scope of practice.

2 Is it possible that you are being asked to undertake duties without proper preparation or without real understanding of the scope of nursing practice?

3 Do any of the comments made about the difficulties of developing roles of perioperative nurses and non-nursing operating department practitioners have significance for the way your own department managers have changed the roles and skill mix in your workplace?

4 Have the disagreements between surgeons, anaesthetists, nurses and ODPs/technicians affected working relationships? What steps can be taken to ensure that each group understands the aspirations and frustrations of the other groups? Do you all recognise the status and expertise of each other?

5 Look around and see if you are aware of a good model for future development of the staffing of operating departments and opportunities for professional development, education and training.

Endnotes

1 i.e. after graduation from nursing college or university and inclusion on a nursing register.

2 See Chapter 4 for further details on the education of Australian nurses working in the operating room.

3 A discussion on links with industry is contained in Chapter 12.

4 Refer to Chapter 6 for further details on perioperative nursing in Europe. Also see Brett, M. 1996 European Common Core Curriculum for Operating Department Nursing (EORNA).

5 Medicare is a compulsory health insurance available to all taxpayers in Australia, the contributions being deducted as part of a personal taxation. This process allows people to access the public health system.

6 The terminology and views expressed here are based on Australian perioperative nursing but can be taken as the general views of perioperative nurses across the world, remembering always that progress towards this ideal is slow and variable.

7 Readers in countries which employ fully trained operating department assistants or practitioners are reminded that Australian operating department practitioners have a comparatively short training and that the legal situation precludes their working as surgeon's assistants.

References

American Association of Nurse Anaesthetists. 1992 *Guidelines and standards for nurse anaesthesia practice.* Chicago, Illinois, AANA.

AORN. 1998 *Delegates forum and House of Delegates agenda – working document on perioperative nursing roles. AORN Journal* January, **67** (1), 51–61.

AORN. 1999 *Standards, recommended practices and guidelines.* Denver, CO, AORN Inc. 100.

Australian and New Zealand College of Anaesthetists. 1998 *The assistant for the anaesthetist.* PS8 1998. Policy Document. Melbourne: Australian and New Zealand College of Anaesthetists.

Baxter, B. 1993 Nurse anaesthetists – can we afford them? *British Journal of Theatre Nursing* 3 (4), 25.

Benner, P. 1984 *From novice to expert.* Menlo Park, CA, Addison-Wesley.

Bevan, P. 1989 *Management and utilisation of operating departments.* London, Department of Health.

Bowey, D. & Caballero, C. 1996 A lead role. *Nursing Times* July 24, **92** (30), 29–31.

Brett, M. 1996 Operating department nurse education in Europe. *British Journal of Theatre Nursing* 6 (4), 5–8.

Busen, N.H. & Engelman, S.G. 1996 The CNS with practitioner preparation: an emerging role in advanced practice nursing. *Clinical Nurse Specialist.* **10** (3), 145–50.

Chopra, V., Bovil, J.G. & Spierdijk, J. 1990 Accidents, near accidents and complications of anaesthesia. *Anaesthesia* **45**, 3–6.

Friend, B. 1996 A risky business. *Nursing Times* July 24, **92**, 30.

Groetzsch, G.A. 1997. RN first assisting – 1997 Canadian update. *Canadian Operating Room Nursing Journal* May/June, 13–17.

Gruendemann, B.J. & Fernsebner, B. 1995 *Comprehensive perioperative nursing,* Vol 1 – Principles. London: Jones & Bartlett, pp.333–58.

Hamilton, H. 1998. Nurse practitioners. (Editorial). *The Collegian* 5 (2), 5.

Henderson, V. 1969. *The basic principles of nursing care,* 5th. edition. Basel, Switzerland, Karger.

Ince, C. 1995. Training non-medical theatre personnel. *Health Trends* **27** (3), 80–85.

International Federation of Nurse Anaesthetists. 1990. *Committee on Education – position on educational standards for preparing nurse anaesthetists.*

Keane, A. & Richmond, T. 1993 Tertiary nurse practitioners. *IMAGE: Journal of Nursing Scholarship* **35** (4), Winter 1993, 281–4.

King, K.B., Parrinello, K.M. & Braggs, J.G. 1996 Collaboration and advanced practice nursing. In: Hickey, J.V. (Ed.) *Advanced practice nursing: changing roles and clinical applications.* Philadelphia, PA, Lippincott-Raven.

Leifer, D. 1996 The future of nursing? *Nursing Standard* July, **10** (41), 13.

Lewin Report. 1970 *The organisation and staffing of operating departments.* London, Department of Health and Social Security, HMSO.

Mitchinson, S. & Goodlad, S. 1996 Changes in the roles and responsibilities of nurses. *Professional Nurse* August **11** (11), 734–6.

NATN. 1993a *The role of the nurse as first assistant to the surgeon in the operating department.* Harrogate, NATN.

NATN. 1993b *The role of the nurse as surgeon's assistant.* Harrogate, NATN.

NHS Executive. 1996 *Professional roles in anaesthetics: a scoping study.* London: NHS Executive.

Nurse Practitioner Project (Stage 3). 1995 *Final report of the Steering Committee.* Sydney, Australia, NSW Department of Health.

Porter-O'Grady, T. 1992 *Implementing shared governance: creating a professional organisation.* St Louis, MO, Mosby Year Book Inc.

Porter-O'Grady, T. 1996. Nurses as advanced practitioners and primary care providers. In: Cohe, E.L. (ed.) *Nursing care management in the 21st century.* St Louis, MO, Mosby, pp.10–12.

Rothrock, J.C. 1997 Ensure your role in the future of perioperative nursing. *AORN Journal* July, **66** (1), 144–5.

Rothrock, J.C. 1998 *The registered nurse first assistant: an expanded perioperative nursing role,* 3rd edition. Philadelphia, PA, J.B. Lippincott.

Staunton, P.J. & Whyburn, B. 1993 *Nursing and the law,* 3rd edition. Sydney, Australia, W B Saunders.

UKCC. 1992 *The scope of professional practice.* London, UKCC.

Vincent, S. 1996 Develop to survive. *Nursing Times* October 2, **92** (40), 59–60.

Woodhead, K. 1995 Assisting the surgeon: the dilemma for nurses. *Nursing Standard* **10** (3), 53–4.

PART TWO

Perioperative nurse education

Educating the perioperative nurse

Menna Davies and Jennifer Cunningham

In this chapter Menna Davies and Jennifer Cunningham review the development of nurse education in Australia, more particularly they concentrate on the development of perioperative nurse education. It is clear that many issues being faced by nurses in Australia are common to nurses worldwide though some solutions are different. Australian nurses were in the vanguard in taking nurse education into higher education and in gaining recognition for nurses as professionals. Yet, even now, they are faced with the same attacks on their status, indeed their future survival, as are nurses in many other countries.

The UKCC developed the concept of the 'knowledgeable doer' which was seen as the epitome of nursing for the future: all patients would be cared for by well-educated, thinking practitioners whose actions would be rooted in a firm knowledge base. This has turned out to be an unreachable ideal. Educated thinking nurses are too expensive for health departments to employ in numbers in the present economic climate. Politicians and managers have resolved the problem by reducing the numbers of qualified, registered nurses and replacing them with a variety of lesser or differently qualified carers and technicians.

In some cases nurses have benefited by increased status and new responsibilities. In others, the changes and demands made on them have proved stressful. Perhaps we should be asking ourselves how well knowledge and practice have been welded together. Is there enough time in a day, or even in a professional life-time, to keep professional knowledge up-to-date whilst still finding time to maintain the competencies needed for quality patient care as a member of the perioperative team? Has there always been a bifurcation between the nurse manager and the nursing or theatre practitioner which we have been reluctant to admit?

Australia is a big country and problems can sometimes be compounded by distance. Nurses often work in small isolated country hospitals. The development of ongoing education and encouragement of new nursing roles raised problems for nurses with family commitments who could not go away to complete courses lasting weeks or months. As nursing goes through a time of major change we are being forced to address many questions about future roles and responsibilities. Menna Davies and Jennifer Cunningham outline how they are addressing the professional issues and the para-doxical situation which faces them. They discuss the way that New South Wales periop-erative nurses addressed the problems following the removal of theatre allocations from student programmes and outline one solution to providing postgraduate perioperative nurse education by the use of distance and computer-assisted learning.

Introduction

Perioperative nurses in Australia currently find themselves in the midst of a battle for survival in a climate of economic rationalism where the health dollar is at a premium and those in charge of the purse strings view the operating theatre as a high spending, technical area. There is also a view that those who work in the operating theatre fulfil a purely technical role, one which could be undertaken by lesser grades of nurses or by non-nurses at greatly reduced cost. The challenges inherent in this scenario are compounded by poor recruitment rates of registered nurses into perioperative nursing.

The response to these challenges must be, firstly, to implement strategies to encourage registered nurses to pursue a career in the specialty and, once they have embarked on their career, to provide educational opportunities. This will not only maintain high standards of nursing care for the surgical patient, but defend against the erosion of the role of the perioperative registered nurse. Some of these strategies have already been implemented and will be discussed in greater detail later in the chapter.

The Australian health care system

To understand the position of the Australian nurse in the perioperative role, it is useful to know a little about Australia and the structure of our health care system. Although Australia is a large land mass, there is a relatively small population;

approximately 18 million in 1996. The country is divided into six States and two Territories which are: Queensland, New South Wales, Victoria, South Australia, Tasmania and Western Australia, the Northern Territory and the Australian Capital Territory (ACT). Each of these have their own State or Territory Governments and Health Departments.

Each of the States and Territories are responsible for administering their own acute hospital and related health services. There is a national public health system, called Medicare (contributed to by the whole population), and numerous private health funds to which people are encouraged to contribute and access the many private health care facilities throughout the country. Policy, funding, administration, regulation, standard setting and monitoring of health is the responsibility of either Federal (national) government, State/Territory government, or a combination of both (National Health Strategy, 1991, p.37). Annual meetings take place between the State/Territory health ministers and the Federal health minister in order to negotiate the Federal government's contribution to each State/Territory health budget.

Each State[1] has its own Nurses Act and Registration Board and nurses pay an annual registration fee in order to maintain their license to practice. Each State has a policy of mutual recognition of registration thus facilitating the movement of nurses wishing to work in different States within Australia. At present there is no requirement for nurses to demonstrate clinical currency in order to renew their registration. However, some States have a 'recency of practice' policy requiring nurses who have not practised for a certain period of time to undertake refresher programmes in order to renew their registration.

Historical background

Nursing in Australia has had an interesting history which highlights its links with England. To address poor standards of nursing care in Sydney in the 19th century, the colonial secretary, Henry Parkes, appealed to Florence Nightingale, considered at the time to be the world authority on nursing care. In 1868 Lucy Osburn, a Nightingale protégée, arrived in New South Wales and took charge of the Sydney Infirmary. This included setting up the first formal training school in Australia, with graduates eventually taking up senior positions throughout the other States (Russell, 1990, p.10).

As a penal colony, Australia looked to Britain for guidance in many areas including health care and nursing. The Florence Nightingale model of nursing was at the forefront of practice during this period, and this model continued to be the major influence in Australian nursing until the 1960s (Russell, 1990, p.15).

Australian nursing quickly became organised into professional groups, the Australasian Trained Nurses' Association (ATNA) being established in 1899. This organisation's aims included scrutinising nurses' qualifications for registration, recognition of training schools and establishing minimum standards for nurses' education (Russell, 1990, p.18). ATNA was eventually superseded by statutory bodies (Nursing Boards) in each state who took over the regulation of nursing registration.

Postbasic training was limited to midwifery and psychiatric nursing as no other courses existed in Australia until 1949. Both The New South Wales College of Nursing and College of Nursing, Australia began to conduct courses in other specialty areas in 1949 and 1950 respectively (Russell, 1990, p.80).

By 1960 nurses could register in six different categories (general, psychiatric, geriatric, mental retardation, midwifery and mothercraft) and the Enrolled Nurse Aide (ENA) position was created to address the shortage of nursing staff (Russell, 1990, pp.53,54). The ENAs underwent a one year training to equip them with skills to carry out routine practical nursing care under the supervision of a registered nurse.

During the 20th century Australia saw a huge increase in its population through planned immigration schemes. With this came a demand for efficient health services which required a review of both basic and postbasic nursing education in order to meet these increased demands.

Education and registration

The hospital-based preregistration training system, based on the Florence Nightingale model, continued in all States of Australia without major changes until the 1960s, when a series of reviews were undertaken and reports made into nurse education. The findings revealed many problems – lack of recruits into nursing, poor educational standards, high attrition rates, staff shortages, the apprenticeship system, no correlation between theory and clinical practice and poor facilities (Russell, 1990, pp.98–101).

It was also becoming increasingly difficult for Australian nurses to register in both the UK and the USA as changes in nurse education occurring in these countries demanded registration requirements with which Australian nurses found it hard to comply because of the Australian nurse training system (Russell, 1990, pp. 153–5).

Possibly the most significant report was the Sax Report in 1978 which recommended that there should be educationally sound programmes for nurses at both preregistration and postgraduate level, in short the education of nurses should be overseen by tertiary educational institutions, rather than by hospitals. Thus, began the movement into the tertiary sector of preregistration nurse education which took place on a variety of timetables specific to each State/Territory, but had attained Bachelor degree status by the late 1980s (Australian Tertiary Education Commission, 1978). Postgraduate nurse education has also developed within the tertiary sector, although a small number of certificate level courses still exist at hospital level. This will be discussed in greater detail later in the chapter.

According to Lublin (1985, p.29) 'tertiary education … is said to be based on respect for intellectual enquiry and to encourage independence and the cultivation of critical and evaluative skills'. A long way from Florence Nightingale and her training schools!

The transfer of nurse education came about not simply as a result of the Sax Report. Changes had occurred within Australian society that affected the role of women during the 1960s and 1970s. Increased interest in professional, educational, political, financial and feminist issues undoubtedly contributed to increasing militancy among nurses, encouraging them to actively seek improvement in wages and conditions of employment (Lublin, 1985, p.18). These often led to marches, industrial unrest and eventual progress in the area of nursing education.

The transfer of nurse education from hospital-based training to tertiary education affected not only the nursing profession and the health care service, but also various governments. Whilst hospital-based, nurse education was the responsibility of State health budgets; this would now become the responsibility of Federal/State education budgets (Cochrane, 1989, p.31).

Changes in health care delivery are dependent on available funding and government economic policy. These changes have obviously had a dramatic impact on nursing with the increase in technology and the increasingly active role of the consumer in decision making being two examples. Health care in Australia, as in other countries, has been moving away from treatment focus towards health promotion and illness prevention. This has challenged registered nurses to be prepared, through appropriate education, to be a part of such changes.

According to Cordery (1995, p.355) recent emphasis on economic rationalism has had a profound impact on Australian health care. Reduced health budgets and pressure to increase efficiency have become facts of life. What this has meant in practical terms is continued pressure to justify the role of nurses, particularly registered nurses in many areas. The operating theatre and the perioperative registered nurse are definitely in the line of fire and role erosion is a very real threat in favour of cheaper grades of nursing and non-nursing staff. Current statistics in NSW, together with anecdotal evidence, show quite clearly a high vacancy rate of perioperative registered nurses – figures which can be extrapolated nationwide with a degree of certainty. Why has this happened? A closer examination of changes in preregistration nursing education provides part of the answer.

Tertiary education

During hospital-based training, the Australian student nurses were generally required (depending on State/Territory regulations) to spend a minimum of 6 weeks in the operating theatre during which time they were required to complete a number of clinical skills assessments. A typical rotation to the operating theatre would include experience in the sterile supply department to 'learn the instruments'; the recovery room; anaesthetics and a final period scouting[2] and scrubbing for a set number of 'major' and 'minor' operations. This experience tended to polarise the student nurses' view of perioperative nursing. Their enthusiasm was either fired or they were scared off, the outcome usually dependent upon the reception they received from senior staff.

Following the transfer of basic nurse education to the tertiary sector exposure to perioperative nursing changed dramatically. More than 18 tertiary institutions currently offer undergraduate nursing programmes throughout Australia, although not all offer exposure to perioperative nursing. Of those that do, the maximum is 2 weeks of clinical experience, and the placements are optional. Exposure to a clinical specialty undoubtedly reduces the probability of new graduates choosing the clinical specialty to pursue later as a career option within nursing.

The perception by both hospital and academic administrators that perioperative nurses perform a primarily technical role, that it is in many ways 'not real nursing' may in part be the reason why clinical rotations to the operating theatre have been largely omitted from undergraduate nursing programmes. Other reasons given are that the 3-year comprehensive curriculum is aimed at producing a beginning level 'general' nurse and the specialty areas should be pursued at postgraduate level. Whilst there may be some merit in this argument, many perioperative nurses maintain that if exposure does not take place at undergraduate level there is likely to be very little motivation to pursue perioperative nursing at postgraduate level. As discussed earlier the lack of registered nurses currently seeking employment in the operating theatre gives some credence to this latter view point. With a little lateral thinking on the part of the universities, many desirable student outcomes could be achieved within the operating theatre whilst maintaining the exposure necessary to entice the students back upon graduation. Allocating clinical practice within the operating theatre environment in the undergraduate programme exposes the student to nursing activities which are of great value and easily transferable to other areas of nursing. These activities include nursing unconscious patients, aseptic technique, infection control, pharmacology, fluid balance, patient assessment, monitoring patients using the latest technologies, communication, positioning patients, an understanding of surgery and related anatomy.

Financial reasons are also given for the lack of undergraduate exposure to the specialty and there is no doubt that the clinical component of the undergraduate programmes forms a huge financial burden for universities which has seen a reduction in clinical exposure across all areas of the curriculum. Other reasons why undergraduates are scarce within the operating theatres could be a lack of academic personnel with the necessary skills and, more importantly, the enthusiasm to promote greater exposure to the specialty. It must also be acknowledged that there have been some operating theatre managers who, although approached by universities to provide clinical placements for students have been less than enthusiastic or cooperative. There is obviously room for further collaboration on these issues.

Promoting the specialty

Faced with the above scenario, perioperative nursing groups throughout Australia have worked hard to find strategies to try and resolve the problems evolving from this lack of exposure to the specialty, in particular the possible consequences for staffing operating theatres in the future. Finding ways to increase exposure to perioperative nursing at undergraduate level remains the challenge for perioperative nurses in each State.

Perioperative nurses in Australia have been organised into State or Territory professional groups for many years. For example the New South Wales Operating Theatre Association Inc (NSW OTA) was founded in 1957 and as with other State groups provides a forum for perioperative nurses to discuss issues related to the specialty. State groups are connected formally through elected councillors from each State group to form the Australian Confederation of Operating Room Nurses (ACORN). This organisation was one of the first national professional groups formed in 1977 and has gained a reputation as being one of the most powerful and well respected of national specialty groups. ACORN has produced standards, guidelines and policy statements, competency standards for perioperative nurses, as well as a national journal published quarterly (ACORN, 1995).

Each State professional perioperative group has been very active over a number of years in attending university open days and successfully lobbying for invitations to speak to undergraduate nurses to promote perioperative nursing experience. Nursing students who showed an interest in the specialty, during these visits, declared their frustration at being unable to access perioperative nursing experience during their undergraduate programmes. They also faced problems upon gaining their registration when attempting to find employment as a perioperative nurse, in that many operating theatres would not accept registered nurses without previous experience. The consequence, as previously indicated, is that these registered nurses may choose another specialty and be lost from perioperative nursing. It became obvious that these students were full of enthusiasm, but needed a mechanism which would provide them with the clinical experience required to assist them in securing employment within the operating theatre.

This was the challenge which encouraged The NSW College of Nursing to design a course specifically for those registered nurses without clinical experience in the operating theatre. Following discussions between the management of the College and the New South Wales Operating Theatre Association the first 'Introduction to Perioperative Nursing Course' was conducted in 1992.

Introduction to perioperative nursing course

The course aims to provide an introduction to the theoretical concepts of perioperative nursing and their practical application. It was decided that the course would be very much a 'hands on', practical experience emphasising the nursing care which perioperative nurses provide.

The course can be conducted in a number of different ways. Initially it was conducted over 8 weeks, one evening a week within a variety of operating theatres in metropolitan Sydney. Operating theatre administrators made their facilities and resources available. Perioperative nurses, who are members of the NSW OTA, provide expertise as clinical facilitators for a number of the practical sessions and specialist educators at the College coordinate the programme as well as actively participate in a number of sessions.

The need for perioperative education was also identified in rural areas of New South Wales who have also been affected by the lack of experienced perioperative nurses or have hospitals which rotate their staff from ward areas into operating theatres. The staff, therefore, have limited experience in the specialty. Such hospitals have taken the initiative to provide staff development in this area, in some cases using government funds specially allocated for orientation programmes to specialty areas. The course has been successfully conducted in several locations in rural NSW with the eight sessions condensed into a shorter time frame of 4 days with the final discussion session of the evening course being replaced by the students being involved in a mock set up, putting together the knowledge and skills covered in the previous sessions.

Course content

The eight sessions begin with an open forum discussion on 'What is perioperative nursing?' An historical review of surgery and the evolution of perioperative nursing is undertaken and the various roles in which perioperative nurses participate are identified. The next five sessions undertaken within various operating theatres environments further explore the knowledge required to carry out the roles identified in the first session and provide the opportunity to practice relevant practical skills. Sessions are conducted on anaesthetics, asepsis, sterilisation, scrubbing, gowning and gloving, positioning, diathermy, prepping and draping, instruments, sutures and needles, recovery room, law and professional issues. The key to the practical sessions is to provide a non-threatening environment for the students. No patients are involved, rather the students act as patients within the operating room environment, gaining an insight into the patient's perioperative experience.

The courses have been well-attended and very successful, although no data exist on actual recruitment rates for the graduates from such courses, anecdotal evidence suggests that many graduates have found work within operating theatres. The course, originally designed for newly graduated registered nurses has also attracted a number of nurses returning to the profession who use the course as a refresher programme. In late 1997 the course was opened up to third year nursing students in NSW whose aim was to find work as perioperative nurses upon graduation. This strategy is a significant move in trying to increase recruitment rates by providing preregistration experience to which they may not normally have access.

The course in NSW has encouraged professional groups in two other States, Queensland and Victoria, to conduct similar courses.

One area which needs serious consideration is the support which the course graduates require upon gaining employment in the operating theatre. The students should and do exit the course with a clear understanding of the many and varied roles of the nurse within the operating theatre. Participation in the course does not, however, produce instant perioperative nurses, despite what some employers might believe. The graduates require nurturing with specific orientation and further education in specialty areas within the operating theatre to become safe and efficient practitioners.

Many hospitals throughout Australia run new graduate programmes, which involve a number of clinical placements during the 12-month programme. This gives the new graduate an opportunity to 'try out' a few different areas before committing to one. Unfortunately, rotation to the operating theatre does not figure prominently in many of these programmes. The reasons for this are similar to those given by universities for not including greater perioperative nursing exposure in their curriculum. Although it appears, in this case, that the reluctance is mainly on the part of hospital nursing administration in denying access to the operating theatre.

Postgraduate education

Currently postgraduate perioperative nurse education is offered in a variety of awards, through a variety of institutions, by a variety of means. A perioperative nurse may gain a Graduate Certificate, Graduate Diploma or Master's Degree in the specialty. Very few hospital-based, certificate award programmes have survived because they are generally expensive to conduct. It is more likely that postgraduate courses will be undertaken through a university via face to face delivery or totally via distance education mode through The New South Wales College of Nursing. There are also universities who are offering some subjects via distance education. Postgraduate courses in specialties such as recovery room and anaesthetic nursing currently available at a few hospitals and, through The New South Wales College of Nursing via distance education, are slowly being developed at diploma level within the tertiary sector.

It is difficult not to be somewhat cynical about the enthusiasm with which universities have developed and embraced postgraduate education in perioperative nursing given the apparent indifference to the specialty at undergraduate level. To be fair it should be stated that the operating theatre is not the only specialty to suffer, intensive care and the emergency department are other areas unable to be accommodated in the undergraduate programme. However, the universities have worked hard in collaboration with members of perioperative professional groups to provide the variety of postgraduate courses currently available. The proliferation of courses at all levels can only be of benefit to a specialty which is constantly challenged to justify its existence. Better educated nurse specialists will be a vital defence against the ever increasing threat posed by external forces of economic rationalism which has, unfortunately, seen many operating theatres look to employing increasing numbers of lesser grades of nurses, namely the enrolled nurse and non-nursing personnel, in particular the anaesthetic technician. More on this issue a little later.

From a distance

As previously discussed there are a variety of courses and modes of delivery available for perioperative registered nurses. The hospital- and university-based programmes are found in large city centres requiring students to attend lectures and obtain clinical experience in participating hospitals, thereby making access to such courses difficult for nurses living and working in rural areas.

In July 1990 The New South Wales College of Nursing embarked on an educational project never before attempted in Australia, namely providing an external course in the clinical specialty of perioperative nursing. The College has been active in providing a wide range of clinical postregistration and continuing education courses since 1949. As well as providing on campus and external courses, it is proactive in the advancement of all aspects of professional nursing, collaborating with a number of government agencies and nursing organisations and enjoying the respect of the profession across Australia.

The prospect of an external course in perioperative nursing was first discussed during the mid 1980s by perioperative nurses in rural western NSW who were concerned at the lack of educational opportunities within their specialty. If registered nurses living in rural areas wished to complete the city-based courses, it meant leaving their job, family and support systems to spend a year away studying. Although a number of perioperative nurses took the plunge and came to the city, they were few in number and the year was often full of homesickness and marital trauma, hardly conditions conducive to learning. An alternative had to be found which allowed students to live and work in their home town whilst providing an opportunity to obtain a specialty qualification in perioperative nursing. A programme conducted by distance education appeared to be the best option.

The idea of a distance education course was brought to the attention of the Executive of the NSW Operating Theatre Association. Having close professional ties with The NSW College of Nursing, they commenced discussions with them on the possibility of such a venture. The NSW Department of Health was approached and funds were made available to get a distance education course in perioperative nursing off the ground. The first certificate course, lasting 12 months, commenced in July 1990 with 52 students, 39 of whom came from rural centres in NSW. The course has expanded over the years to include students from other States and even from New Zealand and Hong Kong. It also increasingly attracts students living in metropolitan areas who prefer the flexibility which studying by distance education allows. A course offered by distance mode is attractive to employers, too, because it negates the need to release students to attend lectures.

The profile of the student group is typically female, ranging in age from mid-twenties to late forties. Despite the increase in metropolitan-based students, the majority of students still come from small rural centres where they have lived and worked for most, if not all, of their lives. Many are married, have two or three children, have not studied since their general training and have anywhere between 2–15 years operating room nursing experience. There is a wide range of skills – some students work in very small hospitals which have only one operating room. They may be the only registered nurse and surgery may take place only 2 or 3 days per week. A cholecystectomy is perhaps the biggest procedure they have to contend with. At the other end of the scale there are students from large city hospitals who participate in major cardiac procedures and neurosurgery. It has been a challenge to provide course material which will cater for this wide range in skills and experience.

The aims of the course are to use the principles of adult learning in order to produce an educational programme which challenges the students to think critically, to problem solve and to make changes in their clinical practice where necessary.

The course is divided into four modules of study. The first module examines the role of the perioperative nurse and some of the economic and professional issues which impact on that role. The student is introduced to theories of nursing and to the use of research in perioperative nursing. 'Relationships within the team' tackles communication issues, for example assertiveness and conflict resolution. Patient advocacy, legal and ethical issues are also addressed.

Module two looks at the operating suite environment – and begins by examining operating theatre design. This is followed by a comprehensive section on asepsis, beginning with a review of microbiology and examining issues such as surgical conscience, prepping and draping, scrubbing procedures and operating theatre apparel. Environmental issues within the operating suite are discussed, for example, electrical, chemical hazards, noise and ergonomics. The student is introduced to management issues, there are sections on clinical teaching, total quality management, instruments and equipment care.

Modules three and four both relate to the perioperative patient, pull together information gained in the other modules and are particularly enjoyed by the students as they include an opportunity for the student to follow a patient through their perioperative experience. There are topics on interviewing skills, assessment and planning for care, pre- and postanaesthetic care, positioning, sutures, needles, haemostasis, prioritising care for emergency surgery and dealing with death in the operating suite.

The course material is mainly print based with the various sections containing guided readings and activities which the students undertake at their own pace. Some sections include the use of audio and video tapes to supplement the written material.

In a course conducted by distance education it is logistically impossible to require students to rotate through all surgical specialties when students are scattered all over Australia. Students who work in rural areas would not have access to a wide variety of surgery nor, it could be argued, would they benefit greatly from experiencing types of complex surgery in, say, a large metropolitan teaching hospital, when they may never be called upon to use those skills in their own hospital. The practical skills of the typical student are well-developed within the range of surgery undertaken at their own hospital. The course aims to build on those skills by exposing the student to a range of educational materials which arouses and actively engages them to explore their role in caring for the perioperative patient and to think critically about practice, using knowledge gained to confirm or change existing practices.

The course emphasises that there is more to being a perioperative nurse than simply standing at the operating table handing instruments to a surgeon. Practical skills are certainly of great importance to the perioperative nurse as a person with this expertise can shorten the length of surgery considerably and is, indeed, an asset to any surgical team. Relying too heavily on promoting technical expertise may, however, lead to comments of 'A trained monkey could do that' or 'You don't need to be a nurse to work in theatre' whilst the spectre of the operating theatre technician looms large, a most unwelcome and threatening prospect to Australian perioperative nurses.

It would appear from student feedback that the course material has acted as a catalyst for changes in practice in the area of practical skills whilst still emphasising the integrity of the patient as a person and how it is imperative to address the total needs of the surgical patient.

Exposure to the course material has certainly changed a number of clinical practices within the students' own workplaces. The rich collaboration of theory and practice has seen many students comment on the greater confidence they now have in their own ability. They now feel less afraid of challenging the status quo, of questioning the ritualistic practices which abound in some operating theatres. The sound theoretical base from which the student now operates and the wealth of research articles now at their disposal have provided the students with evidence which they use to argue their case for change. Many students have felt they now use greater assertiveness to act in the role of patient advocate because they are now more aware of their own rights and those of their patients. They are now more aware of why certain techniques are used and are not afraid to point these out to others who are not complying. Knowledge has empowered many students to take control of their practice.

This Graduate Certificate programme has allowed many perioperative nurses, who never thought they would have the opportunity to gain a qualification in their specialty because of their geographical isolation, the chance to achieve so much. The positive experiences recounted by students of the course and by their colleagues, who frequently comment on the changes in attitude, increase in confidence and practical ability they have witnessed in the students will ensure that this course is operating from a distance for a long time to come.

The success of the perioperative nursing course has seen the College develop further distance education courses related to the specialty. These include operating suite management and anaesthetic and recovery room nursing.

University courses

Many universities offer a whole range of perioperative nursing programmes and over the past 5 years there has been an explosion of educational opportunities for nurses. Courses at Graduate Certificate (one year), Diploma (2 years) and Master's (3 years) level are available in most States. In recent years as the battle for students has heated up, more and more collaboration with hospitals and innovative programming has occurred from which the nurse student can only benefit. Many university-based programmes are linked with specific hospitals, called collaborative partners, where students undertake clinical experience and assessment. Theoretical subjects are undertaken at the university and students enrol in a variety of study modules related to different aspects of perioperative nursing whilst also taking core subjects alongside nurses studying other specialties. Universities are increasingly recognising courses undertaken in other institutions and granting students advance standing, for example a nurse possessing a Graduate Certificate is likely to gain credit when entering a Diploma or Master's programme in the specialty or one which is closely related. Some universities allow simultaneous enrolments of their students in subjects conducted by The NSW College of Nursing. The cost of each course depends on the university, students either pay course fees which can be quite expensive, e.g. approximately A$800 per subject, or they pay into the government's Higher Education Contribution Scheme (HECS) which is less, but not tax deductible as a self-education expense.

The use of technology

In a country the size of Australia the use of multimedia technology is extensive and an essential component of supporting students, particularly those in rural and remote areas. Australia has always been in the forefront of developing technology in order to reduce the isolation of rural and remote communities. Many children in outback Australia receive much of their basic schooling by radio via the 'school of the air' which connects them to central educational institutions. The development of sophisticated computer technology facilitating computer assisted learning programmes, and widespread use of personal computers with CD-ROM facilities and/or connected to the Internet has been an invaluable addition to learning strategies used within educational institutions (Downing, 1993). Students in remote areas who once had problems accessing even the most basic of library facilities can now dial into libraries and search a variety of data bases for the latest in journal articles or 'surf the net' for virtual books and e-journals. For students in remote areas who do not have their own computers some universities, the University of Central Queensland, for example, have computer 'cottages' to which students can travel. Students use e-mail facilities to communicate with course facilitators, forward assignments and 'chat' to other students. In many instances the use of e-mail has surpassed the telephone as the most common method of communication.

More 'traditional' forms of communicating and supporting students are still in use and are welcomed by students still struggling to negotiate their way along the 'information super highway'. Telephone and video conferences are effective and relatively cheap ways of keeping in touch with students. Buying satellite time to conduct tutorials with students gathered in a number of locations is popular in many educational institutions. Television and radio are also used extensively to broadcast university course material to large numbers of students, for example, The Australian Broadcast Commission has used television via its 'Open Learning' programmes since the late 1950s.

Assessing the perioperative nursing student

Students, depending on the institutions conducting postgraduate courses, undertake written assessments many of which allow the student to select topics which are relevant to their own personal and professional needs. The typically used assignments include:

- reviewing perioperative nursing research
- clinical learning contracts
- case studies (either guided or on a patient selected by the student)
- reflective learning journals
- classroom presentations
- clinical simulations.

Some courses require students to complete written examinations, though these are generally in the minority. Progressive assessment together with some form of practical assessment within the work place are the most likely methods of assessment.

One of the most popular assessments has been the participation of the student in a clinical contract. The student selects a topic related to perioperative nursing in which they are interested and in which they wish to expand their knowledge. The topic must also be relevant to the student's own workplace as they will be expected to bring back new knowledge and teach their colleagues. This may involve looking at a specific surgical procedure, staff education or anaesthetics. The clinical contract is individualised to meet each student's needs, they formulate objectives and plan how they will achieve them, which may involve arranging visits to other hospitals to view equipment, participate in the procedures and patient care, acquiring skills which they then pass on to their colleagues back in their own operating theatre.

Verification of having achieved their objectives is forwarded by the students to their course facilitator and generally comes in the form of written resource and procedural material, posters, videos, audiotapes, patient education pamphlets, care plans or critical pathways. Feedback from students has highlighted that they have learnt new skills and networked with expert nurses in different specialties, have increased their interest in the area being studied and have been motivated to share this new found knowledge with their colleagues.

Students undertaking many of the postgraduate courses are asked to reflect on their studies and its application to their workplace by keeping journals. Journalling has become an increasingly popular method of encouraging critical and reflective thinking in a variety of educational settings. The journals contain reflections and startling accounts of changes in practice and in attitudes as a direct result of exposure to the course material. Engaging in reflection on their practice has helped the students make sense of day-to-day issues which confront them (Barnard, 1988; Callister, 1993). It has also required many students to come face-to-face with certain shortcomings, whether these are of a personal or professional nature. This confrontation has been quite daunting to some students as personal inadequacies have been revealed, requiring re-evaluation of their practice and their attitudes. In distance education courses where face-to-face contact with students is usually non-existent, the journal works very well as a way of getting to know the students, their home life, their family and work situation. It also serves as an evaluative tool for course developers to ascertain if the material is meeting the needs of the students.

Case studies are a popular method of integrating theory with practice. A guided case study provides students with clinical scenarios which ask numerous questions on the clinical management of the patient and rationales for actions taken. Another type of case study is one in which the student selects a patient, carries out an assessment and plans for the patient's perioperative experience. An evaluation is made on completion of the perioperative experience in order to review the nursing care given. Students undertaking this type of case study generally feel a great deal of satisfaction from following a patient through their hospital experience – an all too rare experience for many perioperative nurses. Both styles of case study concentrate very heavily on the student rationalising the clinical management and nursing care of the patient.

Research-based practice has come to be seen as an essential component of contemporary nursing practice. For many perioperative nurses the language, and skills associated with 'doing' research are important additions to their clinical knowledge base. Most courses include an assessment which examines perioperative nursing research. This may be in the form of a literature review, critique, annotated bibliography or journal club. The exercise of locating, interpreting and discussing perioperative nursing research can be quite challenging. Many nurses are being exposed to research for the first time in their careers and learning to discriminate between sound and questionable research.[3] Many have used the findings within their clinical areas and have changed practices which have made a substantial difference not only to patient safety, but to the quality of the care they give to their surgical patients. Some examples are:

- introduction of music therapy to reduce patient anxiety and the need for pain relief;
- lobbying for the purchase of warming devices to protect patients from post-operative hypothermia;
- introduction of parental presence within the recovery room.

A number of students have pursued their own research studies and it is pleasing to see more and more Australian research undertaken in the perioperative environment.

Assessing practical skills is an important aspect of Graduate Certificate and Diploma perioperative nursing courses. A series of competency-based clinical skills assessments, are completed by each student, the assessor being a preceptor from the student's own workplace selected collaboratively by the course facilitators, student and the nurse manager. Preceptor workshops are used to prepare each assessor in the university/hospital-based programmes. Due to students in The NSW College of Nursing distance education programme being geographically widespread each workplace preceptor is provided with written guidelines to explain their role and telephone contact is encouraged.

Staffing issues and education

Providing opportunities to educate the registered perioperative nurse is seen as a major strategy against the ever present threat of technicians and increased numbers of enrolled nurses eroding the role of the registered nurse. The educational background of these two groups and the roles they currently fulfil is worthy of discussion in order to place in context the position in which the registered nurses finds themselves.

Australian operating theatres are staffed primarily by registered nurses who may work across all areas, i.e. anaesthetics, scrubbing (instrument) and scouting (circulating), recovery room, depending on the size and needs of operating theatres. In some larger operating theatres nurses tend to specialise in one of these areas, whereas in smaller units, particularly in rural areas, nurses are multiskilled and work in all roles.

Enrolled nurses generally fulfil the roles of anaesthetic nurse or scout (circulating) nurse, though their roles may vary depending on the state regulations. However, as stated in the ACORN Standards, Guidelines and Policy Statements (ACORN, 1995) enrolled nurses carry out their role under the supervision of a registered nurse, thereby limiting their scope of practice. Enrolled nurses have undergone a one year pre-enrolment educational programme conducted by Technical and Further Education Colleges (TAFE) who also conduct specialty education programmes in perioperative nursing. There is no doubt that enrolled nurses perform an important role within the surgical team, in fact many operating theatres could not function without them, particularly in rural areas. There is much ongoing debate on the expansion of the enrolled nurses' role into areas once held sacred by registered nurses, i.e. scrub or instrument nurse. Whilst this does occur in some hospitals, it is not a widespread practice at present. Whilst the scrubbing/instrument nurse should not be seen as the 'be all and end all' of the perioperative nurse's role, there are concerns amongst registered nurses that if hospital managers see enrolled nurses performing roles once the domain of registered nurses there is likely to be a proliferation of the cheaper enrolled nurse across all roles. The role of the registered nurse will not only be eroded, but also devalued. Enrolled nurses have the necessary practical skills to function effectively within the surgical team, but very few have or wish to develop the knowledge base necessary to manage patients in a critical care area. They may be a cheaper option, but are not necessarily the most effective, versatile or safest.

The same can be said about anaesthetic technicians who are found in many Australian operating theatres. Some have a formal anaesthetic technician qualification, though there are very few such courses. A few hospitals use technicians exclusively, whereas other hospitals use all three grades of staff in the anaesthetic assistant's role.

Whilst acknowledging that technicians do have a role to play within the operating theatre, the major concern is that they often undertake roles outside the parameters of their level of educational preparation and industrial award (Peters & Axford, 1995). A research study carried out by Australian nurses Peters and Axford (1995) revealed some quite alarming results. They found that over 74% of operating theatres which employed a Grade 2 technician (under their award they are able to undertake anaesthetic and assistive roles with minimum supervision and guidance) were using them in a capacity which saw them initiating direct patient care activities, for example unsupervised placement of diathermy plates and calf stimulators. In 30% of operating theatres technicians were preparing intravenous equipment and in a small number of theatres they were also transporting Controlled Drugs (15%) and restocking anaesthetic drugs (28%), both roles clearly outside legal parameters of their educational preparation and award. The legal implications and dangers to patients are obvious. However, there are considerable professional implications if there is a continued trend to educate and employ more technicians in roles previously fulfilled by registered nurses. As with the enrolled nurse there are obvious economic attractions which would no doubt be seized upon by embattled health authorities trying to cope with shrinking budgets. But what about the quality of patient care? True, technicians may have the technical expertise necessary to provide an important role, but like the enrolled nurse they certainly lack the versatility and educational preparation of the registered nurse to provide holistic care for the patient at the most crucial periods in the surgical intervention. Peters & Axford (1995) rightly point out that the nursing contribution needs to be demonstrated and articulated to the wider nursing community.

Educational institutions also need to recognise the importance of the anaesthetic nursing role and offer appropriate courses. Some courses already exist and more are planned within the tertiary sector. The debate on skills mix within the operating theatre is ongoing with operating theatre managers battling hard to keep current levels of 'expensive' registered nurses in a tough economic climate when there is a demand that cheaper staffing options be considered. This battle may be futile if operating theatres cannot attract registered nurses into the specialty. There is a need for strong leadership from professional organisations both at State and national level to ensure that the care of the perioperative patient remains within the hands of registered nurses and is not eroded.

Multiskilling v. specialisation – educational challenges

Multiskilling versus specialisation raises some challenging issues with ramifications which are both economic and educational. In many rural and smaller hospitals in Australia there is a very strong push to multiskill staff in order to maximise usage of available nurses of all grades. The luxury which many larger hospitals enjoy of having staff who work in one specialty only cannot be afforded in a hospital which has, for example, 50–60 beds and only operates 2 or 3 days a week. The operating theatres of these hospitals are usually staffed by a permanent perioperative registered nurse who has both clinical and administrative functions and who works in other departments on non-operating days. In addition, there is generally a rotation of staff from ward areas who are rostered to the operating theatre for varying periods of time, anything from 3 to 6 months. These are usually a combination of enrolled nurses who fulfil anaesthetic and scouting roles and registered nurses who concentrate on scrubbing, scouting and recovery room roles. The success of this rotation system varies, depending on the enthusiasm and commitment of the incoming staff, but it is seen by the hospitals as essential and particularly useful in emergency cases where any member of staff from within the hospital can be sent to theatre to assist. In practice this system can cause problems if the staff member's theatre experience is not recent. Delays can be experienced in setting up equipment and carrying out specialised care which would be seen as routine by experienced nurses.

Providing education for staff who rotate into operating theatre for short periods only is often difficult to carry out. Registered nurses from this environment who wish to pursue formal qualifications in the specialty are often hindered by the fact that they will only be rostered for a short period of time, usually insufficient to meet course requirements. Incoming staff generally undergo an orientation to the theatre but very little in the way of ongoing education in perioperative nursing. Although many larger metropolitan operating theatres employ clinical nurse educators to facilitate orientation of new staff and inservice education, in rural areas this is a luxury which operating theatres are unable to afford. In addition to this, continuing education programmes are conducted by various educational institutions usually based in metropolitan areas and, therefore, generally inaccessible to the rural hospitals who would benefit most. Programming of some courses in rural centres does occur through The NSW College of Nursing and professional perioperative groups who are active in providing education days in rural areas. The development of self directed learning packages, such as those facilitated by Curtin University in Western Australia, have assisted rural perioperative nurses in keeping up to date with current practice. The packages are print based study guides and workbooks, supplemented by a series of videos.

The future

The future of educating the perioperative registered nurse depends on a number of factors. Firstly, there must be an ongoing supply of nurses wishing to pursue perioperative nursing as a career, otherwise there will be no one to educate! The strategies discussed earlier in this chapter for encouraging nurses into the specialty need to be increased nationally, not limited to two or three States. Professional perioperative nursing groups, at both national and State level must continue to show strong leadership in lobbying government agencies for funds to facilitate transition programmes into the perioperative specialty and universities to increase exposure to the operating theatre and perioperative care at undergraduate level.

The choices for postgraduate perioperative nursing education are many and varied, providing access to a larger number of registered nurses across Australia than ever before. In a national review of specialty education it is recommended that by 1998 the minimum initial qualification for nursing specialties will be at Graduate Diploma level and by 2003 at Master's level (Russell, *et al.*, 1997, p.xvi). The review supports continuation of the current system using multiple providers of specialty education across the tertiary sector, hospitals and professional nursing groups, but urges the greater articulation of Graduate Certificate awards with higher education awards offered by the university sector. Educational provisions should be adaptable in order to respond to the changing needs of the work force and continue to be offered in a variety of study modes (Russell *et al.*, 1997, p.xx). The review recommends greater flexibility in methods of delivering specialty education. One recommendation is the development of modules of study which could form components of larger courses, for example a course conducted within the tertiary sector could be a component of a course run by a hospital and vice versa. Another recommendation is creating flexibility so that a nurse could commence a course at a hospital or The NSW College of Nursing and then have the option of upgrading the award at a university at a later date (Russell *et al.*, 1997, p.33).

The most significant aspects of the review by Russell *et al.* (1997) are the recommendations related to collaboration between education providers. This already occurs to some extent with universities using hospitals as 'collaborative partners' in the running of specialty courses. The review goes further and recommends joint appointments across the health and university sectors with staff exchange between both settings and the establishment of additional clinical chairs of nursing. Joint involvement in curriculum development, implementation and evaluation and participation by staff from both areas on a range of committees across both university and hospital settings is also recommended.

There are many benefits to the recommendations for closer collaboration between the various education providers, including cost-effectiveness, the sharing of resources, greater understanding of each other's role, formal recognition of the input of professional nursing organisations, the creation of greater opportunities of research and greater incentives for nurses to enter tertiary study (Russell *et al.*, 1997).

Conclusion

This chapter has provided an overview of nursing history in Australia and the progress of perioperative nursing to date. It also reveals current perioperative nursing practice in Australia to be something of a paradox. Never before have there been so many opportunities to increase knowledge in the specialty, whilst at the same time the role of the perioperative registered nurse is being threatened by economic and administrative strategies. Perioperative registered nurses are obviously concerned that together with the erosion of their role will come a decline in the standard of care for the surgical patient. It seems that, to address the latter, we must embrace the former. The most effective strategy for ensuring the survival of the perioperative registered nurse together with the continued high standard of patient care will occur by taking the opportunities to educate ourselves to the highest possible standard. Participation in nursing research is essential in order to demonstrate that registered nurses do make a difference to patient outcomes and that their continued high profile within the surgical team is a matter of necessity not economics.

Reflective activities

This chapter has given a wide view of changes in nursing and the pressures on nurses across Australia. It is sometimes good to make comparisons with the way nurses in another country and different situations are being affected by change and to reflect on why their responses may be the same or different from your own responses or the responses of your managers or your government.

1 It appears that the training of enrolled nurses and technicians is not as intensive as that of their equivalents in the UK. Has this affected the concerns of Australian perioperative nurses?

2 Does it appear to you that perioperative nurses in your country, or even in your hospital, are engaged in a battle for survival? If so, why is it happening?

3 Can you identify with the comments in this chapter and does it give you some insights into:
    • why nursing and nurses are being asked to change;
    • the steps perioperative nurses can take to justify their existence?

4 Are perioperative nurses a valuable, if expensive, resource who have a large part to play in maintaining high standards of patient care before, during and after surgery?

5 Reflect on your nurse education and further steps which you can take to improve your knowledge base for perioperative practice.

6 What is the first thing you are going to do to implement this? If you have not already embarked on further professional development, set a date to start implementing your plans. Write down possibilities and discuss them with your manager or tutor.

7 Make some firm plans and follow them up.

Endnotes

1 The word 'State' will be used to cover both 'State' and 'Territory' from here onwards.

2 Scouting is an Australian term for 'circulating' or 'running'.

3 See Chapter 5 for more information on nursing research.

References

Australian Confederation of Operating Room Nurses. 1995 *Standards, guidelines and policy statements.* ACORN.

Australian Tertiary Education Commission. 1978 *Report from committee of inquiry into nurse education and training (Sax Report).* Canberra, Australian Tertiary Education Commission.

Barnard, P. 1988: The journal as an assessment and evaluation tool in nurse education. *Nurse Education Today* 8, 105–7

Callister, L. 1993 The use of student journals in nursing education: making meaning out of clinical experience. *Journal of Nursing Education* 32 (4), 185–6.

Cochrane, J. 1989 Influencing the politics of health reform. In: Gray, G. & Pratt, R. (eds.) *Issues in Australian nursing* 2. Melbourne, Churchill Livingstone, Chapter 3.

Cordery, C. 1995 Doing more with less: nursing and the politics of economic rationalism in the 1990s. *Issues in Australian Nursing 4.* Melbourne, Churchill Livingstone, Chapter 21.

Downing, T. 1993 *The use of CAL in a distance education context.* Selected Students' Papers. Master of Distance Education. Paper 1. 7–13. Deakin University and University of South Australia.

Lublin, J.R. 1985 Basic nurse education in CAEs; the educational evidence for transfer. *Australian Journal of Advanced Nursing* 2 (2), 18–28.

National Health Strategy. 1991 *The Australian health jigsaw: integration of health care delivery.* Issues paper No.1, July. Canberra, Commonwealth of Australia.

Peters, G. & Axford, R. 1995 The utilisation of technicians in operating suites in Victorian hospitals. *Australian Confederation of Operating Room Nurses Journal* 8 (3), 21–5.

Russell, R.L. 1990 *From Nightingale to now: nurse education in Australia.* Sydney, W.B. Saunders / Balliere Tindall.

Russell. R.L., Gething, L. & Covery, P. 1997 *National review of specialist nurse education.* Canberra, Department of Employment, Education, Training and Youth Affairs.

Acknowledgements

We wish to acknowledge the assistance given by the following perioperative nursing groups in the preparation of this chapter:

Northern Territory Perioperative Nurses.
New South Wales Operating Theatre Association (Inc).
Operating Room Nurses' Association of Western Australia (Inc).
Perioperative Nurses' Association of Queensland.
Victorian Perioperative Nursing Group (Australian Nurses' Federation).
South Australian Perioperative Nurses' Section (Australian Nurses' Federation).
Tasmanian Operating Room Nurses.

Thanks is expressed to numerous colleagues within the university sector for their input into the chapter and to colleagues within The NSW College of Nursing for advice and assistance.

Developing the research basis of perioperative nursing

Colin Rees

Colin Rees is a lecturer in the School of Nursing Studies at the University of Wales. He has published a number of books and articles on nursing research. His current links with perioperative nursing are through the National Association of Theatre Nursing. He has published articles in the British Journal of Theatre Nursing *and is one of the judges for their annual writer's award. He has placed the research process in the context of perioperative nursing, describing the elements of that process. Perhaps, most of all, he encourages his readers to consider nursing research with a critical eye. Each piece of research should be evaluated to establish both good and bad qualities and to identify its value for perioperative practice. Considerable guidance is given on this and on learning how to read and evaluate literature reviews with a view to implementing the lessons of research in practice. Perioperative nurses need to use research as they move forward into evidence based practice and are encouraged to see that it is perioperative nurses who carry it out or they will find themselves dependent on research carried out by others whose priorities may be different from their own.*

The chapter is set very much in a UK context, but it will not be difficult to extrapolate to another national context.

Introduction

Research is now accepted as an important aspect of practice in all areas of nursing. It is also a source of fear, misunderstanding and indifference. Although few perioperative nurses would say research is unnecessary, the extent to which it is used, and particularly talked about, may suggest that this is a problem area that needs closer examination. Perhaps the real problem is that nursing is still in the process of developing a research culture. In the past, clinical decisions were frequently made on the basis of custom and practice, in other words, nursing rituals (Walsh & Ford, 1989). Although there is a certain comfort in following this method of making decisions, there is a danger that many of these rituals have passed their sell-by-date. From a professional credibility point of view, there are also dangers in becoming complacent, and lacking a challenging outlook in the way that services and individual activities are organised. These dangers are clearly emphasised by Walsh & Ford (1989) as follows:

> Traditional nursing is based on many unsubstantiated beliefs, but not so many facts. Qualified staff who do not keep up to date with research findings have little other than intuition, outdated ritual and mythology to guide their practice. While there may be a place for intuition in the art of nursing, there is no place in the science of nursing for ritual and mythology!

A great deal has happened since that was written. Research is more a part of basic nurse education and postbasic courses and modules. More research is also available on which to base practice. The more recent drive towards evidence based practice and clinical governance means that the perioperative nurse will increasingly be required to demonstrate that activities are based on the best evidence available. There are a number of important issues arising from this, which include the following questions:

- What is the role of research in perioperative nursing care?
- Should the emphasis be on the perioperative nurse as the producer or user of research?
- What are the skills required of the perioperative nurse to achieve a better use of research?

We should at this stage make a clear distinction between two potential roles for the perioperative nurse in research. The first is the nurse as the 'doer' of research, and the second is as the 'user' of research. Although some perioperative nurses should carry out research (it would be interesting if you ask yourself how many perioperative nurses you know who have completed a research project), the emphasis here will be on using research as part of perioperative nursing. The aim of this chapter is to clarify the nature and role of research in the work of the perioperative nurse. In order to achieve this the following questions will be answered:

- What is research?
- How can it figure in the work of the perioperative nurse?
- How is research structured?
- How can we make better use of the research available?
- What is the way ahead for the perioperative nurse and research?

What is research?

Many nurses have their own mental picture of what research is and the way it is conducted. This may include the 'mad professor' working in a laboratory, or the person stopping you in the street with a clipboard. Within the health service, the view of research is often coloured by medical research which appears very statistical and often full of incomprehensible jargon. Although it is possible to find examples which confirm these stereotypes, it is important to realise there is more to research than these negative images. Research is integral to nursing activity. Although nursing can take advantage of medical research, there is a need to carry out and utilise what is best described as 'nursing research'. This can be defined as research carried out by nurses, which examines questions relevant to nurses, and which directly, or indirectly enhances patient care. Parahoo (1997) defines nursing research in these terms:

> Nursing research is an umbrella term for all research into nursing practice and issues related to it. It can be defined as the systematic and rigorous collection and analysis of data on the organisation, delivery, uses and outcomes of nursing care for the purpose of enhancing clients' health. It is not only about what nurses do, but also about clients' behaviour, knowledge, beliefs, attitudes, perceptions and other factors influencing how they make use of, and experience, care and treatment.

This emphasises that nursing research can examine aspects relating to both patients and the nurse, what they do, and the way they interact with each other as well as other health workers. So how do we define 'research'? One of the classic definitions is the following by Macleod Clark & Hockey (1989) who say it is:

> An attempt to increase the sum of what is known, usually referred to as a 'body of knowledge', by the discovery of new facts or relationships through a process of systematic scientific enquiry, the research process.

It is worth stressing that sometimes research reveals something we knew all along. In other words, it doesn't always seem to be new knowledge. When this happens, research has provided firmer evidence that will allow us to use the knowledge more confidently in our practice. Most definitions of research will contain two main elements; firstly the knowledge that is produced through research, and secondly the process involved. So, for example, Parahoo (1997) suggests that:

> Research is a systematic way of knowing and lays bare its methods for all to see.

It is this holding up for scrutiny that is important, as we can see how the knowledge has been produced. This differentiates research knowledge from other forms of decision making, such as custom and practice or role modelling, where the rationale on which it is based is not clear or open to scrutiny. Finally, Rees (1997) suggests that:

> Research consists of extending knowledge and understanding through a carefully structured systematic process of collecting information, which answers a specific question in a way that is as objective and accurate as possible.

This definition emphasises the purpose of research, and the way it helps in decision making by providing answers to the questions important to the perioperative nurse.

It is worth making the distinction at this point between research and audit as there is often some confusion as to whether they are the same or different. Whereas research seeks to increase our knowledge and understanding of a topic, audit is more limited. It merely quantifies an aspect of service performance and allows comparisons to be made with previous measurements, a baseline or standard. It tells us what is happening, but not why or how. It does not increase our understanding of that topic. Malby (1995) draws out the relationship between audit and research by saying that while audit is not research, much of the data collection relies on research tools. Hence, there is confusion as to whether they are part of the same activity. It can also be added that both should be carried out in the same systematic and rigorous way. We can end this section by listing some of the ways in which research differs from other sources of knowledge (Box 5.1). This is based on a collection of definitions of research and considers some of the common features found in them.

Box 5.1   Research is characterised by:

- An orderly and systematic process of gathering information
- Control over the process in which the information is gathered
- Objective evidence of a 'factual nature' taken from real situations (empirical evidence)
- Absence of individual bias
- Use of logic in analysing the information
- Can be applied to other settings (generalisability).

Source: Rees 1997.

Although useful, it is important to note that research does vary a great deal in its design, and so some of the features above will be more evident in certain types of research than others.

How can research figure in the work of the perioperative nurse?

The starting point for this section is that the perioperative nurse must first accept that research is an important part of providing care. Whereas, in the past it may have been possible to provide care without reference to research, professional accountability now includes accepting responsibility for the knowledge base that informs individual practice. This essential aspect of being research minded is brought out by Smith (1997), who presented the following, almost stern, warning for all nurses:

> The current climate *demands* that nurses become research minded. The whole 'evidence-based practice' movement has changed the environment in which we now work in health care. Research mindedness is no longer a luxury, an 'add-on' extra, but has to be an essential component of our day-to-day practice.

In other words, research knowledge must be a conscious aspect of care delivery, where the nurse is continually questioning the basis of her or his actions. To achieve this, the following are three crucial challenges which should be asked as frequently as possible each time an activity is carried out:

- Why do I do this in this way?
- Has this way of doing things passed its 'sell-by-date'?
- Is there a better way of doing this?

These questions suggest a close relationship between research and reflective practice. Where the perioperative nurse reflects on performance, which would include questions such as those above, it may become evident that research findings need to be accessed. So, in which specific areas of clinical practice can research play a part? It is easy to stereotype research as concerning only clinical trials involving patients. We must remember, however, that we are concerned with nursing research which should be the major concern of the perioperative nurse. That is not to say that medical research is irrelevant but that it is only a part of the picture. The range of topics covered by nursing research can be illustrated in Box 5.2 below.

Box 5.2 Broad areas examined by nursing research

- Accepted perioperative practices
- New techniques and practices
- Specific patient groups and the problems they present for the perioperative nurse
- Communication with patients, relatives, as well as other nursing and health professional groups
- The role of the perioperative nurse
- The training of the perioperative nurse
- The working environment of the perioperative nurse.

This provides a far wider canvas to consider than just clinical trials and illustrates the usefulness of research in all aspects of the perioperative nurse's activities. However, we must consider what is required to make full use of this material. White (1997) suggests that where nurses are trying to use research to answer a clinical question, the following criteria need to be met:

1 Access to the literature must be reasonably straightforward.

2 The person trying to answer the question should have literature searching skills.

3 Research on the question being posed must be available in the literature.

This is just the beginning, as we can add a number of further considerations, such as the possession of critiquing skills, negotiating skills, and the skill of introducing change. One important element is knowing what to look for in a research article. So, before we go further, we need to consider the basic stages in the research process.

The research process

Research is not carried out in a haphazard way. It would be a disaster if it was, as it would be totally unreliable as a basis for decision making. There is a basic framework which researchers follow in carrying out a study – the research process. In essence, this is very similar to following a recipe, in that although people may have personal variations in the way they produce the same dish, there will be basic similarities that give the outcome its distinctive appearance and taste. We also need to acknowledge that the research process will differ depending on the broad research approach followed. So for instance, quantitative research, which is concerned with numerical accuracy, starts from clear assumptions or hypotheses, and is different from qualitative research. Qualitative research is more concerned with how those in a study define what is important to them. Issues and categories which form the analysis of qualitative research emerge only once the data has been collected. There is no prior attempt to construct categories that will form the basis of data collection. It is recommended that you consult Holloway & Wheeler (1996) for more details of qualitative design. For simplicity, the quantitative design is used to illustrate this chapter. If we are to make sense of research, we must understand the basic elements in the research process. These are shown in Box 5.3 below. The outline shows a standard quantitative design.

Box 5.3   Stages in the research process

1 Develop the research question, and produce as an aim or 'terms of reference'.

2 Review the relevant literature to provide the rationale for the study.

3 Plan the method of investigation.

This includes:

- the broad design i.e. descriptive, experimental, action research, etc.
- the characteristics of the sample, sample size, sampling method

- the information to be gathered to answer the research question
- the tool of data collection
- the method of data analysis and presentation
- the way in which the ethical issues relating to any study will be addressed.

4 Carry out a pilot study to test data gathering tool and method of analysis.

5 Collect the data.

6 Analyse the results.

7 Develop conclusions and recommendations.

8 Communicate the findings in terms of a verbal presentation, report or journal article.

There is a wonderful logic to this process, which helps it to 'hang together'. It is worth looking at the detail of the process so this can be highlighted.

1 THE RESEARCH QUESTION

The starting point for any piece of research is a question which the researcher wants to answer. This could be 'Is the day surgery nurse giving preoperative information based on assessment of individual patient need?', 'What kinds of courses do perioperative nurses see as important?', 'Are postoperative telephone calls carried out by perioperative nurses useful?' These are usually turned into a research aim, or 'terms of reference', which is a statement of what the researcher is trying to achieve. So the above questions may be developed into the following terms of reference:

- To identify if nurses employed in a day surgery unit assess the individual informational needs of patients in their care (Reid, 1997)
- To determine the kinds of courses perioperative nurses see as important
- To establish whether the relatives of patients undergoing coronary bypass surgery would benefit, in terms of reducing their anxiety, from a telephoned progress report (Driver, 1997).

It is sometimes felt that every research question must have a hypothesis. This is not true. A hypothesis, which is a prediction about the relationship between two or more variables (LoBiondo-Woods & Haber, 1998), is only needed in experimental designs. So, for instance, the example of providing telephone reports to relatives of patients (Driver, 1997), could have been undertaken as a randomised control trial (RCT). Relatives could have been randomly allocated to either the phone, or non-phone group, and the hypothesis could have been something like this:

Relatives who receive a telephone call regarding the outcome of surgery of a patient undergoing coronary bypass surgery, will score lower on an anxiety scale about the operation, than those who do not receive a call.

This suggests that there is a relationship between anxiety levels, which is here the dependent variable, and the telephone information system, which is the independent variable. The study would then be conducted to establish if the researcher should accept or reject the hypothesis. Researchers do not talk about proving or disproving a hypothesis, as it is difficult within the confines of any one study to talk about something as definitive as proof. The important point is that there is a very close relationship between the research question and the method chosen to answer it. Where the researcher is looking for cause and effect relationships (in this instance: will telephone information produce a lower level of anxiety?) then an experimental approach is needed to rule out the possible influence of other variables which might explain the results.

2 REVIEW OF THE LITERATURE

Studies should not be carried out in isolation from what is already known about a topic. The researcher must provide the reader with a review of the literature which helps to locate the study within the context of previous knowledge. The style of the review should be a critical analysis, and should not simply be a summary of previous work. For this reason when we read research reports we should expect the writer to quickly put us in the picture of previous research, or government reports or policies, to illustrate that the literature has been accessed, and taken into account when designing the study.

3 PLANNING THE METHOD OF INVESTIGATION

The essence of good research is planning. The researcher needs to draw up a clear plan of action in the form of a research protocol. This is an outline of the study which details the reason for the study, the research question, and how it will be answered. This protocol allows the researcher to consider the implications of the methodological decisions made. This can quickly reveal any flaws in the process. It also provides a detailed plan that can be used for an ethics committee or to gain approval from those who are important in providing access to the data. The details that need to be considered cover a number of important areas and include the following considerations:

(a) The broad design

We have already touched upon one of the major broad designs in health service research, that of the experimental design or randomised control trial. It has been emphasised that this approach is important where the researcher wants to establish cause and effect relationships. This is frequently the purpose of medical research, so not surprisingly for many it has become the 'gold standard' of research. This is illustrated by the fact that when an application is made to an ethics committee, it is not unusual for them to send the would-be researcher a form to complete which is laid out as if the research was to be a randomised control trial. There are other broad approaches, just as relevant to the perioperative nurse. One example is descriptive research where, as the term implies, the intention is to paint a descriptive picture of a situation to answer the question 'what is going on?'. The answer is frequently in the form of numbers and so comes under the heading of quantitative research. This design, which is similar to a government census, is often referred to as a survey design. An example of descriptive research is the work of Willmer *et al.* (1997) which looked at the reuse of single use instruments. Their terms of reference were to determine:

- The number and grade of staff who had reused or been asked to reuse a single use instrument.
- The initiator of the request.
- Whether one type of instrument above others was being resterilised.
- Whether the issue was specific to one type of hospital, or relevant to all.

This research raises a number of important issues because of the safety and legal aspects of reusing items that have been designated single use. The descriptive approach was clearly the right choice. It is also important to say that this form of research is very close to that of audit which looks at present service activities against previous time periods or standards. A further broad category is evaluative research where the purpose is to describe whether a particular activity is meeting its objectives, or the purpose that was seen as a potential benefit. The work by Driver (1997) on postoperative telephone notifications discussed above would be an example of evaluative research. This set out to establish whether there was a viable role for the theatre nurse in carrying out this activity. There are other broad forms of research that are used less often such as action research and historical research.

Action research has been seen as ideal for nursing as, according to Webb (1996) it is so highly suited to the kind of problem-solving and evaluation research which the profession needs. It involves trying out a new activity or form of delivering a service. It is highly participatory and involves those in the setting working as a team with the researcher. A clearer picture of how this operates is given by Webb (1996) as follows:

> Action research is a way of doing research and working on, solving a problem at the same time. Researcher and participants work together to analyse the situation they wish to change: this may include doing some baseline measures using questionnaires, observation or other research methods. After this assessment they can then plan the desired change, set their objectives, and decide how to bring about the change. While they are putting their plans into action, they continue to monitor progress, changing their plans if this is judged appropriate. At the completion of the change process, they will make a final assessment and draw conclusions, perhaps writing a report on the project for themselves and/or others.

This seems an ideal way to reduce the resistance to both research and change, as it involves contributions from those working in the situation. Surprisingly, it remains an under-utilised method in nursing research generally.

The same can be said of historical research, which at first sight may appear to have little to offer the perioperative nurse. However, this would not be a fair assumption. We must remember that experiences from the past are very powerful in shaping our reactions to the events and activities of today, and in planning for tomorrow. As perioperative nursing is just developing its political profile, historical research which looks at the role of the nurse in theatres could produce guidelines on what should be encouraged, and what should be avoided.

Finally, an important approach that seems to have been neglected within perioperative nursing is that of qualitative research. This is not the same as gathering qualitative data, which are basically the comments to open questions in a questionnaire, which could be part of quantitative research. It is more a philosophical way of thinking about research. Under qualitative research the aim is to start from where the respondent is, and not enforce the researcher's definition of the situation or the factors which they feel are important to study. Qualitative research typically consists of in-depth accounts from a small number of respondents who describe a situation, such as living with a condition, or experience a situation such as receiving a life-threatening diagnosis. The findings are presented under themes or categories, and the data takes the form of quotes or dialogue. No numeric tables or bar charts are used to summarise findings. The intention of such research is to sensitise others to that experience; to raise issues that may have to be addressed in providing care, and to increase understanding from the participant's point of view. It remains to be seen whether perioperative nursing will develop an interest in this potentially useful approach to research in the future.

(b) The sample

At the design stage, the researcher must choose the source of the information to be collected, in other words, the sample. This could be people, things, such as pieces of equipment, or events. So, for instance Carthew (1997) tape-recorded 20 teaching sessions to explore the use of a clinical practice suite in the acquisition of clinical skills. The three points that must be addressed by the researcher in regard to the sample are:

- Who or what will make up the sample?
- How many will be included?
- How will they be chosen?

To answer the first question, the researcher frequently states the inclusion and exclusion criteria used to select those in the study. The characteristics of those felt to be typical of the study group – the inclusion criteria – must be identified, along with those characteristics that may either put individuals at clinical risk, or which may introduce bias – the exclusion criteria. Although it is difficult to gain the perfect sample, an attempt should be made to make it as typical as possible. Those reading research reports also need these details to allow them to judge whether they can apply the results to their own clinical area.

Perhaps the hardest part of sampling is to plan the sample size. A great deal of the credibility of most studies is related to this aspect of a study. The researcher can gain some idea of what would be a reasonable number to include by considering the sample size of other studies in the literature. However, the following principle from Polit & Hungler (1997) is good advice.

Although there is no simple equation that can automatically answer the question of how large a sample is needed, quantitative researchers are generally advised to use the largest sample possible. The larger the sample, the more representative of the population it is likely to be.

It is not only the number that the researcher starts with that is important, it is also the number they end with that needs careful scrutiny. In clinical trials it is important to be aware if the composition of the groups changes for any reason, such as people dropping out of a study. This may make it difficult to carry on comparing experimental and control groups, as they may no longer be similar once a number of people have dropped out of the study.

Similarly for surveys, it is not the number of questionnaires sent out which is important, but the numbers returned and the proportion they represent of the total. Response rates of under 50% are obviously a problem, as those who did not return their questionnaires could vary from those who did respond. This could make the results suspect. Response rates of over 60% provide more assurances concerning the typicality of the replies.

Finally, in regard to choosing the sample, there are a whole range of methods from which the researcher can choose. Although some of these will be familiar to you, it is easy to confuse some of them. There are two main sampling approaches. These are:

- Probability sampling methods
- Non-probability methods.

The difference between them is the extent to which the sample can be said to be typical of the larger group which they are taken to stand for, or represent. How do we know how typical they are? The answer is whether the researcher has selected those involved in such a way that it is possible to calculate whether everyone had an equal, or at least calculable, chance of being included in the study.

Using probability sampling methods, the researcher conducting a randomised control trial can take all patients on the operating list and number them to form a sampling frame. Then, using a table of random numbers or computer generated random numbers, pick say 20 numbers to form the experimental group and 20 to form the control group. Whoever corresponds with the chosen numbers on the sampling frame would be in the appropriate group. Using this method, there is no way of foreseeing who will be in which group, so avoiding any influence from the researcher, or anyone else. Everyone, theoretically has an equal chance of being selected using this method. This is called a simple random sample.

One variation of this is where characteristics such as age, sex, condition, or grade of staff, etc. are felt to be important, i.e. the stratified sample. This is where different sampling frames based on these criteria are first of all constructed, and then those within them are numbered. The table of random numbers is then used to pick out so many numbers. This may be an equal number from each group or could be proportionate to the size of each group. Those who correspond with the numbers in the selected lists are chosen. In this way there is a representative spread of the factors felt to have an influence on the 'representativeness' of the results.

Where it is not possible to know in advance who may be included in the study, for instance in a prospective study of patients who have yet to be admitted, a different method is used. Numbered sealed envelopes are used where random numbers have been used to allocate people to the experimental or control groups. An example would be that of a situation where it was planned to have a total of 60 patients in a trial with 30 in each of the control and experimental groups. Sixty envelopes would be numbered consecutively. The researcher would then choose 30 numbers from the random number table between 1 and 60, and those envelopes which corresponded with the 30 numbers selected, would form the experimental group. Instructions would then be placed in the envelope corresponding with those numbers saying that the person was in the experimental group. The remaining envelopes would receive the instruction to allocate the person to the control group.

The advantage of these sampling methods is that sophisticated statistical techniques can be used on the results which allow inferences to be made on the extent to which any variations between the outcomes could have happened by chance. This allows some calculation to be made of whether a cause and effect relationship could be demonstrated in the study.

Non-probability sampling methods are not as sophisticated, which means that it is not possible to suggest that the findings may have wider applicability. One common technique that can be mistaken for a 'random sample' is the opportunity or convenience sample. This takes the form of those people or things that just happen to be at the right place at the right time for the researcher's purposes.

The accuracy of a study based on this type of sample is unknown. This begs the question 'Why use this method?' The answer is that it is easy to conduct and, although we do not know how typical the answers are, we can argue that by the same token we do not know how untypical they are. They may be as good as something far more elaborate. The real question is what is at stake if the interpretation of the results is wrong? Where the consequences are a matter of life or death, this method of sampling is inappropriate. Where the purpose is to gain an impression of views or experiences, then it may be acceptable. The larger the sample the more convincing the results, particularly where the characteristics of the sample seem reasonably typical.

The researcher can try and increase the representativeness of the convenience sample by quota sampling, which is trying to ensure that so many from each group are included using such criteria as sex, age, experience, etc. This may then give a fairly typical cross-section of respondents.

Finally, it is possible to use a purposive sample, where the individuals are hand picked on the basis of the researcher's knowledge of whether they are typical. This is a useful technique where the sample is likely to be small, such as in qualitative research which, because of the depth involved, tends to have small samples. In this case the researcher tries to ensure that those with representative characteristics are included.

(c)   The information to be gathered

The essence of any project is to answer the aim of the study. The researcher must be clear at the outset what information will need to be collected, and the form in which it will be collected. In this respect the definition of the terms used in the aims have to be clearly explained. This can cause problems where the researcher wants to examine patient 'satisfaction', 'comfort', or 'anxiety'. The questions that always need to be answered first are:

- How will you know it when you see it (how can you describe its defining characteristics)?
- How can it be measured (how can you tell to what extent it is present)?

Again, consulting the literature will give some indication of how others have answered these questions convincingly.

(d)   The tool of data collection

Designing the research protocol is a matter of considering the options for the way the information could be collected. The rationale for each choice must be examined, taking into account the study aim, and the sample selected. The most frequently used methods in health service research are:

- Questionnaires
- Interviews
- Observation
- Documentary methods
- Experimental methods (physiological measures, swabs, etc).

As each one of these methods will have their advantages and disadvantages, it is important that the researcher takes account of these and justifies their selection. So, for instance, questionnaires are frequently used by nurses in perioperative research as they can reach a large group of potential respondents. They are also cheap and quick. However, they frequently have a poor response rate, and tend to produce fairly superficial data. They are also based on reading and writing skills which due to illness and surgery may be problematic for some potential respondents.

Interviews have a greater advantage over questionnaires in that there is a greater depth to replies. The interviewer can check that respondents have understood the question and they can also clarify any answers. However, because of the time taken, interviews are more costly, and the face-to-face situation can encourage respondents to give socially acceptable answers, or answers respondents feel the interviewer wants to hear.

Both interviews and questionnaires fall into the category of self-reports, that is, the researcher has to accept that people do what they say they do. We know that this may not always be the case. With both of these methods there will always be a margin of error in the accuracy of the results.

Observation does not depend on self-report data, as the researcher sees first hand for themselves the behaviour in which they are interested. However, where people know they are being observed, there is always the concern that this will influence their activities and so make the observations unreliable.

Documentary methods which include the use of records, similarly have their advantages and disadvantages. They will not be influenced by the presence of the researcher but they are likely to be fairly limited in the detail they have about a particular aspect of perioperative nursing. They are good in identifying the extent to which activities are carried out, and in identifying trends over time, which makes them useful in audit.

Finally, experimental methods are crucial if we are trying to establish causal relationships. They have a great currency within the health service, and have become a kind of 'gold standard' for the conduct of research. However, they have as many problems attached to them as the other methods of data collection. One example is that there is such a tight control over the way the study is conducted that we may not encounter such situations in every day clinical practice. This means that the application of the results to other situations may be very tenuous.

There are also a number of other problems for the perioperative nurse in carrying out experiments. This includes the ability to have total control over the situation in which the study is being conducted, and the ethical problems in withholding treatments or procedures from individuals. Experimental designs also require high levels of statistical knowledge. The special facilities required for an experimental design also makes them a costly method of research. As yet, nursing research does not seem to attract the same kind of funding in comparison to, say, medical research.

Given that each method has its strengths and limitations, it is possible to combine more than one method in a single study. This is called triangulation. So, for instance, the researcher may interview perioperative nurses regarding what they do, and then observe to see if there is a correspondence between what they say they do and what happens in practice.

(e)   Data analysis and presentation

It is important at the planning stage to consider how the results are to be analysed and then presented to others to make sense of them. Responses have to be grouped, counted or classified in a way that makes it easier to understand the overall picture. Examining previous research as part of the review of the literature will provide some ideas on the options of presentation. In preparation for the analysis, the researcher should get advice at the very start to ensure that data is collected in a suitable form. It is rarely possible to correct mistakes once the data has been gathered. One very readable book which outlines statistical concepts and principles that should be consulted for more information is Clegg (1982). Although this was published some time ago it is still widely available.

(f)   Ethical considerations

Research is not just about the collection and analysis of data, it is also about how the researchers conduct themselves and the relationship they form with those who provide them with data. This is the concern of ethics in research, which Polit & Hungler (1997) define as:

> A system of moral values that is concerned with the degree to which research procedures adhere to professional, legal and social obligations to the study participants.

Above all, the researcher must attend to issues of the safety of those involved in the study, to ensure that they do not suffer any harm (non-maleficence). In the theatre situation there is the possibility of direct physical harm, but ethics also considers psychological and social harm. We must remember that even tools such as questionnaires are an invasion of people's privacy, and could evoke feelings of regret, anxiety and fear. It is right then, that great care should be taken when carrying out research and that the researcher accepts responsibility to protect those who take part in a study.

Most people acknowledge that informed consent is an important element in respecting someone's autonomy. This relates to their right to make decisions for themselves, and to have the right not to take part in research, or pull out at any time, without any consequences for the care they receive or the relationship they have with health professionals. But what does the researcher have to do to ensure that the consent given is 'informed'? If we are going to really achieve this, then anyone invited to take part in a study must be given the information outlined in Box 5.4.

Box 5.4   Information to be provided to individuals in order to achieve informed consent

- The purpose of the study.
- The identification of the researcher and their organisation.
- The nature of the participation (what will happen over what period of time).
- Possible risks or implications of participating, and any anticipated benefits.
- Assurance of confidentiality.
- Informed they need not volunteer.
- Assured they have the right to withdraw at any time.
- Offered the opportunity to ask questions.

Source: Rees (1997)

Other ethical issues include confidentiality, which is the trusting relationship built up between the researcher and their subjects. One of the most important ways that this is exercised is in the safekeeping of information about individuals. Health professionals are already bound under their professional codes by this aspect and so no further details are included here. It is worth emphasising that many people confuse confidentiality with anonymity, which is another way in which confidentiality is maintained. This basically protects the identity of individuals and also includes identifying characteristics.

One element that is not always considered under the principle of justice is that of coercion. This is an issue in two ways; firstly, those undergoing or having just undergone surgery are vulnerable and may not, when asked to take part in research, make the same decision that they would under different circumstances. Here the coercion is subtle, as people are not in a position to refuse although that is not always apparent. The second way in which coercion can occur is where the researcher is a perioperative nurse who may already have a relationship with individuals invited to take part in the study. Under these circumstances it is very difficult for the individual to give a refusal to someone to whom they may feel a debt of gratitude. This, then becomes close to exploitation. One way around this is to get a third party to ask the individual to participate so that a refusal is not given directly to the researcher.

Finally, in cases where the study cannot be seen as audit, permission to undertake it may have to be given by an ethics committee or Local Research Ethics Committee (LREC). These are available in every Trust or Health Authority. Their role is to consider the ethical implications of all research involving both patients and staff. Where in doubt, the researcher should seek advice from senior nursing staff, or the secretary of the LREC.

4   PILOT STUDY

A study is only as good as the accuracy of the tool of data collection. Before a study is carried out, the researcher should ensure that there are no unanticipated problems in gaining access to the data and that the tool of data collection does work. This is the role of the pilot study which Polit & Hungler (1997) define as a small-scale version, or trial run, of the major study. Although its purpose is usually thought to relate to checking the accuracy of the data collection tool, it should be used to consider a range of factors. The whole feasibility of the study in terms of the resources, time, the availability of the sample, willingness to participate and the support required from others, needs to be assessed before a total and perhaps expensive commitment to the study is made.

In addition, the data gathered in the pilot should be processed in order to ensure that the method of analysis will work smoothly. This is important whether analysis will be by hand or computer. The major purpose of the pilot is to assess the reliability of the method of data collection and to provide the researcher with experience and practice in using it. Refinements can then be made which will allow the main study to progress as smoothly as possible. In this way the pilot study is very much like a dress-rehearsal which allows all the elements in the study to be tested and adjustments made before the opening night.

5   COLLECTING THE DATA

This is the most exciting part of research. It can have its pitfalls and the researcher may need to make corrections to the original intention despite a pilot study as conditions for collecting data can change rapidly. This can range from the sudden closure of theatres to postal strikes. On the whole, however, the researcher should follow the terms of reference and the research protocol as closely as possible.

The period of data collection can vary considerably from a short period such as an afternoon to several months. Care needs to be taken to monitor all aspects of the study, and to record any changes in plans. It can be difficult at the end of a study to remember why things look so different from the original intentions.

6 ANALYSIS OF THE RESULTS

Although many people can feel overwhelmed by the data produced in a study, this is the real part of the study, which is finding out the answer to the terms of reference. Where the results require statistical analysis it is important to get advice from someone competent in statistics at the planning stage. It is also a good idea to check the literature and see how others have presented their findings.

7 CONCLUSION AND RECOMMENDATIONS

So what does it all mean and where do we go from here? At this point the researcher has to decide what is the answer to the terms of reference, using the results to make a clear statement. Following the conclusion, what recommendations could now be made? These should be concrete and specify who should do what, and how.

8 COMMUNICATION OF THE RESEARCH

Research is only of use if it is communicated. This could be in the form of a report, a verbal presentation, or an article for a professional journal. The format of all of these will be very similar and is outlined in Box 5.5.

Box 5.5 Format for reporting research

- What the researcher set out to achieve (the aim/terms of reference).
- Why they did it (what the literature says/local needs/problems).
- How they did it (methods).
- What they found (results).
- What it all means (discussion of the issues raised by the results and conclusion).
- What should happen now (recommendations).

The research process is a very logical series of steps. This framework allows the researcher to plan a study and also allows those reading research reports to ensure that the study has been undertaken in the right way. It should be emphasised again that this outline relates to quantitative research, true qualitative research does vary from this. Like all frameworks, this is meant to provide a clear guideline for the conduct of research. The implementation of this into practice may produce some slight variations. Although it is presented as a linear progression, some of the processes may be carried out in parallel or there may be some jumping back and forth. For most situations, however, this should be a reasonable guide to follow.

How can we make the best use of research?

Following the last section, there are clearly a number of essential elements we need to understand if we are to make the best use of research. One of the most frequently asked questions about published research is 'How do we know if it is any good or not?' By this is meant how can the reader tell if a particular piece of research has produced trustworthy findings? Although research is a difficult enterprise, we should expect it to stand up to external criticism if those using it are to feel it is a reasonable basis for making decisions. There are four concepts that will help us in this task. These are:

- Reliability
- Validity
- Bias
- Rigour.

Taking these one at a time, reliability relates to the method that is being used to collect the data and refers to the accuracy and consistency of the measurements generated by a particular method. If someone had measured the area of an operating theatre using a metre length of elastic, we would be very sceptical about the accuracy of the results. Reliability, then, is to do with the consistency of the measurement tool. Polit & Hungler (1997) define this as:

> The degree of consistency or dependability with which an instrument measures the attribute it is designed to measure.

Validity is concerned with what is being measured, and is an attempt to ensure that the research tool is really measuring what the researcher believes it is measuring. So, for instance, we might think we were measuring satisfaction with the outcome of surgery, but were we really measuring the quality of the relationship with nursing staff, and the extent to which they allayed fears concerning the outcome of the visit to theatre? Although reliability is usually amenable to checking, and may be tested with a pilot study, validity is far more difficult to confirm.

The degree of accuracy in the results of a study will be influenced by the amount of bias contained in the research process. Bias has been defined by Polit & Hungler (1997) as any influence that produces a distortion in the information collected. This can take a number of different forms. There could be distortion in the way the research question has been constructed. Bias could relate to the selectivity in the literature reviewed as part of the study. It could also relate to the sample of people or things included in the study which may not be typical. All of these influence the accuracy of the findings and the extent to which sound decisions can be made on the basis of the research.

Finally, rigour relates to the overall planning and implementation of the research design. It is concerned with whether the researcher has carried out the study in a logical, systematic way and paid attention to factors that may influence the accuracy of the results. Burns & Grove (1995) suggest that rigour is the 'striving for excellence' in research and involves discipline, adherence to detail, and strict accuracy. They argue that a rigorously conducted study has precise measurement tools, a representative sample, and a tightly controlled study design.

Once we are familiar with these four concepts we are in a better position to judge the value of not only what has been done but how well it has been done. This helps the perioperative nurse to avoid taking research reports at face value, and to become a more informed consumer of research.

The skill of critiquing

One of the most important ways in which the perioperative nurse can make better use of research is by developing the skill of critiquing. This section will cover the process of critiquing research reports. Critiquing means considering a piece of research fairly, balancing both the strengths of the study and any weaknesses or limitations. Whatever weaknesses we find, we should always consider what positive element can we gain? For example, how has it helped raise our awareness of a topic, or how has it helped us consider alternatives to the kinds of procedures we currently carry out? However, critiquing is a skill, and like many activities expected of the perioperative nurse, it does not necessarily develop automatically. This has been identified by Kirkevold (1997) who comments:

> Many clinical nurses find reading and critiquing research reports difficult. They lack the qualifications necessary to understand and critically evaluate research. Even if they try they will frequently find that different research reports about the same topic will draw different conclusions. They are then faced with the question of what conclusions to believe or how to overcome the inconsistencies in the literature.
>
> The danger of this situation is that nursing research is not considered a resource of relevant knowledge by clinical nurses to help them better understand observed phenomena in practice, or to solve problems they encounter. Another danger is that individual studies, the ones clinical nurses happen to read and understand, make an unreasonable impact on practice, an impact that may be unwarranted, given the quality of the studies.

This suggests that the relationship between the perioperative nurse and written research reports can be a source of problems. There is a suggestion that nurses do not see research as important in decision making, although this may come from their difficulty in making sense of the way research is written. It has to be said that research reports are not the easiest of reading material. The wordy and jargonistic way some research reports are written acts as a barrier to many who could potentially benefit from research. This problem has been identified by Casteldine (1997) who warns that research findings do not tend to come in neat, consistent, easy-to-find packages.

In addition, Walsh (1997) found that one of the common obstacles for the majority of nurses in his study was the statistical presentation of findings in research reports. There are, then, a number of personal and organisational barriers that must be overcome, such as access to journals, libraries and literature search facilities. Here, we will concentrate on helping you to critique research in a systematic and useful way, which does not require too much prior knowledge of research. The process of critiquing can be simplified to a three stage process of:

- Comprehension
- Evaluation
- Application.

The first stage of comprehension is understanding the basic 'story line' of the article – what is going on? This concentrates on the subject content. The second stage of evaluation is concerned with the way the study has been conducted and factors related to the methodology. This is the process element and requires an examination of the study in relation to rigour, bias, reliability and validity. In other words we should satisfy ourselves that the study is sound.

Application considers the question: what use can we make of the research? This does not necessarily mean we have to put the findings immediately into practice. We are still applying the knowledge if we reflect on our current activities and find that our outcomes are just as successful as those suggested in the study. We would be justified to maintain our current practice but we would have some measure of its success and, also, have an alternative should the need arise. Similarly, we may be interested in a new procedure, but want to wait until further evidence of its effectiveness became available. All of these are ways in which we can apply research knowledge.

There are a number of critiquing frameworks that can be used to help us with this process. The one included below in Box 5.6 is a straightforward example that has been successfully used by many students on a variety of courses. It is suggested that you photocopy this and try it out on a number of articles. As you go through the headings underline on your research article what you feel relates to each heading and write the heading in the margin, i.e. focus, terms of reference, main finding, etc. These can be abbreviated to suit yourself. Critiquing is more useful if you can carry it out with a colleague, or group and compare what you found and discuss the implication for practice.

Box 5.6 Framework for critiquing quantitive research
(It is suggested that you photocopy this box, and use it when reading relevant articles)

---

1 Focus
What would you say is the theme of the article? What are the key words that sum this up? E.g. preoperative visiting, parents in the operating theatre. Is the title a clue to the focus? How important is this for the profession/practice?

2 Background
What is the rationale for examining this topic? Is previous literature presented? Are gaps in the literature or inadequacies with previous methods highlighted? Are local problems or changes that justify the study described? Is there a trigger that answers the question 'why did they do it then?'

3 Terms of reference

What is the aim of the research? This will usually start with the word 'to', e.g. the aim of this research was to examine/determine/compare/establish/etc. If relevant, is there a hypothesis?

4 Study design

What is the broad research approach? Is it experimental? Descriptive? Action research or audit? Is it quantitative, or qualitative? Is the study design appropriate to the terms of reference?

5 Data collection method

Which tool of data collection has been used? Has a single method been used or triangulation? Has the researcher addressed the issues of reliability and validity? Has a pilot study been conducted? Have any limitations of the tool been recognised?

6 Ethical considerations

Were the issues of informed consent, confidentiality, addressed? Was any harm or discomfort to individuals balanced against any benefits? Was coercion avoided? Was the study considered by an ethics committee?

7 Sample

Who or what makes up the sample? Are there clear inclusion and exclusion criteria? What method of sampling was used? Are those in the sample typical and representative? Are there any obvious elements of bias? On how many people/items/events are the results based?

8 Data presentation

How are the results presented; tables, bar-graphs, pie-charts, raw figures, percentages? Does the researcher explain and comment on these? Can you make sense of the way the results have been presented, or could the author have provided more explanation?

9 Main findings

Which are the most important results that relate to the terms of reference? (If you were to put the results in priority order, which is the most important result followed by the next most important result, etc.) There may only be a small number of these.

10 Conclusion and recommendations

Using the author's own words, what is the answer to the terms of reference? If relevant, is the hypothesis accepted or rejected? Are the conclusions based on, and supported by the results? What recommendations are made for practice? Are these relevant, specific and feasible?

11 Readability

How readable is it? Is it written in a clear, interesting style? Does it assume a lot of technical knowledge about the subject and/or research procedures (i.e. is there much jargon)? Is it complete, or are there some missing details?

12 Practice implications

Once you have read it, what is the answer to the question 'so what?' Was it worth doing and publishing? How can you relate it to practice? Who might find it relevant and in what way? What questions does it raise for practice or further study?

Source: Based on Rees (1997)

Reviewing the literature

The final suggestion for making the best use of research is to develop the skill of reviewing the literature. This is not an academic exercise limited to courses and modules. With the introduction of audit, evidence based practice and clinical governance, practitioners need to agree on best practice for their clinical area, based on the literature available. A review of the literature is therefore essential to establish what is the current evidence on which standards and best practice can be based. Many people mistakenly believe that a review of the literature is a summary of what has been published by others. Reviews following this principle turn out to be a story of who said what. To be useful a review must be a critical review of the literature, which is a careful evaluation of a large selection of latest evidence on a particular topic. In other words it should be an analysis of what different people have found and the strength of that evidence. When faced with writing a review it is useful to keep in mind their purpose. According to LoBiondo-Woods & Haber (1998) the written review should:

1 Determine what is known and not known about a subject, concept, or problem.

2 Determine gaps, consistencies, and inconsistencies in the literature about a subject, concept, or problem.

3 Discover unanswered questions about a subject, concept, or problem.

4 Discover conceptual traditions used to examine problems.

5 Uncover a new practice intervention(s), or gain support for current practice intervention(s).

6 Promote development of new or revised practice protocols, policies, and projects/activities related to nursing practice and the discipline.

7 Generate useful research questions and hypotheses for the discipline.

8 Describe the strengths and weaknesses of designs/ methods of inquiry and instruments used in earlier works.

9 Determine an appropriate research design/method (instruments, data collection and analysis methods) for answering the research question.

10 Determine the need for replication of a well-designed study or refinement of a study.

There are now increasing attempts to make the method of selecting articles for reviews more stringent. This is particularly true of systematic reviews of the literature. In these, only articles that are based on randomised control trials are used and care is taken in terms of the rigour that has been used by the researchers included in the review. This is to ensure that the conclusion is based on the highest quality information currently available. This will frequently include unpublished research (so called 'grey literature' as it is not yet on published white paper) conference papers and personal contact with researchers, to ensure that as much up-to-date information as possible is included. At the moment, systematic reviews are mainly carried out by such bodies as the NHS Centre for Reviews and Dissemination at the University of York and the Cochrane data base.

The increasing use of the Internet does allow a better access to published work, and subject interest groups on the web with access to 'notice boards' allow people to ask for information from others all around the world. There is a wealth of websites in this country that may be useful to the perioperative nurse, including the NATN (www.natn.org.uk), as well as America, with sites such as the Association of Operating Room Nurses (AORN) (www.aorn.org/).

It is important that perioperative nurses conduct their own reviews of the literature and these should be as comprehensive as possible. It should be emphasised that a review is not a series of critiques put back to back, nor is it an essay that says what you would like with selected quotes to back up your views. It should be a balanced assessment of different perspectives which allows the reader to feel confident that your recommendations are based on a fair assessment of the literature. As a way of judging reviews, the following assessment guidelines are offered to ensure that your reviews stand up to scrutiny (Box 5.7). The check-list is also useful in evaluating some of the published reviews currently available.

Box 5.7 Checklist of elements in a review of the literature

- Is there a clearly stated aim for the review which is specific rather than general (e.g. to review the literature on ...)?
- Is there a stated source of articles in terms of time period covered, and countries included in the search?
- Are any inclusion and exclusion criteria for articles stated?
- Is the method of searching for the literature outlined (e.g. electronic databases such as CINAHL, MEDLINE, etc)?
- Does the author appear to include up-to-date material as well as any 'classic' work on the subject?
- Is the literature presented under appropriate themes and subheadings?
- Does the author critically analyse the literature or merely summarise it?
- Are consistencies and differences between authors identified?
- Are there comments on the quality of research articles, and identification of methodological issues?
- Are both strengths and weaknesses of work identified?
- Are the analytical comments balanced and free from individual bias?
- Is there a use of summary tables to make it easier for the reader to compare different authors?
- Is there a summary of main points?
- Are the implications for practice presented?
- Do you feel that the review makes a clear contribution to perioperative nursing knowledge and practice, and allows justifiable changes to practice to be made?

The way ahead

In this chapter we have examined one of the important tools for perioperative nurses to continue to develop their professional role – the application of research to practice. The emphasis has been on the use of published research as a way of demonstrating clinical effectiveness. This is a highly skilled activity. There is a need, first of all, to feel that research is important to clinical and professional practice. At the moment, too much research is being under-utilised by the perioperative nurse. There are a number of reasons for this, as many barriers exist to the use of research.

An attempt has been made to increase both knowledge and skills. Firstly, an essential element in using research is knowing how it is conducted, so that some assessment can be made of the rigour that has been followed by those producing the research. The research process has been outlined to help you feel comfortable with the framework involved. In keeping with the current emphasis in health care this has focused on quantitative research approaches. Increasingly in nursing, generally, there is a growing use of qualitative methods that give a more complete picture of situations, particularly from the patient perspective. It is recommended that you seek to increase your depth of knowledge by referring to other texts on this subject (e.g. Holloway & Wheeler, 1996).

There are essential skills that the perioperative nurse must possess, and they include critiquing and producing a critical review of the literature. These are both practical skills that need practise. There must be a purpose in their use, and so it is recommended that, if not already in existence, research interest groups should be set up, or journal clubs where the latest research can be discussed and related to practice. If the UK Government's strategy for clinical governance as outlined in the White Paper *A First Class Service: Quality in the New NHS* (DOH, 1998) is to become a reality, clinical areas will have to produce evidence that they have developed their own assessment of what is best practice. These skills will then be paramount if perioperative nurses are to play a proactive role in clinical developments. Perioperative nursing must also develop a strategy for encouraging research activity by nurses working in the theatre setting. This should not be everyone's responsibility, but someone will have to do it. One of the intentions of this chapter has been to demonstrate that research is a reasonably straightforward and logical activity that can be carried out by perioperative nurses with support. The consequence of ignoring the need to produce nursing research in this area is that it will be other forms of research that will dictate the organisation of services. It seems sensible, therefore, that rather than let that happen, perioperative nurses should contribute to the clinical agenda themselves.

If these points are acted upon, then we can look forwards to a dynamic and proactive clinical and professional area which is built on a solid foundation of research, staffed by research minded and skilled practitioners. Research is a tool – use it!

Reflective activities

If you are embarking on postgraduate studies you will almost certainly be preparing to read and evaluate perioperative nursing research. If you are already a qualified perioperative nurse, in whatever capacity, there is something useful for you in this chapter.

1 If you are embarking on nursing research or considering which way to set up a study of your own, reflect on the elements of the nursing process outlined in this chapter. You may like to extend your knowledge by using one or more of the books in the suggested 'Further reading' list.

2 Read a report on a piece of perioperative nursing research, perhaps one with which you are already familiar and critique it, or re-evaluate it, using the guidance in this chapter. You might find it particularly instructive to do this with a colleague.

3 Do you have a journal club in your department? Why not start one? Whether or not you are able to do this it would be particularly valuable to use the guidance offered in this chapter to critique several literature reviews. Are the reviews critiqued by the reviewer in a way that gives you some idea of the value of the research?

References

Burns, N. & Grove, S. 1995 *Understanding nursing research.* Philadelphia, W.B. Saunders.

Carthew, L. 1997 The role of the clinical practice suite in skills acquisition in the Common Foundation Programme. *British Journal of Theatre Nursing* **7** (6), 31.

Casteldine, G. 1997 'Evidence-based nursing: where is the evidence?' *British Journal of Nursing* **6** (5), 290.

Clegg, F. 1982 *Simple statistics.* Cambridge, Cambridge University Press.

DOH. 1998 *A first class service: quality in the new NHS.* London, DOH.

Driver, J. 1997 Post-operative telephone notification: A theatre nurse's role? *British Journal of Theatre Nursing* **7** (6), 27–30.

Holloway, I. & Wheeler, S. 1996 *Qualitative research for nursing.* Oxford, Blackwell Science.

Kirkevold, M. 1997 Integrative nursing research – an important strategy to further the development of nursing science and nursing practice. *Journal of Advanced Nursing* **25** (5), 977–84.

LoBiondo-Wood, G. & Haber, J. 1998 *Nursing research: methods, critical appraisal, and utilisation,* 4th edition. St. Louis, Mosby.

Macleod Clark, J. & Hockey, L. 1989 *Further research for nursing.* London, Scutari.

Malby, B. (ed.) 1995 Clinical audit for nurses and therapists. London, Scutari Press.

Parahoo, K. 1997 *Nursing research: principles, process and issues.* Basingstoke, Macmillan.

Polit, D. & Hungler, B. 1997 *Essentials of nursing research: methods, appraisal, and utilisation,* 4th edition. Philadelphia, J.B. Lippincott.

Rees, C. 1997 *An introduction to research for midwives.* Hale, Books for Midwives.

Reid, J. 1997 Meeting the informational needs of patients in a day surgery setting – an exploratory level study. *British Journal of Theatre Nursing* **7** (4), 19–24.

Smith, P. 1997 *Research mindedness for practice.* New York, Churchill Livingstone.

Walsh, M. 1997 How nurses perceive barriers to research implementation. *Nursing Standard* 11 (29), 34–9.

Walsh, M. & Ford, P. 1989 *Nursing rituals, research and rational actions.* Oxford, Butterworth-Heinemann.

Webb, C. 1996 Action research. In: Cormack, D. (ed.) *The research process in nursing,* 3rd edition. Oxford, Blackwell Science.

White, S. 1997 Evidence-based practice and nursing; the new panacea?' *British Journal of Nursing* 6 (3), 175–8.

Willmer, S., Willson, P., McEnteggart, K. & Rogers, J. 1997 Reuse of single use items in minimal surgery. *British Journal of Theatre Nursing* 7 (3), 11–13.

Further reading

Holloway, I. & Wheeler, S. 1996 *Qualitative research for nursing.* Oxford, Blackwell Science.

DOH. 1998 *Achieving effective practice: a clinical effectiveness and research information pack for nurses.* Abridged version included with *Nursing Times* July 15 1998, 94 (28).

LoBiondo-Wood, G. & Haber, J. 1998 *Nursing research: methods, critical appraisal, and utilisation,* 4th edition. St. Louis, Mosby.

Parahoo, K. 1997 *Nursing research: principles, process and issues.* Basingstoke, Macmillan.

Rees, C. 1997 *An introduction to research for midwives.* Hale, Books for Midwives.

Polit, D. & Hungler, B. 1997 *Essentials of nursing research: methods, appraisal, and utilisation,* 4th edition. Philadelphia, J.B.Lippincott.

Appendix: Perioperative nursing research

Chapter 5 has been largely concerned with discussing the research process rather than referring to specific pieces of perioperative nursing research. This is not because there is little research in the area. On the contrary, a great deal of research in operating departments, on perioperative practice and on and by perioperative nurses has been carried out. Much research has also been carried out by professional researchers employed elsewhere and focusing on, for example, the spread and control of infection. To give some idea of the range of perioperative nursing research a selection of reports from the *British Journal of Theatre Nursing* are referred to here.

If we turn back to the early Royal College of Nursing research papers there are several pieces of nursing research directly related to what we now know as perioperative nursing:

Boore, J. 1978 *Prescription for Recovery.* London, RCN.
Hayward, J. 1975 Information – *A prescription against pain.* London, RCN.
Hamilton Smith, S. 1972 *Nil by mouth.* London, RCN.

These well-known pieces of research have been much quoted and encouraged theatre nurses to become research minded. Surgical research and government working parties have always taken place in operating departments and also contributed to making perioperative nurses interested in using research methods in their work. The Bevan Report was itself based on research carried out on the work in 12 different theatres:

Bevan, P.G. 1989 *Management and utilisation of operating departments.* London, NHS Management Executive: Value for Money Unit.

Two topics which have been extensively researched by theatre nurses over the years are directly related to patient care. These are inadvertent hypothermia during surgery and the incidence of intraoperative pressure injuries. Turning to recent research papers on these topics reveals a considerable bibliography of previous studies utilising research methods in a variety of ways, ranging from local studies to PhD research:

McNeil, B.A. 1998. Addressing the problems of inadvertent hypothermia in surgical patients. Parts 1 & 2. *British Journal of Theatre Nursing* **8** (4), 8–14 and **8** (5), 25–33.

Scott, E. 1998 Hospital pressure sores as an indicator of quality. *British Journal of Theatre Nursing* **8** (5), 19–24.

The Audit Commission, too has carried out considerable research into such an expensive and rapidly changing area as the operating department:

Audit Commission. 1992 *All in a day's work – an audit of day surgery in England and Wales.* London, HMSO.

Perhaps one of the most significant pieces of research carried out on perioperative nurses was one element of the PhD study completed by Bernice West in 1994. The researcher is not only a nurse but also an educationalist and clinical psychologist and she studied the caring component of nursing in a cardiothoracic unit from two points of view, caring for the patient and caring for colleagues. The results showed that the majority of nurses are 'sacrificers' who elicit only sufficient information to enable them to deal with the somatic aspects of care. A few nurses, notably graduate nurses, seek further information to enable them to ensure the physical, psychological and social wellbeing of their patients.

The study concluded that the psychological aspect of care was not well-understood by all groups of nurses. Turning specifically to perioperative nurses, West concluded that nursing in operating departments was so dynamic and fast-moving that it was difficult to articulate its holistic nature but that the wellbeing of the patient was central to all the nurses' concerns.

The transition from novice to expert involved equal consideration of technical competence and the emotional aspects of caring.

> The reality of nursing in the operating department is that the nurse must be the labourer, the craftsperson and the artist at all times and for all people.

West, B.J. 1994 Caring: the essence of theatre nursing. (A paper delivered at NATN Congress.) *British Journal of Theatre Nursing* **3** (9), 15–24.

Another research topic which is regularly re-visited by both perioperative nurses and surgeons is mask-wearing. A small-scale study was carried out when the wearing of visors was being assessed during the development of precautions against viral infections:

Norman, A. 1995 A comparison of face-masks and visors for the scrub team. *British Journal of Theatre Nursing* 5 (2), 10–13.

Lloyd-Jones, H. 1995 Attitudes of nurses to donor organ retrieval. *British Journal of Theatre Nursing* 5 (11), 28–32.

The above source considers nurses' communication skills and was read as a paper at a world conference before publication.

A final example of perioperative nursing research which has been published recently is also a study of the quality of patient care:

Reid, J. 1997 Meeting the informational needs of patients in a day surgery setting. An exploratory level study. *British Journal of Theatre Nursing* 7 (4), 19–24.

This is a very small selection of perioperative research in the UK, but it does give some idea of the breadth of interests which are covered and the uses which are made of research methods in assessing and evaluating the quality of care in perioperative practice.

6 Perioperative nursing across Europe

Margaret Brett

When Margaret Brett wrote this article she was the President of the European Operating Room Nursing Association (EORNA) following several years during which she had been an active representative at their meetings and had led the work on the common core curriculum. It was during her presidency that EORNA held the first European conference. As a result of this she has great insights into the advantages and disadvantages of working across national boundaries with nurses from different cultural backgrounds. This chapter discusses how perioperative nursing has developed and can now view the future from a broader perspective. Making contacts with other countries and working within the European Union has opened up new opportunities. However, working with nurses from many European countries, not all yet members of the Union, has shown that not all are starting from the same point economically, politically or culturally. Once again we are reminded of how perioperative nurses in all countries are facing many of the same problems and are being encouraged to become involved nationally and internationally in attempting to solve the problems and take the lead in implementing change. Taking such an initiative will ensure that the voice of nursing across Europe will be heard in the setting of nursing priorities.

Introduction

In reviewing books and articles relating to the history of nursing one finds constant reference to the varying status of nursing throughout its development (Baly, 1995; Dolan, 1968). Nightingale in her *Notes on Nursing* (Skeet, 1980), refers to the importance of the individual in maintaining that status. Later years found her and Mrs Bedford Fenwick at odds with each other over the issue of registration for nurses because Nightingale thought this would affect the status of nursing. In more recent years we have often looked to colleagues oversees to see whether they had anything to offer us in our fight to become recognised as a true profession in our own right. I'm sure few of us ever anticipated that there would be a day when somebody outside our own homeland would dictate what nursing should be about. We have moved through a continuum of being the doctor's assistant, or even servant, to our current state in which we would like to think we are valued practitioners in our own right working as an equal part of the team. We have looked to our national bodies for the guidance as to the way forward for the profession often, perhaps, feeling frustrated that even they at times appeared distant from the real life situation of the nurse within her clinical area.

We now have an even more distant controlling body in the form of the European Commission which has already laid down firm rules for general nursing throughout all member states of the Union. Currently postregistration nurse education has escaped its attention mainly because there is no clear agreement about what constitutes postbasic or continuing education and, indeed, in many countries there is no formal recognition of postbasic qualifications. You may think this lack of attention is a blessing in disguise, however there are issues to be considered in relation to the implementation of EC Directives which require us to accept colleagues from within Europe to work within our environments. As the portfolio of European legislation increases there are certain to be many areas which will affect theatre nurses either directly or indirectly. Such areas already include aspects of product handling and packaging, of consumer protection, working times, equal opportunities, health and safety and technology.

This chapter aims to explore this new Europe and to define the potential effects of it upon the profession of perioperative nursing. In using the development of the European Operating Room Nursing Association (EORNA) as an example it is hoped to raise an awareness of some of the benefits and difficulties in establishing and working with European groups. Whatever our personal wishes, there is no turning back now and, therefore, it is important that we, as nurses, recognise and utilise every opportunity to raise the awareness and voice of nursing so that many of the future developments will actually be nurse-led.

Most of us in nursing have given little attention to the organisation of the European Union. We perhaps recall that a few years ago there was a reorganisation of general nurse training based upon the agreed formula for a common period of education to be recognised throughout Europe. Whilst most of us will be aware of the impact of the Project 2000 nurse training here in the UK, we may forget that even that programme is underpinned by European legislation on nurse training for the general nurse.

European nurses are first recorded as meeting together in 1946 and an early Western Nursing European group was established in 1953 (Brett, 1996). The production in 1967 by the Council of Europe of the document *The European Agreement on the Instruction and Education of Nurses* followed the first formal contacts between nurses and the Commission in 1961. This was followed by the first EC Directives on the training of nurses responsible for general care in 1977, together with the establishment of the Advisory Committee on Training for Nurses (ACTN) which held its first meeting in 1979. It was the work of this group, containing three professionals from each country, which led to the amendments of the Training Directive to give attention to the balance between theory and practice in general nursing. These directives are seen by nurses as invaluable guidelines in setting up training programmes in countries in central and eastern Europe and for lobbying for standards of health care in their own regions.

In order for nurses to have any influence over the future developments within the profession there is a need to target representative members of the ACTN group with firm proposals and ideas as this is one of the main forums through which nurses can obtain direct access to the ears of the Commission. Lack of funds has reduced this particular group's meetings to one a year, and it is, therefore, vital that we seek ways to ensure that it remains as a voice. We need to think about our own specialty of perioperative nursing from a European perspective and ensure that members of ACTN are provided with relevant information to relay to the commission thus ensuring the value of this forum.

At European level, the 'PCN' forum consists of nursing leaders from its European member countries, yet as a group, even there we cannot agree on something as simple as a name. For some countries it is known as the Permanent Committee of Nursing (PCN) whilst for others it is the Standing Committee of Nurses. If we cannot agree a name are we truly united in a cause? Since its inception in 1971 PCN has worked consistently to establish direct dialogue with the Commission, and has recently opened its own office in Brussels to reinforce its image as a truly European organisation. The PCN has now acknowledged the importance of the growing number of specialty groups which are developing across Europe and has recognised the need to bring them into the forum if there is to be a truly united European nursing representation with one voice.

Boundaries of Europe

For many people during their lifetime the concept of the word Europe was simply interpreted as the name of a continent – one of the five great sections of the world to which we were introduced during our school days. For the more enthusiastic followers of geography it had a number of specific features which linked its member countries and which differentiated it from the other four divisions. As individuals, we may well have recognised our own position as one of its member constituents, but I suspect few of us would ever have dreamt of its significance in relation to the future developments of our lifestyles both in our daily living and in our employment.

Geographically, Europe consists of territory between Finland and Cyprus on a north-south axis, with an east-west perspective covering Iceland to Russia. However, definitions and borders of 'Europe' vary depending upon which organisation is referring to it. The European region of the World Health Organization (WHO) actually incorporates 50 countries within its boundaries whilst the European Union (in 1998) embodies just 15 countries – with 410 million people – as its members but with others awaiting entry. European borders also vary for sports organisations and, indeed, for the Eurovision song contest. The issue of establishing borders for membership of any European group can in itself be a major topic of discussion as one considers the principles of equal access to all members of 'Europe' against the manageable size of any working group of representatives. Who has the right to refuse another country membership if it is to be called a European Association? Within the European Operating Room Nursing Association (EORNA) this was found to be a very delicate situation and eventually it was necessary to confirm that any country had the right to apply and that representation may need to be reduced from the customary two per country to only one if the group becomes too large.

Historically, our main links with Europe were not focused towards developing permanent relationships with our neighbours residing in those countries, but more on accessing resources or features of their part of this large land mass such as fashion, romance, fame or fortune. It has been seen as fitting for young ladies to travel Europe in order to further their education and development when some parts of Europe were seen to offer a far superior 'finishing' to the education of gentleladies than that of our own native parts.

Nowadays, however, many of those early dreams of holidays and wealth in Europe have become everyday realities as developments in transport have brought us luxury ferries, speedy hovercrafts and, more recently, the famous Channel Tunnel to enable those of us in the UK to easily access colleagues on the other side of the water. Similarly, an increase in air traffic with a corresponding decrease in costs has made access to more distant parts of Europe easier. Individual cultures have become blurred as small communities establish themselves in countries other than their own and adopt part of the host culture whilst retaining their own traditions. This freedom to visit, together with the experiencing of other cultures within our own environment, has brought greater understanding of the ways of others within Europe and, indeed, the world.

The development of the European Union

The European Union (EU) previously known as the European Economic Community (EEC) started as just that, an economic activity. The question as to who actually started the ball rolling for a European wide approach to trade and industry will receive varying answers according to which country you are in when you ask that question. Although many consider it all started with the Treaty of Paris (1951) which established the European Coal and Steel

Community (ECSC) this was actually preceded by the rarely mentioned Benelux agreement between Holland, Luxembourg and Belgium which had existed since 1947. The ECSC started with just six members, Belgium, France, Germany, Holland, Italy and Luxembourg. Following on from Paris was the establishment in 1957 of the EEC and the European Atomic Energy Community (EAEC) through the Treaties of Rome. Britain, Norway and Ireland were initially refused membership but eventually Britain joined in 1973 along with Ireland and Denmark, whilst the people of Norway now declined.

The European Monetary Systems, denied by the British, appeared in 1979 as did the first direct elections to the European parliament. Membership rose to 12 after Greece joined in 1981 and the signing of the Treaty of Accession by Spain and Portugal in June 1985. The addition of Austria, Finland and Sweden in 1995 brought the membership to the current figure of 15, but with the frequently used word 'enlargement' indicating potential new additions for the future.The removal of all restraints on trade by 31 December 1991, the single European act of 1986 prepared the way for the single market and the 'Open Europe'.

The Treaties of European Union, commonly known as the Maastricht Treaty, was eventually agreed in May 1993 following an initial denial by Denmark. The Maastricht Treaty agreed full economic and monetary union. The Europe of which we now speak has, therefore, arisen from the concerns of business and economy and, although it still sits within the borders of the geographical Europe, it usually refers to a much smaller part of that territory included in the EU. Its development has been that of gradual infiltration rather than sudden impact upon our daily lives.

Much of the trade effects have been attributed to general growth and change in the market place rather than specifically seen as a result of the European trade networks. Farcical tales bringing supposed threats to our cultural features such as our red buses and our British sausage have perhaps aroused more awareness of the influence of Europe than has the gradual appearance of a greater variety of fruits, vegetables and cheeses in our supermarkets. The food mountains, the quotas and trading restrictions within the Common Agricultural Policy are a real live feature of today, as is the problem of British beef. The traditional British Sunday lunch may well find itself in the archives with the pounds, shillings and pence; the feet, inches and yards and the stones, pounds and ounces. Heated internal arguments about identification cards see countries fighting to retain their own systems, whilst already the idea of a European driving license has received approval (European Parliament, 1996b). As a general rule nurses have paid little attention to the developments within European legislation yet if we are to have a say in the future of our profession we need to be alert to the way in which the new Europe now functions.

The structure of the European Union

The structure of the European Union comprises of a number of institutions. The Council of Ministers comprising representatives of the governments of member states is the decision making body for issues debated at the European summit. In relation to health, it attempts to achieve common health policy throughout Europe and retain responsibility for health promotion and prevention of ill health. Issues such as standardisation of tissue typing techniques for organ transplant, drug abuse and trafficking, rehabilitation and socialisation for disabled persons and nursing research and education are all part of its activities.

The civil service style European Commission, which has 23 directorates, uses its powers of initiative in developing and bringing forward legislation and in acting as the guardian of the Treaties. Health issues are spread across several of the Directorate Generals. For example, DG5 is about Health and Safety, Health targets etc; DG15 is about nurse education. This means that all but the most determined explorer of a health issue would be easily discouraged from the search. What is interesting is that there are actually very few resident commissioners within the commission.

Directorates function through liaising with the experts within a profession or trade to obtain relevant information. This offers excellent opportunities for nursing to find its way into the more influential aspects of the Commission. Once individual nursing groups become known to the commissioner, they are seen as a source of expert advice available for consultation. This again reinforces the need for nurses to stand up and declare their presence and let people know they exist. After only 3 years as an official organisation EORNA was invited to join discussions at the Commission on specialist nurses. This invitation was due to the constant approaches by the Association for recognition of the specialism and the organisation.

The European Parliament, whose members serve for a period of 5 years, is responsible for approving proposals before their adoption, and modifies legislation as it sees fit. It is interesting to note that the annual report from the Union is produced not by the specific departments but by the Court of Auditors who closely monitor activity and waste within the organisation. The Committee of the Regions advises both the council and the commission on public health following liaison with regional and local authorities. It is hoped that this process will lead to a more integrated 'citizen's Europe' as people take ownership of its development.

European law

Most of us will be familiar with the name of the European Court of Justice as it regularly features in our news headlines. People who have been unsuccessful in gaining satisfaction through their own legal system can appeal to the 13 European judges if the issue is included within European legislation. Its main role is the interpretation of EC treaties and agreements in relation to individual member country situations. In real life terms, this means that the legal system within any member country can be over-ridden by the Law of the Community which takes precedence over national law.

Community law was established in the Treaty of Rome (1957) and has been expanded through the regulations, directives and decisions adopted by the

Council, Commission and, to a lesser extent, the parliament of the Union. Those of us in health care are likely to be affected by community rules governing free movement of goods, persons, capital and services. One of the fundamental rights that the Treaty gives is the right to pursue one's professional activities anywhere in the member states of the Community. This movement is controlled through directives.

Whilst a European Regulation is binding to both member states and individuals, thus establishing a uniform law throughout the community, a Directive simply requires an amendment to national law to support a common obligation rather than stipulating common law. Directives are further divided into General Directives and Sectoral Directives.

The sectoral system directives governing the criteria of training programmes for a specific profession are established through 'harmonisation' – the agreement between representatives of that profession from each member state. This, unfortunately, tends to be a very slow and tedious process. For example, it took nearly 15 years for nursing directives to be agreed and engineers had still not achieved agreement after 18 years. However, the Commission believes strongly that such decisions should be reached through negotiation with relevant professionals/experts before any directive becomes part of the enforcement towards facilitating the free movement of individuals within that specific profession.

Several of us involved in the development of the European Common Core Curriculum for Operating Room Nursing (Brett, 1996) have felt that the 4-year period involved in the development of that programme has been a lifetime but, judging by these standards, we have done extremely well.

General Directives require that each individual person is considered on the basis of their personal qualifications. Of the two directives the first considers those with a university or equivalent qualification of 3 years and above, and the second is for those with formal qualifications of less than 3 years. General Nurses fall into the former category under Directive 89/48/ EEC. A competent authority in each country assesses the qualifications and either issues instant permission to practice or requests the applicant to undergo further training or an aptitude test. Here, in the UK the relevant body for nursing is the United Kingdom Central Council (UKCC), which has to respond according to whether the applicant is to be considered under a general or a sectoral directive. Language is an issue within this system. It invokes national requirements and insisting upon applicants having competence in the English language here in UK could potentially contradict terms of the Sectoral Directive which does not apportion such powers of selection.

Movement of nurses to and from the UK

In 1995 the UKCC reported that, of the 7000 or 8000 applications for new registration each year, only 10% come from Europe and 85% of these come from Southern Ireland so, currently, movement to the UK is very small (Wallace, 1995). The big factor which may influence the similarly small number of nurses wishing to work overseas may well be that as a nation we are lazy when it comes to languages. This is unfortunately perpetuated by the ability of many of our European colleagues to speak fluent English.

In health care circles it is vital that one is able to converse fluently with patients and clients in their own natural tongue. European nurses from other countries wishing to work in the UK would be required to produce evidence from the nursing body of the country in which they trained that they have completed the relevant qualification and/or worked as a nurse for 3 out of the previous 5 years. It would also be necessary to confirm that the programme of training/education meets the requirements of European law (UKCC, 1995). A certificate of good character, together with a photocopy of passport or identity card, must be sent to the UKCC along with the nursing diploma and all must be translated into English with confirmation that it is an authentic translation. Movement of nurses is governed by EC Directive 77/452/EC whilst midwives fall under directive 80/154/EC.

Midwives are also required to notify the local supervising authority if undertaking temporary registration here and intending to practice (ENB, 1995). Midwives who have undertaken an 18-month training must have completed an additional 12 months of professional practice unless they entered midwifery without any formal qualifications suitable for entry into higher education. If this is the case, they must have completed 2 years of professional practice (UKCC, 1996).

European nurses wishing to work here on a temporary basis may not need to register with the UKCC providing they are currently employed within their own country but they must still inform the UKCC of their intention to practice within the UK. A temporary registration is also available for nurses wishing to undertake postbasic courses in the UK. Those students undergoing first level qualifications need to be aware of new immigration rules, as of October 1994, which require them to satisfy entry clearance or immigration officers that they will return to their own land once qualified. It is not now possible to move into work permit employment and remain in the UK once qualified.

For a nurse who holds a specialist qualification as his/her first form of registration there can be some difficulty when he or she wishes to work in a country which does not recognise that area as a specialty. An example would be a nurse who possesses psychiatric or mental illness training without a general training to accompany it. The recognition of the profession is through a similar diploma within the host country so, if no such diploma exists, there is no facility for recognition. In 1995, the Commission undertook discussions and consultations on a proposal for a new directive which would cover these specialist practice areas. Its intention was that specialist nurses should receive the same consideration as any other professional moving through Europe. In other words, the ability to deliver health care should be assessed on an individual basis in relation to the post for which the nurse is applying (EC, 1996).

Within the field of perioperative nursing the limitations of the existing directive mean that people from countries such as Holland, Germany and Switzerland who are qualified technicians cannot work as a qualified person in their own right in some of the member countries due to the lack of registration for this group in other countries. In many countries in southern Europe there remains a strong refusal by nurses to employ any persons other than qualified nurses within operating departments. For others, the concept of non-nursing operating department practitioners is gradually being introduced by managers but still carries great resentment from nurses.

Perioperative nurses who were not primarily general trained, but had undertaken a core programme leading to operating department nursing specialism were also limited in their ability to move freely. This was seen as a form of discrimination where people possess a qualification which may well be of equal standing to that of the host country. A simple addition to General Directive 2, confirmed that they also must be considered on an individual basis, and offered an entrance test and/or the necessary further education. Perioperative nurses, such as our own here in the UK, are able to move on the basis of their general qualification. However, we would also be subject to the above criteria when applying to work specifically within operating departments within Europe.

The majority of the 6000 persons who had acknowledgement of their diplomas by the UK through Directive 89/48/EEC between 1981 and 1994 were teachers (EC, 1996). Only 11 000 in total throughout Europe were acknowledged during this time, with just 5% being refused free movement. One of the factors affecting free movement at any time has to be the number of the professionals currently available within the host country. Hospital Trusts from the UK can often be found offering interview and consultation days in other countries in the hope of recruiting nurses to areas which are desperately short here in the UK. In the past the main focus has been Ireland where there should be few problems with the language. However, as overseas countries focus more upon the English language we find the activity spreading to Sweden and Finland. Currently, the time frame for negotiating access within Europe can be up to one year. This should reduce as host countries become familiar with overseas qualifications and can easily recognise their comparability with their own criteria. It is for this reason that the Commission is very supportive of the development of European wide professional groups who will themselves establish acceptable standards and levels. The development of common core curricula such as that developed by EORNA is seen as extremely valuable by the Commission as documents such as these will provide 'professional passports' for individuals within a specific profession.

The inclusion of a section on health in the Maastricht Treaty poses an opportunity for nurses to step forward and play a fundamental role in developing future health care (Pritchard, 1995). With a united voice we surely must be in a position to raise our suggestions and play an active role in shaping the implementation of health care strategies. Those of us in the west are having to cope with the introduction of new diseases whilst our colleagues in the east are experiencing changes in disease patterns (Richards, 1992). Aspects of disease training within educational programmes are being revived as it was thought the diseases themselves were a thing of the past. A very good example is that of diphtheria which is gradually reappearing across the continent and nurses are finding themselves unfamiliar with its presentation and treatment.

Clinical responsibilities vary greatly in different European countries mainly because there is no coordinated approach to health care. There is no minister of health within the Commission who might take responsibility for ensuring comparability and standardisation across the delivery of European health care. We now have a Competence for Health but, at this time, many departments are involved on an individual basis in the future shaping of health care.

Nursing's biggest disadvantage, certainly here in the UK is that we have a reputation of being doers not sayers, of being reactive rather than proactive, compliant rather than debative and accepting rather than negotiating what is really required. Until we can demonstrate the ability to be active participants in instigating change we will never be in a position to dictate our own future or use our knowledge and experience to direct future health care standards for ourselves or our patients. Once individual nurses become known to national organisations there is the potential for their involvement at both national and international level around the debating table. European nursing groups must also take every step to raise their own profile within the Commission. This does not happen overnight, it needs persistence at every opportunity. When any issue is being considered send in your contribution, ask for reports, show your interest and let them know you are there and are capable of participating in such discussions.

We need to present ourselves as a sound investment which will reap future benefits rather than an expensive short term activity which could easily be replaced by cheaper options. Here in the UK, our biggest weakness remains that we have failed to come together as one voice. We do not have one single organisation which truly represents all nurses within the UK. Whilst the National Association of Theatre Nurses (NATN) has seen a rapid growth in membership over recent years, even as perioperative nurses we do not all belong to one group which could speak for all theatre specialists. If we cannot be seen to be united into one group on basic points how can we expect to receive credibility in our fight for essential issues?

The influence of European legislation

As nurses, we have already experienced a number of ways in which the influence of Europe has impinged upon our working environment. In 1990 a directive was drafted on the minimum Health and Safety requirements for the Manual Handling of Loads, Directive 90/269/ EEC, laying the ground for the adoption of Manual Handling Operations Regulations by 1993. All of you who are in regular employment will be familiar with the requirement for an annual update on 'Lifting and Moving' as it is sometimes called. This, at last, brought perioperative nurses' concerns about training in this area to the forefront as, previously, the focus had been upon obvious area of wards and awake patients. The operating theatre was often left to make its own interpretations of the stated requirements but trainers were now required to assess the situation in all areas and to work closely with employees to design specific training programmes to meet the needs of those particular people as well.

In January 1995 the European Medicines Evaluation Agency (EMEA) was formally inaugurated here in the UK at the Canary Wharf in London, its main remit being to facilitate a more speedy introduction of new products onto the market whilst ensuring levels of safety were maintained to ensure protection of the patients through the reinforcement of high standards of safety, quality and efficacy.

Although a European environment agency was set up in Copenhagen in 1994 it has no formal mechanism or powers to guarantee enforcement of commonly agreed legislation and therefore tends to be a monitoring rather than reinforcing body. Activities by members of NATN through the *British Journal of Theatre Nursing* have, however, focused upon such legislation in identifying what is relevant to the disposal of medical waste – a subject very pertinent in operating departments.

Our partners in industry are also experiencing the burden of European legislation regarding both production and packaging of products. The Producer Responsibility Obligations (PRO) require businesses who handle more than 50 tonnes of packaging per year to recover and recycle packaging waste. This can be either done by themselves, through the individual route, or by joining a registered compliance scheme which, for a fee, takes care of the waste on their behalf. Here in the UK, VALPAK is one such compliance scheme. In Holland, systems for this have existed for some time whilst Germany runs a system known as the Green Dot Code which identifies recycling and disposal variations for different waste materials.

By mid-1997 all relevant companies had to be registered, either independently or with a compliance scheme. This must ultimately mean that an even closer look will be taken at packaging materials and presentation. As consumers, we need to monitor developments closely. We need to consider whether refusal of what appears to be a simple request from us to the users may be prohibited by legislation rather than an unwillingness of industry to oblige. New products require rigorous testing and full documentation of all aspects before receiving the prized quality standard which permits production. Nursing organisations need, therefore, to establish links with national groups to provide a forum for the nursing voice rather than simply leaving all the decisions to industry.

EORNA has been invited to join one of the Commission's working groups discussing standards of production for disposable gowns and drapes. This group is part of the wider European committee for standardisation – The Commité Européen de Normalisation (CEN). Access to such a committee is normally through the national body responsible for standards, in our case the British Standards Institute. Each country holds its own meetings and submits proposals and discussion responses to the European group through its three nominated experts who sit on the CEN committee. The CEN is broken down into various Technical Committees (TCs) who in turn have smaller workgroups (WGs).

EORNA has been admitted as advisor to the CEN/TC205/WG14. Although they have no direct voting rights they are free to join in the discussion thus influencing those who do have freedom to vote. Access for EORNA was achieved through the persistence of its representatives who constantly address the Commission, and through the support of companies who are party to the organisation of the committee. At national level, other organisations should themselves explore what European committees are relevant to their field of work and seek to gain entry so that nursing has a voice in future production and activity.

Another important feature of products will be the CE marking which will already be familiar to most people both at work and in the home. This marking confirms that the device carrying it conforms to the relevant Directives (Medical Devices Directorate (MDD), 1992) and that it may be freely marketed anywhere in the community without further control. Beware! This does not necessarily mean that it is of the same high pattern as that of the national standard in some countries. Reclassification of products is under way and although we may not instantly attribute relevance to this, its importance increases when for any reason we need to explore that product further. The existing Medical Devices Agency (MDA) here in the UK continues to be the main monitoring centre for all medical devices. It remains responsible for the checking of all devices and for processing and exploring all complaints and for issuing the necessary hazard warnings. Again, the MDA is very much dependant upon users such as ourselves advising them of potential problems when using equipment.

Consumer information legislation brings further implications for nurses. Within this section consumers must not be given any false or misleading information, even verbally. The information can relate to quantities, capacities, method and place of manufacture, packaging, conformity to standards for sterilisation and /or appropriate use. The fundamental issue underlying this is a breach of safety and those who recklessly or knowingly mislead individuals are subject to legal accountability. Nurses are most commonly the ones to develop information packages for patients and relatives and it is, therefore, crucial that extra attention is given to every detail included in those packages.

In relation to shift patterns another potential influence upon nurses and nursing comes from the European Directive on working time established in November 1996 following Directive 93/104/EC, itself introduced in 1993. This seeks to standardise patterns of working hours by stipulating maximum hours per shift and week, together with minimum weekly and daily rest periods. Not surprisingly, a study by the University of Sheffield (Bivand, 1994) revealed nurses to be well over the permitted stipulations. The maximum 48-hour week criteria was not met by half of the nurses sampled in 21% of the weeks worked. The highest weekly recording of 84.25 hours was by a night nurse! The government can apply for deregulation in relation to hospitals but employees are to be given equivalent periods of compensatory rest or the appropriate protection.

Scope of Practice

Here in the UK the Expanded Scope of Practice provides a constant challenge to nurses and provides a formal framework in which many activities which have been custom and practice over the years can now be recognised.

Currently, the discussions considering nurse anaesthetists is based very much upon what happens in other countries. One hears the constant mutterings of colleagues: 'They do it in Sweden and other countries in Europe. Why not here?' It was interesting to listen to the chairman of the nurse anaesthetists of France recently (Maroudy, 1995), when he relayed to a meeting on European nursing that, for many years, any qualified nurse or midwife could administer an anaesthetic in France. Over the last few years formal training for that role has been approved and is now a requirement for the nurse anaesthetist.

Some recent articles in nursing journals and conference papers (Moore, 1996) have questioned whether the difficulty of such developments over here might simply be the inclusion of the word 'nurse' and suggest that we may need to move to a global term, something like 'health care professional' and erase the terms 'nurse' and 'doctor'. That, in itself, could provide an interesting discussion for the rest of the chapter. Orthopaedic assistants have existed for several years now. Many of those are nurses, yet no outcry has accompanied their participation in surgical activities. Is this because they are not using the term nurse assistant?

The profession across Europe

I am not sure that George Evers (1996), a Belgian Professor of Nursing Science, would receive total support for his recent classification of the perfect European. Nevertheless it makes interesting reading to hear of that person being:

> as humble as a Spaniard, as controlled as an Italian, cooking like a Brit, driving like a Frenchman, as organised as a Greek, sober as the Irish, humorous as a German, generous as a Dutchman, discrete as a Dane, famous as a Luxembourger, technical as a Portuguese and as available as a Belgian.

Aside from this light hearted appreciation of our individual characteristics there should be a recognition of the diverse backgrounds from which any European group of professionals arises and a need for acceptance of that fact when attempting to seek common understanding and agreement.

Few would dispute the acknowledged differences in health and social situations between those in eastern and those in western Europe. Across Europe there are increasing structural differences with high non-wage labour costs, disincentives to work and a lack of qualifications (Kunst & Mackenbach, 1994). As part of those differences nurses also receive varying levels of respect and autonomy and, until we can establish the value of nursing throughout Europe, we will have little chance of making any real headway in moving the profession forward. For example, in Portugal only 17% of the total figure of full time employees in hospital health care are registered nurses (Brett, 1997).

Within EORNA we are advised of the struggles operating room nurses are having to establish themselves as a profession there. At a recent meeting of the European group of operating room nurses, colleagues from Portugal formally requested the help of theatre nurses throughout Europe in combating an intention by hospital managers in Portugal to place two operating tables in each operating room so that two sets of surgery could be completed at the same time. Although EORNA carries no authorised responsibility or jurisdiction in such situations it was rewarding to see the idea was dropped following the receipt by the health managers of many letters from around Europe highlighting the dangers and implications of such action. It is a good example of what nurses can achieve when they unite with one voice.

In France, nursing costs comprise just 19% of the total hospital budget compared with our own high of 57%. Such discrepancies within nations have to be considered before we set unrealistic targets for the profession. Those of us who have established our credence must now help our colleagues obtain theirs, whilst at the same time looking to the place of nursing in the future.

The development of EORNA and the common core curriculum

The formation of the European Operating Room Nursing Association (EORNA) has, in itself, not been an easy development. Initially a small group of representatives from four countries met informally at theatre nursing conferences around the world. Gradually others joined this gathering until it established itself as a networking link group. As the developments of the new Europe took place the group recognised the likely impact of this new organisation and legislation upon nursing, and, therefore, agreed to formalise itself into a recognised group representing theatre nurses across Europe. With a membership of 15 countries, by this time it was one of the largest European groups outside of the Permanent Committee of Nurses (PCN). In restricting its membership to the national organisations representing perioperative nurses it was a truly distinctive organisation.

An initial sharing within the group of the current mode of delivery of health care and the state of nursing in countries throughout Europe revealed a long continuum running from low profile, low esteem areas such as Russia and some parts of Greece through to the higher status found in the northern parts and Scandinavia. Perioperative nurse education varied also from no training in southern and eastern parts across to the in-depth 3 or 5 years of some of the more northern territories. These programmes varied according to whether one did or did not have a previous nursing qualification or whether this needed to be built into the overall programme. With the prospect of free movement of persons, once the gates of Europe were thrown open wide, it was recognised that this could provide the opportunity to pursue recognition of perioperative nursing as an acknowledged career and to establish essential standards of care within the operating rooms throughout Europe.

The introduction of a common core curriculum for operating department nursing was seen as the way to encourage the introduction of training programmes in those countries which currently lacked any such provision. It was also hoped the programme itself would be seen as a theatre nurse's passport throughout Europe. The intention was that once all countries became familiar with the curriculum, managers who received applications from persons outside the host country who possessed the EORNA Certificate would instantly be aware of the educational programme undertaken by that individual. By applying the rules of the Directive, the manager would be able to establish whether the person was suitable for immediate employment within that individual country's criteria or whether they needed to sit an entrance test or undergo further education or experience to meet the requirements of the host country. In areas such as Spain and Portugal there are current discussions around the introduction of the curriculum, thus establishing for the first time the relevance of operating department nurses there.

The development of the EORNA curriculum is unique in that it has maintained full involvement of every member country at every stage of its progress. Similar programmes established for groups such as the cancer nurses have arisen from a small working group which alone has decided the programme and then simply presented it to the larger group for adoption. True, this is a much simpler approach, assuming you have a good working group which is truly representative of all countries but the advantage of the EORNA programme is that every member country can identify an area of the finalised document which contains their contribution. This gave value to the efforts of all participants, even those less well-developed in the field of operating room nursing. It has also brought a greater degree of understanding of the completed programme and an eagerness for its success. It would have been very easy to establish a working group from the very strong countries who at times tended to monopolise the debate and participation but by encouraging equal participation from all there is a common ownership of the project.

As a leader of that kind of working group one finds one's interpersonal skills stretched to the limit at times. You can feel the frustration of both those who wish to run on ahead and those who are struggling behind. The provision of a very accepting and safe environment in which all feel able to contribute is essential for this kind of group to succeed. The work is labour intensive and can appear unwieldy and never ending at times but the fruits are worth waiting for when you see the pride on the faces of all participants as the project is launched.

Specific areas of the curriculum presented considerable difficulty in reaching an agreement. Never underestimate the influence of culture, politics and language in such discussions. Major issues included the form and style of assessment and the minimum hours which should be stated for the programme. The issue of assessment became a problem because of the different interpretations and types of assessment in different countries and here language was a major agent. The question of minimum hours was difficult to decide because those countries who already possessed longer programmes were concerned that their own allotted times would be cut if a shorter time was allocated elsewhere, whereas those without any programmes were looking to a shorter time to support their introduction of education.

Throughout its development, two major issues have repeatedly reared their head during meetings of the group. The first is that of language. Although it was agreed early on that English would be the language of the organisation

Loan Receipt
Liverpool John Moores University
Library and Student Support

Borrower ID: 21111147178115
Loan Date: 06/11/2009
Loan Time: 11:06 am

Understanding perioperative nursing /
1111010457362

Due Date: 27/11/2009 23:59

Please keep your receipt
in case of dispute

items. In modern units the old-fashioned hopper or sluice does not always exist so it may be the staff toilet as the flushing mechanism or a difficult decision as to whom are we permitted to give those drugs. Are we a handler if we give them to the patient, a receiver if we keep them or are we breaking a confidentiality code by talking to the waiting policeman? It is at times such as this that the problem solving approach needs to take on a true team spirit.

Currently, although there are efforts to standardise products, there is very little attempt to come to an agreement regarding specific issues in health care and it is, therefore, important that nurses intending to work in other countries clarify the situation regarding difficult ethical issues within their own country. Two such issues relevant to perioperative nurses are organ donation and euthanasia. Here in the UK, we run a system of allowing people to opt into organ donation if they so wish whereas in Belgium the individual must state if they do NOT wish to have their organs donated. Theirs could, therefore, be considered as an opt out system. In Holland, the legal system is looking to accept euthanasia under special circumstances whilst here in the UK it is still taboo.

The agreement between the European Union and the World Health Organization on targets for health is heavily biased towards promotion of health and health education and could be argued to exclude perioperative nurses as an active group in achieving those targets. National targets have a similar slant. Are we, therefore, going to accept that health is only about prevention and promotion? Are there not going to be ill people as well in this new world – people who need our expertise to overcome current illness before they can consider how to become or remain healthy? Is there not an equally important need to emphasise areas such as early diagnostic procedures in which we can play a leading role and which will also have a radical impact upon health statistics? The oncology nurses have played an active role in bringing and keeping cancer in the forefront,yet are there special programmes for surgery against cancer? Where is the mention of the perioperative nurses in this field of care?

Day surgery is on the increase, so why are we not up there proposing and agreeing the way in which the future of day surgery should be established throughout Europe? As perioperative nurses we have continued to grumble and to resist what others are imposing upon us yet had we the forethought to anticipate future climates we could probably have decided a response to current needs which would have allowed us to set the ground rules.

For years nursing as a profession has been the subject of change by other people's decisions and wishes. Management function needs to return to those who do the caring. The first time round nurses were ill-prepared, but we have learned from our mistakes. There is now a wider field for us to impregnate if we wish to have some say in our future. The new Europe is still young and still growing and that means that, before it becomes firmly rooted in its traditions and controls, perioperative nurses need to stand up and be counted as a profession which knows where it is going.

From a variety of different human cultures we assemble as one nursing culture in which we all possess the same basic skills, who share the same knowledge and attitudes and use a common language centred around patients and caring. We are all concerned about skill mix and roles within the multidisciplinary team, about the constant apparent underfunding of our departments and about the legal and ethical challenges which surround us. Whatever else might vary, when nurses across the spectrum meet, our one common language and conversation unites us in an impassioned concern for the welfare of patients. Territorial cultures, languages and political influences can all be lost against the deep rooted culture of nursing which has no boundaries but unites individuals in the ultimate goal of appropriately equal health care for all. It is, nevertheless, important that within that exchange an atmosphere of reality is maintained. The saying is that the grass is always greener on the other side of the fence but perhaps that is because we often do not look down at our own feet at the grass upon which we are walking. We often neglect to identify what is good and profound about our own situation and slip into thinking that good news is no news, whereas the bad is always worthy of discussion. Objective evaluation sometimes needs to separate perfection of values and protocols from the reality of life. That is not to say we should give up aiming for our goals, but we should look carefully at what we realistically can achieve and select one or two areas at a time to work towards in the same way as we set our patients their short and long-term goals. We cannot conquer the world in a day but, like the slow and persistent tortoise, we can map out where we wish to go and set ourselves daily targets which all lead towards the final standard.

The future of nursing within Europe

With the integration of nurse education into higher education it was felt that nursing research would develop alongside traditional university research as nursing teachers would be required to fulfil that side of their role in the same way as other university lecturers. In real life, however, there needs to be considerable change in the mode of delivery of nursing courses if the true university philosophy is to be adopted as in other European countries.

There is a tendency to simply declare nurse education as part of a university yet retain the culture of a school of nursing. Managers, who are purchasers of nurse education, are showing how ill-prepared they are for this new system. Many still see nurse teachers as an extension of hospital life and require courses to be ongoing in a regular pattern which does not fit into an academic discipline. As nurses, we have a fixation regarding hours and content and fail to recognise other variables which can effect outcomes. Unlike several of our European colleagues, nurse teachers in the UK have failed to utilise university systems to secure the opportunities for academic freedom. In other territories, such as Scandinavia, we find our colleagues constantly pushing forward in nursing research, often utilising existing works but continuing to test those theories through application on a regular basis. Even during the Year of Lifelong Learning, European monies to promote liaison between countries (EC, 1995) were only partly utilised. The writer herself was host to 13 Finnish nursing students who spent 2 months at the local hospital earlier that year. Other ongoing exchange and joint educational programmes exist around the UK. The opportunities were there for the taking, and still are if you are prepared to make the effort.

A European Educational and Research Foundation will soon be available through EORNA, thanks again to our colleagues in industry. The First European Conference of Operating Room Nursing in Brussels in 1997 offered great opportunity to compare and contrast perioperative nursing across Europe. The attendance consisted of more than 2000 perioperative nurses with a further 500 being turned away. This emphasises the need for such activities.

For those countries developing educational programmes for the first time there is a great sense of achievement. Those of us who already have such programmes also need to be looking at future goals. Where do we want the profession to be in another 100 years? Must we wait for others to decide our fate? Bodies such as WHO are providing us with the necessary landmarks to help us find our way to developing a profession which will form a crucial part in the decision making process of future health care. A very apt statement from a Korean nurse, cited by Professor Alexander from WHO, says it all:

> There is nothing around us to reverse the direction of development and change ... thus we are posed with the question of being master of these changes or their servant. Whether we can adequately meet this challenge depends upon our own ability.
>
> Kim (WHO, 1995).

Our profession has a long-standing history of nursing cooperation across borders and boundaries. We need to keep this tradition and to show that whatever the future of our continent, nurses and nursing need to be at the forefront in strategy planning and implementation. As perioperative nurses, what do you do across Europe that only you can do in the manner that requires your special expertise? Who else is made aware of that fact? The Permanent Committee of Nursing (PCN) has recognised that, if it is to be the truly representative voice of nursing when it approaches the European Commission, it must embrace all the new nursing specialist groups which have sprung up across Europe. It now invites representatives of those groups to come together with PCN twice a year. It has also invited one member of the International Committee of Nursing (ICN) to be present as an observer to maintain links with that group. This larger group is currently developing a strategic plan to ensure it has access to the ears of the Commission and secures participation in all future discussions on areas likely to affect nursing. Their activities do not absolve us as individuals of the responsibility for furthering the development of our own specialty.

While there are countries in which postregistration education is not considered essential for nurses, we will be limited in our efforts to gain recognition of specialist nursing roles. Those of us who have already demonstrated the benefits of an educated workforce need to look at how we can help our colleagues in poorer areas to gain that acknowledgement also.

The European Union recognises that more countries will be seeking integration in the coming years and accepts that the influence of those countries may well affect the rate of economic development proposed for the future. They acknowledge that the establishment of a strong political identity with a firm policy is essential to maintain the intended programme.

Nursing should be looking at establishing a similar positive target of achievement for the future of our profession. Our approach needs to be three-dimensional. Firstly, we need to maintain recognition of the role and requirements of the specialist nurses in practice in our own country and anticipate their needs for the future in line with developments within health care delivery. Secondly, we need to offer necessary support and guidance to colleagues in countries where nursing is in the earlier stages of development. A cautious note here – in offering that help we must not seek to impose our standards and criteria upon a culture whose systems are not conducive to working within our kind of framework. Our help should consist in providing guidance when requested and in seeking ways in which to help the natural residents to identify approaches which would be appropriate for their own development. That is very different from imposing a 'We know best – you should do it this way' approach which is likely to fail due to its unrealistic focus within a differing health care delivery system.

Thirdly, our approach needs to be as a united perioperative nursing voice across Europe. This will be both as a specialist group which has developed a broader understanding of the needs of all its individual members and as a combined voice across the whole sphere of nursing. It is not sufficient to leave this responsibility to the ranks of a group of senior nurses who may well have moved far away from the clinical delivery of care. As current practitioners, we need to use both local groups and national forums to voice our ideas and concerns. Nurses in the UK have repeatedly been urged at conferences to become political and target national parliamentary members in order to influence health care (Moore, 1996). This need is now even greater and our targeting must also include those European ministers who represent us within the Commission. Whilst the European Union is still in its infancy we must make sure that nursing is firmly embedded in its policies and that nurses themselves are part of the discussions from which these policies arise. The development of the European Union has provided a golden opportunity for nurses to step forward and contribute first hand to the development of nursing throughout that Union. Failure to do so can only be attributed to lack of professional responsibility on the part of all of us who are practising nurses.

Reflective activities

1 Has this chapter given you new understanding of how international contacts between groups of nurses can throw new light onto changes in society, in health care and in nursing and suggested new ways in which change can be addressed?

2 Can international groupings of professionals such as perioperative nurses help them to exert their influence at a political level?

3 Reflect on whether nursing has the same skills, knowledge and attitudes wherever it is practised.

4 Have you seen the European common core curriculum? Does the training that you received meet the demands of the common core curriculum? How can you relate this common core to the nurse education and the training to work in theatres currently being received by the nurses working in your operating department?

5 Are you a member of a professional nursing organisation? If you are, what do you give to it and what benefits do you receive? If not, reflect on the advantages to you and to your profession of such organisations.

References

Baly, M. 1995 *Nursing and social change.* London, Routledge.

Bivand, P. 1994 *Nurses' shifts and the European directive on working time.* Euroforum, Spring No.1.

Brett, M. 1996 *European common core curriculum for operating department nursing.* European Operating Room Nurses' Association.

Brett, M. 1997 The European influence. *British Journal Theatre Nursing,* February.

Dolan, J. 1968 *History of nursing.* London: WB Saunders.

English National Board. 1995 *Information for nurses and midwives qualified overseas.* London, ENB Leaflet OQN/NOV.

European Commission. 1993 *The European directive on working time.* Council Directive, 93/104/EC. Brussels, EC.

European Commission. 1995 *Decision of the European Parliament and of the Council establishing the community action programme Socrates.* Brussels, EC.

European Commission. 1996 *Report to the European Parliament and the Council on the state of the application of the general system for the recognition of higher education diplomas.* Brussels, EC.

European Parliament. 1996 Green light for driving license. *EP News,* June.

Evers, G. 1996 *The future role of nurses and nursing within the European Union.* Unpublished Conference Paper.

Kunst, A.E. & Mackenbach, J.P. 1994 *Measuring socioeconomic inequalities in health.* Copenhagen, WHO Regional Office for Europe.

Maroudy, D. 1995 *The nurse anaesthetist in France. Development, preparation and current practice.* Masterclass on Europe Paper.

Medical Devices Directorate. 1992 The CE marking. *Directives Bulletin,* July.

Moore, Y. 1996 A Strategy for Operating Department Nursing. *British Journal Theatre Nursing,* December.

Pritchard, P. 1995 *The European Union structures, processes and opportunities for nursing.* Masterclass on Europe, unpublished paper.

Richards, T. 1992 *Medicine in Europe.* London, British Medical Journal Publishers.

Skeet, M. 1980 *Florence Nightingale's notes on nursing.* Edinburgh, Churchill Livingstone.

United Kingdom Central Council. 1995 *Statistical analysis of the Council's Professional Register.* April 1994–March 1995.

Wallace, M. 1995 *European Directives: what they mean for us.* Masterclass on Europe, unpublished paper.

World Health Organization. 1995 *The World Health Report: Bridging the gaps.* Geneva, Report of the Director-General WHO.

Further reading

The following booklet is available from the European Commission offices and provides a very simple outline to the European Union and its legislation and organisation.

Weidenfeld, W. & Wessels, W. 1997 Europe from A–Z: a guide to European integration. ISBN 92–827–9419–9.

PART THREE

Management issues

Leadership for theatre managers

7

Libby Campbell

This chapter has been written by a nurse manager who has a very special interest, not only in nurse management but in leadership and nurse leadership in particular. Libby Campbell has spoken on the topic at theatre nursing conferences around the world. She has a particular interest in aspects of leadership concerned with personal and professional empowerment. She also places the issue of leadership into a broader background than merely considering the management of operating departments.

As a true nursing leader, in a nursing speciality and as a national leader in her own country of Scotland Libby Campbell's comments reflect her own distinctive views on management and leadership. Whilst repeating some of the messages of management training and education, this chapter should be read as a commentary on how effective leaders incorporate management techniques into their own leadership strategies. It is a broad ranging essay which also considers how nursing leaders have to operate within the political and organisational processes and structures of the health services. This was actually written at a time when a change of government was expected to change the political perspective from a business approach to health care, utilising an internal market with purchasers and providers, to a more people-centred ethic.

Introduction

> If you ask me what I have come to do in this world ... I will reply: I am
> here to live my life out loud.
>
> Zola (1997).

In the UK, there have been many books and articles written about leadership;
some about individual leaders and their attributes (Adair, 1989; Crainer, 1996;
Gardner, 1996) and some about the applications of theory to practice (Bennis &
Townsend, 1995; Mant, 1983; Tappen, 1989). There are probably even more
books about management and the various theories to augment that practice.
Indeed, throughout the world the number will be considerable, particularly in
the USA where leadership and management theories emerge frequently and
often with sophisticated marketing. Many of these will concentrate on the
management of businesses and people will transfer appropriate theories to try
to make sense of their own situation.

Recently, there has been a bit of a sea-change and books on management are
emerging that recognise the complexity of some organisations, and the needs
of the people who work in them (Carnegie, 1993; Handy, 1994; Paulson, 1991).
Mind you, there are even more books that seem to depend less on theoretical
and logical argument than on fantastic marketing skills. Even I was persuaded
to buy the latest management 'guru' diatribe and regretted the departing of the
£20, whilst recognising the excellence of the marketing strategy. And, of course,
there is always the possibility that there might be the odd helpful phrase ...

The plethora of books and theoretic output doesn't always provide too much
help to health care organisations, however, partly because these organisations
are usually very complex and, although some business organisations are big,
they are not usually as complex as health care 'families'. Recently, there have
been more articles about leadership in nursing although there are few on leadership within operating theatre practice or perioperative nursing. To be fair, the
principles of leadership are universal, but there is something about the challenges and opportunities offered within operating theatre nursing that
warrant attention. It is often only when one has left the operating theatre environment that one realises what special challenges and opportunities are
offered there. Without specific attention, and even with it, knowledge about
leadership within perioperative nursing may depend upon exposure to individuals, locally or nationally, who have influenced one's life, one's practice or
one's view of the future.

How many of these influencers are nurses and how many are doctors or
managers? Actually, I have no view about whether there should or shouldn't
be other clinicians or other managers but I do despair about the number of
speakers at conferences who are invited simply because they are doctors or
senior managers as opposed to being asked because they have something to
offer intelligent minds.

Nurses are as likely to be influenced by dysfunctional leadership as by good
practice and they will recognise lack of leadership as much as good leadership.
They will have a view on positional leaders as opposed to charismatic leaders

and they will have a view on everything these individuals do, whether or not they have the facts.

Now, I've written several paragraphs without too much supporting data and I have given you the benefit of my opinion, with which you may or may not agree, but that is what this chapter is all about. You can read as much as you like in the journals and in well-advertised 'guru' books but you and I know that the way that we view leaders is as much to do with the way we see things as the way that people fit into a theory or meet the criteria laid down for a so-called good leader.

We do not see things as they are; we see them as we are.

All of that said, there are ways in which one can recognise the likelihood of someone developing well as a leader and it is those coming forward now that must be nurtured and educated to lead in the future.

There are different levels at which leadership can be exercised and the effect will be greater on others depending upon the level within the organisation. For example, the nurse who leads the patient through uncharted territory such as a surgical procedure under local anaesthetic will have tremendous influence over the patient during that period of care. A wrong word or a missed opportunity can change an anxious moment into a terrifying experience and so it is extremely important to get it right. The effect on others will not necessarily be as great as might be in other circumstances, but that is a matter of scope rather than importance. On the other hand, to lead through a development of professional practice, such as the introduction of the role of surgeon's assistant, will have a wide-ranging effect upon many others within the organisation and possibly even within other organisations.

Maybe the NHS is not the place to nurture leaders as it is so hard to be entrepreneurial in such a complex environment. Indeed, the recent views within the White Paper (NHS in Scotland, 1997) indicate a more centralist approach despite this government's objective to remove the internal market. I have the greatest admiration for the nurse managers of today who work to deliver effective services in the most demanding of situations. It is said that 'If you can manage in the NHS, you can manage anywhere'. With the clear intention to introduce 'clinical governance', individual clinical staff are set to become more influential in decision-making within Trusts.

We need a vision though; there is clearly no point in developing leaders if there is nowhere for them to lead. I read a quote in that respect; a poem by Roger McGough, called 'The Leader':

> I wanna be the leader
> I wanna be the leader
> Can I be the leader?
> Can I? I can?
> Yippee, I'm the leader
> OK, what shall we do?

I do realise that there are still those people in positions of leadership who do not have the right skills and who should probably not be encouraged. I refer, occasionally, to the fact that 'the scum also rises' and read an interesting book on the subject (Mant, 1983). The dilemma is to encourage the one and to offer alternatives to the other.

So, from all of this pontificating, the main themes of this chapter will be those that have emerged over a number of years both by being led and from trying to lead others through such an extremely complex organisation, the National Health Service within the UK. I will promote a number of hypotheses and attempt to support them with some evidence, even if it is only anecdotal. After all, is not the management guru stuff similarly drawn together?

1 Leaders and leadership – so what is it all about?

2 Roles and modelling – or lead by example but don't do everything yourself.

3 Chance and challenges – or take those opportunities.

4 Verve and versatility – action must change within different situations and probably all at the same time.

5 Clues and credibility – have knowledge and plenty of credibility.

6 Communication – communicate, communicate and communicate.

7 Sense and sensitivity – but be selective about taking advice.

8 Decision-making – I think – therefore I am.

9 Values.

10 How do you know – or tools and measurability.

Leaders and leadership

> A leader has to be one of two things: he either has to be a brilliant visionary himself, a truly creative strategist, in which case he can do what he likes and get away with it; or else she has to be a true entrepreneur, who can bring out the best in others.
>
> Mintzberg (1997).

This section is about what leadership is and how it is described. As is the way with such things, it is generally easier to describe what it is not or when it is absent than when it is present. However, it is important to describe what effective leaders do and what leadership is, especially when it comes to recognising the emerging leader so that they may be encouraged and developed.

Leadership is not management, although that is part of leadership as some of the skills are relevant but some people simply do not have the 'extras' that make the successful leader. They do not change opinion, influence values, stop and make you think or make you listen, or light a spark. They are more likely to control; to stop rather than make you stop and think.

Leadership doesn't have an end point which, once reached, means that you can say you've achieved it. There are leadership styles, of course, and people describe these.

Equally, I'm not sure that you can describe a model and then expect it to just happen. There are many, many books about the subject (Adair, Mant, Carnegie, Handy, Tappen) indeed, every book about leadership will list qualities or explore behaviours and the impact of those behaviours on others. I have picked out a number of issues for this chapter that I believe are important when considering the future of leadership in the NHS.

I believe that effective leadership depends upon a combination of individual qualities (characteristics), along with developed skills (competencies) and experience (confidence) within a context and a time framework.

Characteristics

The characteristics are the personal qualities that can be recognised by others, the 'what I am' traits that are sometimes perceived to be innate. They are, in no particular order of importance:

- Personal values – these are covered in more detail later in the chapter but an effective leader's values will be those which inspire trust and will be consistent.
- Sensitivity – effective leaders are sensitive to others' needs and to how individuals will be affected.
- Intelligence – people who have been successful have usually been intelligent and people of wit and intuition.
- Interpersonal skills – effective leaders are said to have excellent interpersonal skills and have a questioning and direct open-minded attitude.
- Enthusiasm – effective leaders have enthusiasm for whatever they are doing and have the energy to persevere towards what they want with exceptional tenacity.
- Decisiveness – effective leaders are usually found to be assertive and action-orientated.

Competencies

The areas of competence which I have identified are the skills or tasks in which the effective leader is competent. The 'what I do well' attributes which can be taught and which can develop over time. These areas are covered in detail later in the chapter.

- Communication – it does help if the leader already has good communication skills to build on but development is always possible with articulateness, listening skills, receiving communication feedback, presentation skills and in areas of networking with others.
- Thinking – I perceive the thinking skills to be on three levels; problem solving or 'decision thinking', policy and planning or 'critical thinking' and

vision or 'innovative thinking'. In addition, effective leaders recognise the possibilities of linkages between thinking skills to develop strategies.

- Knowledge – a sound knowledge of the theories of management and leadership is important. Change management, goal setting, motivational studies, public relations and teamwork are all noted but there are many others. Equally important is a sound professional knowledge or credibility and this includes areas such as development of one's own area of practice; clinical, educational, managerial or leadership.

Confidence

Effective leaders always take every opportunity to develop themselves and learn a great deal from every leadership experience. It is not related to length of time in an area of practice but is about meeting challenges, maturity and personal growth; the 'what I have learnt' aspects of leadership that help to build confidence.

- Adaptability – leaders are at ease in different situations and have become versatile. They will have developed strategies to cope with various contexts and will use a combination of strategies as the occasion demands.
- Resilience – effective leaders cope well with challenges, learn to overcome setbacks and cope well with stressful situations.
- Recognition – the effective leader will learn to recognise when it is sensible to take advice and when it is wiser to ignore it or when it is time to stop arguing and to move on.
- Persuasion – effective leaders usually have confidence in their power of persuasion; of making effective arguments and they will have the will to influence others.
- Awareness – effective leaders will be aware of alternative options and possibilities and will have the ability to predict the effect of policy.
- Self-awareness – leaders also need to develop a sense of self-awareness in order to recognise their strengths and development needs.

Context and time frame

There is a fourth aspect which is relevant and that is a combination of context issues and getting one's timing right. In terms of context, effective leadership needs a combination of qualities such as those described above, but it needs to take place in an acceptable emotional context and organisational context.

- Emotional context – this refers to the environment which might be calm or busy and which will influence the effect of the skills brought to play in the situation which might be an environment of conflict which will also necessitate the use of appropriate strategies.
- Organisational context – the values or common purpose of the organisation in which the leader works will have a fundamental effect and the organisation's encouragement of education or development of emergent leaders will be important issues for the leader.

The fifth dimension

At the risk of sounding daft, the fifth dimension is to me the thing that sets people apart; the behaviours that stamp people as effective or emergent leaders. These behaviours are usually described with action verbs so I see these behaviours manifest in the person who:

- initiates action
- confronts problems
- enables and facilitates
- analyses and evaluates
- mobilises support
- plans and organises
- takes risks
- inspires others
- attracts respect
- recognises others.

It is a combination, then, of characteristics, competencies and confidence within a context and time framework but with the fifth dimension – that 'sets people apart'.

> You see things; and you say 'why'. But I dream things that never were; and I say 'why not?'

George Bernard Shaw,
in *Back to Methuselah*, Part 1, Act 1(1921).

There are views about how one can acquire some of these qualities or skills and a fairly well-accepted, if somewhat cynical view is that it is 60% image, 30% exposure and 10% ability. I don't know if that concept has been examined, but for theatre nurses it is quite an interesting prospect.

Image can be difficult if people still see them in the handmaiden image, and perception of nurses in theatre is an interesting phenomenon. Theatre nurses are frequently, and quite rightly, accused of remaining behind the theatre doors at all costs and if they are not exposed to other areas, and the staff from other areas do not meet them, views will not change. Take the risk and get out there to accept the challenges and opportunities of change. Ability is only apparently required to be 10%, although I question that, but if you don't have credibility, you'll soon be found out.

So how do you start?

Roles and modelling

> If the best of me can make more of you
> then the best of you will reflect on me.

Josefowitz (1983).

Most people have role models of one sort or another; people they want to emulate as well as people whose attributes they will make it their life's ambition to avoid. In nursing there will always be those practitioners who elicit admiration and those who do quite the opposite. They will be your role models and you will, maybe even unconsciously, mould yourself on their behaviour.

Some talk of having 'heroes' although I have some difficulty with that expression since most heroes have turned out to have 'feet of clay'. Actually, I'm quite happy that that is the case as we, mere mortals, have a fighting chance of succeeding ourselves. I prefer the thought that we admire people when they act heroically or whose behaviour is to be admired.

I found a quote some years ago that epitomises my thoughts:

> Our lack of heroes is an indication of the maturity of our age. A realisation that every man has come into his own and has the capacity of making a success out of his life. Of being able to say, 'I have found my hero, and he is me.'
>
> Dr G. Sheenan.

So be realistic and don't expect too much of your mentors, preceptors, role models or heroes.

What is a slightly more terrifying thought is that you might well be a role model for someone else without even realising it. In fact, it's not usually a choice, as people regard you as a role model whether you like it or not. Beware, it could just as easily be as a poor example as a good role model. My, what a responsibility!

Having been around for as long as I have, I am occasionally reminded that the reason someone took up nursing, or became registered and took their district nurse training, was the result of something I said about 20 years ago. No doubt there is a balance of people at the other end of the continuum, but it's very good to see protégés or people in whose development you have played a part, do well. So be generous to others and give them every chance and opportunity to develop.

Find a role model

For the emergent leader, it is important to find a role model. It is always interesting to think about what aspects of the role model it is that you admire or recognise. That will be important as you try to develop skills in that direction but be careful that you appreciate all aspects of the admirable quality. It is fine to be articulate and persuasive but if it takes excessive preparation or it is so stressful that it's debilitating, it may just not be worth it.

Do remember though that you will never be that person you so admire; people frequently say that they would like to be that other person but it is neither possible nor advisable. You can develop some of the skills though, and rather than learn to be them, you can learn to be you, but better. Leading by example takes some attention as the standards demanded are high.

Delegation

Whilst you are leading by example, though, it is not a requirement that you do everything yourself so you need to delegate. Is there someone to whom to delegate? There usually is. Take a chance with people you normally make an exception. Obviously, it has to be in a carefully considered situation, but you may be surprised and will often boost the other person's confidence. They may blossom and then they are on the 'can be approached again' list.

I have always tried to follow the principle that I should only really ask people to do the things that I have done myself. Clearly, there are notable exceptions where the opportunities were not available, but there has probably been a similar situation. I did not have the opportunity to develop my clinical practice into administration of intravenous drugs or defibrillation for example, but I do know about accountability for my own clinical practice, whatever the procedure, and how it feels when that accountability is tested.

There was a television programme recently about a chief executive being a nursing auxiliary for a week, which was similar to many programmes where an individual swaps jobs with another. Many people commented to me about how good it was for a chief executive to be a nursing auxiliary to see what it was like. I thought their comments quite interesting because, of course, all senior nurses have done that sort of thing in the past, and so it is not unusual for them to appreciate the realities of ward life. Other senior colleagues have not normally had that experience, and it was interesting to see that they learnt so much from the exercise. Unfortunately, being a nursing auxiliary is inevitably task-oriented and nursing is not, so it wouldn't do for people to think that one aspect covers all situations. Then, of course, it is not exactly a swap unless the nursing auxiliary becomes a chief executive for a week ... now that would really be interesting!

You cannot do everything yourself; you will almost certainly not have the time; you are unlikely to have the energy required to do it all well; you are equally unlikely to be good at everything and it probably creates too much stress and pressure. If you are not to do everything yourself then you have to learn to prioritise what it is important to do, what it is important to do yourself, what it is appropriate to delegate and what is not important. Then you have to learn to say 'No' occasionally.

Chances and challenges

> You can't do anything about the length of your life, but you can do something about its width and depth.
>
> Esar, in Weber (1991).

If asked, I'll admit that one of my greatest weaknesses is an inability to say 'No'. Clearly, there are exceptions but when it comes to accepting various commissions such as those of speaking, writing and so on, I seem unable to set aside the opportunity. It can be tough but the rewards are incalculable and the experience is incredible. It is also undeniable logic that one simply can't do everything. For everything you do, there is something that you don't do. So choose your opportunities carefully.

Be careful about getting everything you want, you might just get it and it doesn't always bring the best of everything with it. You can get everything you want so be careful about what you want. One of the interesting things about writing so much down is that you write what you know to be the case and you realise that you have rarely followed it throughout your life.

So learn to take the opportunities – I have learnt many things that way. Examples include a momentous decision when I became a nursing officer many years ago and I was given the opportunity to cover the hospital in addition to my management of theatre areas and I decided to do so. It was the experience that led me to more senior management with a much wider experience than I would otherwise have had if I had only covered the theatre areas.

I also took the opportunity to join the Editorial Board of the *British Journal of Theatre Nursing*, the journal of the National Association of Theatre Nurses, and that led not only to my learning a great deal but also to becoming National Chairman in due course.

So take opportunities – create them if you can but take them when they happen. This, at the very least, requires energy so don't tackle the things for which you have no enthusiasm.

Which leads us to versatility.

Verve and versatility

Masters of change do three things right – they sense the right moment to initiate the plan, they find supporters for their ideas and they have vision.

Bruning (1993).

Unless you have been hiding away for a while, you will know that change is all around. Actually, if you have been away for a while you are in for quite a shock. For those people who may not believe how much has changed, or worse, those who hope that it will all go away and stop bothering them, you need only think about what nursing was like when you began your training compared with now. Equipment in theatre, for example, has developed beyond measure and some of what can now be achieved could not have been envisaged over 20 years ago, or whenever.

Dynamism and change is the life-blood of influence and development but it needs to be planned change, or we will merely be affected by it and not in control of it. Some of the uncontrolled change is inevitable and we cannot control everything so we need to plan as far as is possible, to be as adaptable as possible in order to cope with the rest.

Adaptability

I believe that nurses are particularly adaptable and have continued to develop practice to meet patients' needs. Kane (1992) talks about the range of skills that nurses have:

The ability to remove obstacles, manage dwindling resources and provide vision while empowering staff requires the skills of a juggler, diplomat and clairvoyant.

I have found that the emergent leaders who succeed are those who can adapt well and who are able to manage a number of different projects, can think on different levels, take on new ideas and challenges without being overwhelmed and without returning to their comfort zones too often. I frequently advise people to have strings to their bow to add to their expertise to prepare them better for each new situation.

Coping mechanisms

Alvin Toffler wrote about the shock to the system of immense change as:

> 'Future shock' … the shattering stress and disorientation that we induce in individuals by subjecting them to too much change in too short a time.
> Toffler (1970).

People need coping mechanisms and they need them as much in health care situations as in every part of their lives. Some people love the buzz and one may find that they change jobs frequently to get a new perspective on the work. That is different, of course, from those who do so in order to avoid dealing with the results of their tenure. It is not a requirement to change everything all the time and many would prefer to see a change from the 'disposable society' to a more stable environment.

You may have heard of the Holmes & Rahe Stress Scale (1967) which lists events, such as family changes, work changes and domestic changes, and attaches a stress value score against each event. The score of events which have occurred over a short time are added together to reach the total. Studies have shown that people who have accumulated more than 200 points in a year have a higher risk of physical or psychological stress-related illnesses. Occupational health staff will tell you that even greater numbers of health care workers now report with stress-related illnesses and, although not all will be a result of work stress, the pressure under which people are working must contribute.

Leaders need to know how to cope with stress themselves and how to help others cope.

Some current changes

We are in the midst of changes that will emerge following discussions about the change to Trusts following the White Paper *Designed to Care* published in December 1997 (NHS in Scotland, 1997). There were different papers in separate UK countries and I am only really familiar with the thoughts in the Scottish Paper. But whichever paper you require to follow, there will be changes. I plan to make sure that people understand the implications of various challenges and opportunities and I plan to influence potential moves for better patient-care and for better nurse-care, but I have no doubt that not every nuance of change will be acceptable and I know I will have to ensure that poor outcome or poor effect on patients and staff is minimised.

We educate the preregistration students so that they can deliver care in any environment; we are currently educating or even re-educating postregistration staff to deliver care in any environment; so as leaders we must prepare ourselves to lead in any environment and do it well in any environment. As long as you have all the other skills, it should not matter where you are functioning only that you are functioning well in a supported environment.

> Wise statesmen are those who foresee what changes time is bringing, and try to shape institutions and to mould men's thoughts and purpose, in accordance with the changes that are silently surrounding them.
>
> Morley, in Margach (1979).

Clues and credibility

> If you think education is expensive – try ignorance.
>
> Derek Bok, President, Harvard University.

The leader has to have a sound knowledge base and the eagerness to extend and develop it, but knowledge and education is more than the acquisition of facts. It is about how to apply learning and how to build on what is already learnt to develop in the current context. It is about opening your mind and using your knowledge wisely. It may even be about unlearning aspects of what you have already learnt in order to re-learn some new ideas.

> The illiterate of the future are not those who cannot read or write but those who cannot learn, unlearn and relearn.
>
> Toffler (1970).

Clinical knowledge

Clinical knowledge is a desirable attribute, particularly in the current NHS environment where 'clinical governance' is a focus for many current strategies. The White Papers published by the UK government in December 1997 set out the agenda for health for the next few years. The input from clinical staff, crucial to achieve the aims of this government, has been recognised and tremendous opportunities are offered for clinical leaders. As some have wryly remarked the need is for 'white coats rather than grey suits'.

This is also a challenge for senior nurses, especially executive nursing directors, as with fewer Trusts there will be fewer executive nurses at the Trust Boards. Clinical governance, however, is not all about doctors or about executive nurses. People with a clinical background, at whatever level of the NHS, will have the opportunity to contribute to the future shape of patient-focused health care.

Few senior nurse managers and even fewer executive nurses are likely to be in post without at least a degree and all are likely to have considerable education and experience in management. In a recent survey reported by the Royal College of Nursing (RCN) in the UK (1998) 71% of 238 nurse executives in England had a diploma or above, of whom 37% had a Master's degree or a Doctorate (Girvan, 1998). Education programmes have been of mixed value over the developing years of nurse management, but the experience that nurses have had in the practical application of management and leadership is both invaluable and, in my view, exceeds that of non-nurse managers. However, all nurse executives have to meet both clinical and managerial, if not leadership, requirements.

Credibility

All of this knowledge, whether academic or acquired, is useless if you don't know what to do with it. All of the other qualities, skills or attributes have to work in concert with the theory in order to succeed either as an effective manager or successful leader. The thing that sets you apart is not just the applied theory but the credibility. Credibility can be personal, professional and/or managerial and concerns image, visibility and networking.

Communication

> I know you think you understand what you thought I said, but I am not sure what you heard is what I thought I meant.

Effective communication is to a leader what sunshine is to a plant. Neither can succeed or grow well without it, and illumination is involved with both. Some will adapt to cope with lack of it, but few of either will flourish. Communication issues are mentioned in every list of attributes that good leaders have. It is identified as one of the fundamental skills to be acquired and the behaviour of effective leaders is manifest in excellent communication.

What is meant by effective communication?

There are libraries full of books that describe effective communication and, certainly, all of the books on leadership and management will have a chapter dedicated to it. It is a complex business, as we all know in everyday life, and is littered with misunderstandings and mistakes. Nevertheless there are 'top tips' for emergent leaders to consider.

First, however, the basics. In every communication exchange there will be a sender, a receiver and a message to be sent. It is, rarely, a one-way exchange, it will be between at least two people and the interaction between the sender and receiver is crucial. There is, often, what is called 'communication noise' which interrupts or otherwise affects the exchange. That can be caused by the environment, by perceptions and by the experience of those involved in the exchange or by verbal and non-verbal messages.

Even within the exchange itself, there are said to be two aspects to consider (Watzlawick et al., 1967); 'content', or the explicit aspect of the message, and the aspect of 'metacommunication' which I take to be the messages that are 'written between the lines' as it were.

Communication is a complex business and, in order to be effective, it is important to establish that the message is not only effectively imparted or sent but that it is understood. Hence, the opening quote which introduces the concept of feedback in effective communication.

Communication is the life-blood of nursing and is, actually, something we do effectively in clinical practice most of the time. There are some notable exceptions and in the operating theatre, there are some interesting, special challenges to effective communication so it is always worth thinking about carefully.

Verbal communication

Speaking is fraught with difficulty; you may be someone who speaks a lot or you may be someone who hears a lot, but you will have views about how it is all said. You will know that quantity does not guarantee quality of content; you will know that the use of fashionable, jargon words often indicates more arrogance than accuracy and you will know that frequently used expressions or 'ums' and 'ers' cause more counting than concentration.

Words are still fascinating, though. The way that they develop, especially within health care, and the way that people use them fascinates me. After all, language is really only a series of grunts developed by common consent to have meaning attached (Pluckhan, 1978).

It can also be quite amusing and Bill Bryson (1997) in his wonderful book *Mother Tongue* quotes many examples of the pitfalls of English. He highlights the plight of foreigners learning English who, for example, have to tackle the number of different meanings for one word. One example he gives is the word 'fly' which can mean '… an annoying insect, a means of travel, and a critical part of a gentleman's apparel …', clearly asking for trouble. He notes, too, that in English when a person says to you, 'How do you do?' he will be taken aback if you reply, with impeccable logic, 'How do I do what?' The whole book is an amusing treatise on the development and current use of English and includes, of course, comment on the use of jargon and waffle.

The NHS is full of jargon and waffle especially when it comes to 'management-speak' and for the leader to be effective, they must not only recognise the rubbish but develop an effective style of their own. Equally, many nurses are either managing services as well as, or working with, non-nurse managers and it is important to understand the meaning of the language that is used. So whether you are working with management, carrying out management tasks or developing leadership skills from a sound management focus, it is sensible to try to recognise how it is used.

In an article (Hewison, 1997) in which the challenges of management language are explored, perceptions of nurses about its use are noted. One study (Goodall, 1993) found the belief that managers used language '… as a weapon to confuse and suffocate nurses and that the "soggy verbiage" they employ reflects the transition from a concern of caring to one of business.'

That said, part of the problem is that nurses have not articulated well what is described as the 'emotional labour of nursing' (Smith, 1992). It certainly is difficult to reduce the complexity of care into 'management-speak' but perhaps that is another clue to the need for 'translators' in the nursing leadership port-folio; to translate for managers. You are probably saying that it should all be made simpler and that managers should get to know 'care-speak' and effective leaders do succeed in doing that to a degree. I do believe, however, that that position will change with this notion of 'clinical governance' and effective translators will come into their own.

Volume, tone of voice and rate of speaking also affect meaning and we can all think of examples when these non-language aspects of speech affect the perceptions of meaning: whispering is unlikely to attract attention; when people say 'I believe you' when they quite obviously don't or when people speak so slowly, or with huge pauses, that you have long since forgotten what was at the beginning of the sentence by the end of it. People bring their own perceptions to bear by using particular words, either consciously or uncon-sciously and it is interesting to consider why they are using one word or phrase as opposed to another, for example, 'leadership' when they mean 'management', 'patient' when they might have used 'client', 'business-speak' when they might have used 'care-speak' and so on.

Tappen quotes Mehrabian (1971) who found that facial expression had the greatest impact (55%) and tone of voice second (38%). The actual words used had a surprisingly weak effect (7%) unless backed up with appropriate and confirming facial expressions. There needs, therefore, to be congruency between your verbal and non-verbal messages.

Non-verbal communication

Even if you are using words or pictures to convey meaning, you will also be giving off non-verbal messages. Just being somewhere or with someone will be giving off a message. Design consultants know this well and, for every colour used or logo designed, there will be a message along with it. Not everyone sees colours in the same way (not everyone even spells colours the same way!) but it is generally reckoned that red is associated with risk, yellow is thought of as cheerful, green refreshing and blue, cool. Most food labels are red if they are meant at some point to be hot and green if they are vegetables or meant to be fresh. It is thought that at least 80% of communication is non-verbal so it is worth thinking about the impressions you are making. It is less easily controlled than verbal communi-cation, however, and you know when you think people are not telling the truth.

No mortal can keep a secret. If his lips are silent, he chatters with his fingertips ... betrayal oozes out of him at every pore.

Freud.

I am sure it is not quite as easy to recognise as that, otherwise how would actors be convincing, but for the majority of communication relationships it is true.

Other aspects of non-verbal communication that are of interest to theatre nurses are those described by Argyle (1972) as bodily contact, proximity, orientation, appearance, posture, head-nods, facial expressions, gestures, looking and non-verbal aspects of speech. Proximity of people around the operating table, for example, is close whether one prefers that proximity or not. The angle at which people stand around the table is not usually one of choice, but determined by roles and the interrelationships thus affected. Facial expressions are limited by masks if they are worn and looking becomes one of the most effective ways in which people in theatres communicate. Fascinating stuff to consider, especially if a leader is to be sensitive to what is happening.

Noise

Clearly the environment must be suitable for good communication; not only the lack of decibels so that people can speak and hear, but making sure they feel comfortable about doing so. Privacy might be important to them and people need help if they are nervous. Be careful about interpretation as you could be wrong, so check your perceptions to avoid misunderstanding. You would think that the more often you communicate with specific people the less the possibility of misinterpretation, but it is wise not to assume that. Individuals change and develop so check your perceptions from time to time.

Listening

Paying attention or listening to the entire process is so important; it will give you feedback on how you are being understood and, if you really listen, people will tell you what they need from you. It is not merely waiting for a moment to butt in.

> Listening does not mean simply maintaining a polite silence while you are rehearsing in your mind the speech you are going to make the next time you can grab a conversational opening.
>
> Hayakawa.

You should try something we had to try at a leadership session and you'll see how hard it is to listen without interrupting. Someone is asked to speak about a problem that they have and they are to talk about it for 10 minutes without interruption from anyone. By the time they have finished, they have probably solved the problem as they have had the time to talk the problem through. You on the other hand have probably found that you have a problem in that you found not interrupting extremely difficult.

People just coming into a new environment, whether a new position of leadership or a new place, often have problems with attention as they are overcome by the situation; either by the people, the event or the surroundings. It is important to minimise the effect of that and as you grow in skills you learn the little tricks to overcome it all more quickly.

- You might arrive early to get used to the new place – finding it in order to avoid coming in at the last minute or, worse still, late.
- You might choose to sit in a place where you can see everyone, especially the person chairing the meeting, clearly.
- You should always have your own introduction ready in case you have to introduce yourself and either suddenly get a mental blank when it is your turn, or become so anxious about introducing yourself that you completely miss everyone else's introduction.
- You must prepare with extra care for a new agenda so that information is available to you, even if it is not used.

New technology

There is a Chinese proverb:

Never write a letter when you are angry.

I thoroughly agree and have even waited, on a number of occasions, for a couple of days before responding with some of my better letters. But to the Chinese proverb I would add – and be very, very careful about how you respond to your e-mails as well. It is tempting to respond quickly, but do remember that there is a potential for a great many people to have access to it. Or as Edward Fitzgerald (1859) said, in a much more poetic style:

The moving finger writes; and having writ,
Moves on: nor all thy pity nor wit
Shall lure it back to cancel half a line,
Nor all thy tears wash out a word of it.

Prepare, prepare, prepare

If you are going to be able to persuade others or to present views or to give an account of events, you have to prepare well. What do people want to know, what do they need to know, what questions might they ask, how do they want to have the information presented? And so on. In preparing people for presentations, I usually say that there are only three things that you need to do well for excellent presentation and that is prepare, prepare and prepare. And then I go on to studiously work hard at doing almost exactly the opposite and rush everything at the last minute.

Sense and sensitivity

All I really need to know I learned at Kindergarten.

Fulghum (1986).

If you read as much as I do about management and leadership or attend as many sessions as I have, all over the world, you will read and hear a great many pieces of advice. You need to be selective about it all and some people just do not like the sort of expressions of leadership that do not fit the culture. If you are working with people, they may bring with them ideas that you have to consider. You may hear about how the workforce can be re-engineered along some miraculous lines and we will all be saved. Not necessarily so, I'm afraid. The leader needs to learn when to take advice and when to reconsider the possibilities more carefully.

Enthusiasm is the life-blood of effective leadership. Although it wouldn't do to disregard everything, be selective and try to find out more if you can. That is the one thing about 'good practice' about which one needs to be careful. It will not necessarily be easy to localise elsewhere. Be careful, as even good leaders have what are called 'envious attacks' (Klein, 1975). Klein talks about the danger that a 'good idea which one cannot bear because it is not one's own, may be turned into something bad, which then becomes a threat through having one's hostility projected onto it.'

How many times have you sat in study sessions and someone has been telling you about some practice and you say to yourself – we have been doing that for years. Maybe, but have you measured its success or have you written about it? Or you might say 'It'll never work.' Maybe not 'as is', but if the outcomes are worthy of further thought, perhaps some of the work is worth following up. Or you might just say 'That's a thought.' It is not the whole thought but the start of the thinking that sets you apart. And don't worry if the time isn't right to do what you think is possible. Keep the thought alive until the time does seem right and, without reminding everyone that you actually had the thought 10 years ago, swing into action.

It is said that you can call yourself an expert if you have travelled a long way and have slides or, nowadays, Powerpoint. Do remember to listen to so-called experts with some degree of objective thinking. You'll no doubt be wanting to know what Robert Fulghum learnt in kindergarten. These are the things he learnt:

- share everything
- play fair
- don't hit people
- put things back where you found them
- clean up your own mess
- don't take things that aren't yours
- say you're sorry when you hurt somebody
- wash your hands before you eat
- flush
- warm cookies and cold milk are good for you
- live a balanced life – learn some and think some and draw and paint and sing and dance and play and work every day some
- take a nap every afternoon
- when you go out into the world, watch out for traffic, hold hands and stick together
- be aware of wonder.

I wonder!

Decision-making

We shall not cease from exploration
And the end of all our exploring
Will be to arrive where we started
And know the place for the first time.

Elliot (1944).

Nurses are involved in decision-making all the time; they are usually making the decisions themselves, about patient-care, about technical requirements and about management issues, or they will be involved in team decision-making. As the frame of reference gets wider and the time-scale gets longer, one's capacity for judgement expands and, as with other experiences, the more that you have the opportunity to practice, the easier is becomes. You gain in both competence and confidence.

Decision thinking

Every day and all day, most people are making decisions of one sort or another. In nursing there is constant decision-making and although much can follow protocols or be planned ahead of time, many decisions have to be made quickly. Emergency situations are an obvious example and, increasingly, nurses are the first people on-site to make decisions about triage or initial treatment.

Decisions are also required in management at all levels and it can be relatively simple, like staff holidays, or the more complex management decisions which are those which require either a wider range of options or a longer-term action frame. The process is the same in most situations and is along the lines of the nursing care process; collect the data, diagnose the problem, design the plan of action, implement it and evaluate the action taken. The 'thinking' part of the process is related to the first two parts of that process and how the evaluation affects future decision-making and, as with nursing practice, the action may not be carried out by you but by others, so there is even more need to justify the thinking that leads to any decision. Also, as with the nursing process, people often carry out parts of the sequence of events without thinking in detail about each aspect but it is useful to go through the process, especially if you are having trouble reaching a decision.

COLLECT THE DATA

All relevant data may be easily available, but be sure the right data is there and if not, get it. Audit might be a useful way to collect data but it may be a matter of asking the right people the right questions.

DIAGNOSE THE PROBLEM

This may be evident or require a bit of consideration to make sure you have the right problem identified. When people are involved, there are always about six ways to look at a problem. Nevertheless, options have to be considered and suggestions for solutions examined.

EVALUATE

For evaluation to happen, there needs to be feedback. We learn from every decision we make and, in that way, judgement can be honed as each decision is taken. Some people seem to find it difficult to learn but the leader will eagerly seek feedback so that they can adjust thinking on future occasions.

INTUITION

The intuitive leader is frequently described in relation to decision-making and particularly in crises or when decisions must take immediate effect. This is as true in war situations as in crises in health care, which seems somewhat incongruous. In books about famous leaders, people like Churchill, Montgomery and Nelson will be described and will have made excellent decisions in the face of apparent and available logic as voiced by strategist colleagues (Adair, 1989; Crainer, 1996; Gardner, 1997; Adair, 1997). Intuition has also been described in relation to clinical practice (King & Appleton, 1997; Cioffi, 1997) and acknowledges how nurses link qualitative changes and perceptions to predict future outcomes in patient care.

In a previous paper on power (Campbell, 1987), I remember some very interesting discussions with people then in positions of leadership about whether or not there is such a thing as intuition or instinctive decision-making. Looking at it now, I realise that some of the difficulty in reaching a consensus may have been because I was talking with a mixture of health care leaders and business leaders and the business leaders did not appear to think in the same way about making those very rapid decisions that appear to fly in the face of logic.

Critical thinking

As the leader becomes more involved with longer-term planning or more wide-ranging or complex strategies, their judgement is required to be more sophisticated. There might be a need to review a report or give an opinion about a suggested strategy for manpower planning or give a view about transferability of an area of good practice or review a policy. In those situations you have to think more carefully about the implications of action or inaction and acceptability to others. You may need to apply a number of criteria, from quality to funding to ethics, and on those occasions you need to give yourself time to think through the more complex aspects of the issues. Critical thinking is as much about attitude and approach (Tappen, 1989) and it is necessary to understand your approach to an issue, or your attitude about people, as it is to understand other people's approaches and attitudes. People will question the resulting decisions and they often do so with a sense of personal disappointment so it is important to be able to account for your judgement. I occasionally use a fairly unsatisfactory phrase, 'If it was that easy, anyone could do it' but, often, planning and strategy involve some complex and detailed thinking so the leader needs to employ objective critical thinking.

There is, though, a point at which people have to stop thinking and get on with taking action or reaching a view or finishing writing. John Adair (1989) refers to 'paralysis but analysis' and that it absolutely right. It is also tempting to think that, if you think something should happen, then that's what everyone else will think but that is simply not the way that life is. The reality may be harsh and your excellent logic and seriously considered recommendations are not accepted. The leader must be able to recognise when the time has come to give up for the moment and regroup to fight another day.

Innovative thinking

I was once told that there was no such thing as original thought. Despite my reaction that 'Well, I haven't thought it before', which I thought was perfectly reasonable, it is true that if you are thinking it then it is likely that others are thinking it too. Having said that it is important for leaders to take time out to think about issues and to make new connections between ideas so that fresh thinking contributes to the development of practice. That is innovative thinking which means that you have to have thinking time. Sometimes people seem to be able to set time aside to think things through, in a very logical process but I've never been able to do that, or at least not very often. I do, however, seem to be able to hear one idea and to connect with others to create something else. That is one reason why I like to be involved in areas of development or at the start of projects because it is actually quite exciting to be part of something as it develops. You also need an extra amount of thinking time if you are going to present a case, present a paper or influence people.

It also helps to think things through with others.

> Truth springs from argument amongst friends. Even if we don't convince friends, we often help ourselves to see things in a new way as we look for new angles in the argument.
>
> Hume, in Hardy (1989).

It is helpful to discuss issues with people of like minds, and that is why conferences such as those arranged by professional associations such as the National Association of Theatre Nurses (NATN) are so important to share thinking in both the formal environment of presentations and the informal environment of speaking to people. Networking with others is well-recognised as a skill that leaders use to develop their thinking and to get to know others as well as to get themselves better known. That can work both ways, I suppose, because people will get to know your good ideas as well as your bad ideas but at least it makes people think.

It's also important to test your theories with others who may be less convinced. When I was doing my Master's degree at University I was seconded from my job of the time as nurse manager in a busy theatre suite. I constantly had to hear about how 'We don't need nurses in theatre' but it did hone my arguments quite well and certainly tested my powers of persuasion.

More likely it will be a constant harassment of the same thoughts that suddenly come together and make sense. It really is like a light coming on in your head and there is a need to write it down to see if it still makes sense.

I often sit through study sessions and either something I hear makes me think differently, or I am reasonably relaxed and letting my mind wander a bit when something hits me. No, not the speaker who feels that I'm not paying attention, but something just seems to make sense. That is also the time to write it down. One needs a strong grip on reality though, and there is little use in rhetoric if it does not have an aspect of reality.

Vision

There is not a list about leadership qualities that does not refer to vision. It is the consideration of it and the translation of it to others, a wide variety of others, that is crucial to a leader. In the current environment of rapid change, or 'chaos' as it has been described by many, this is thought to be even more difficult but some writers see that as a positive necessity.

> Creativity and new ideas come from messy, not controlled situations.
>
> Neubauer (1997).

In the absence of some manifestation of 'vision', like a blinding flash possibly, we are liable to think that the gradual development of thoughts is of no value. I dare say there are moments when everything seems to come together in some describable sense, but this 'incrementalism' is as important and likely to be more accessible, certainly at the start of one's leadership journey.

> If one wants to be successful, one must think until it hurts. One must worry a problem in one's mind until it seems there cannot be another aspect of it that hasn't been considered.
>
> Lord Thomson of Fleet, in Adair (1989).

To inspire others to follow it is the important bit, and you can't do that without thinking.

Values

> If you don't believe in the messenger, you won't believe the message.
>
> Hesselbein *et al.*, (1996).

Values and beliefs that people hold will be reflected in their attitudes and behaviours. For leaders this means that they not only require to be in touch with their own values, but that they also need to recognise the values held by others so that they may recognise the reasons for manifest behaviours.

Writers quote leaders' values as being important to the public perception and their success. They also look at the values and beliefs of leaders who have initially succeeded and subsequently failed. It is complex of course but one writer (Mant, 1983) describes his theories of 'raiders' and of 'builders' which differentiates between those who break things down in their efforts towards self-aggrandisement and those who build constructively with others, to achieve success for the whole organisation or team. Much of that is grounded in the value-systems of the individuals, and I have always found it encouraging that those who rise to positions of leadership without acceptable values fall again for the same reason. Indeed, I have noted earlier that 'the scum also rises' and it is comforting to know that it can also sink.

Those who deal with complaints from patients have noticed that patients' expectations have altered over the years. Nowadays, behaviour from some professional staff, manifested all too frequently in aloofness or arrogance, is no longer acceptable. And on an individual basis, people can see through sham and lies, maybe not right away but they do eventually, and leaders need to consider their longer term future in this respect.

So I have looked at values at three levels; from an organisational perspective, from a professional group perspective, and from an individual perspective. Many of the principles are the same and I have no intention of defining lists of acceptable behaviour or 'good things to be' but it is interesting to see the value being placed on values – if you know what I mean.

From an organisational perspective

Some organisations, usually businesses, have mission statements or 'credos' which are regarded as extremely important. They are seen as giving out a strong message about the collective values of the people who work in that organisation.

> Credo values represent the foundation stone upon which leadership is built ... you cannot be a good leader if you don't believe in and try to live up to the Credo.
>
> Larsen (1996).

Many NHS Trusts have also placed value on developing mission statements and the Patient's Charter (1991) describes for patients the values that embody the common purpose of the NHS. The National Health Service reached its 50th Anniversary in June 1998 and this has resulted in a number of articles and books dedicated to looking back before looking forward.

The present labour government came into power in May 1997 and, in line with its election promises, has taken the opportunity to replace the internal market and the competition that it was felt characterised the NHS under the previous conservative government. The new regime has recognised the importance of repositioning values at the top of the agenda, manifest in the clearing out of bureaucracy and the reaffirmation of high quality care for patients. In a recent article, one writer (Giddens, 1991) is quoted as suggesting that this may reflect the current 'obsessive self-absorption that characterises a society anxiously approaching the year 2000.' Whatever the reason, there is clearly an opportunity to see less of the financial imperatives on high-level agendas and more of the clinical quality issues.

Organisational values are important for everyone in that organisation as they will fundamentally affect how the groups within that organisation work. Actually, one could argue that the reason many clinical staff have experienced such stress over recent years is precisely because they have been out of step with the organisational values maintaining their own professional and individual values in the face of great difficulty. It would be daft to think that financial imperatives have disappeared, but it is good to know that the relativities have changed. One project, entitled the 'Living Values' project and set up by the King's Fund, will look at values informing present-day health care practice. That work will report to a conference later this year (1998) and is likely to reflect some of the changes over the years, particularly the changes of the welfare state.

From a professional group perspective

All nurses, midwives and health visitors are bound by the Code of Conduct published by the United Kingdom Central Council (UKCC) in 1992. The UKCC is the statutory body that regulates the professions and thus we are all professionally accountable for our practice and behaviour. People tend to forget that the opening paragraphs include reference to the fact that it is expected that nurses, midwives and health visitors will 'behave at all times in such a manner that ...' and I would stress the 'at all times'. If they behave in an unacceptable way, even though not at that time on health care business, and it is brought to the attention of the UKCC, the UKCC will have a view.

There is also a regulatory body for doctors and dentists but, as yet, there is no statutory register onto which other health care practitioners can be placed and from which they may be struck off. That is of particular interest to nurses working in areas of care where they may be accountable for tasks carried out by others who are not registered. We are familiar with this situation in operating theatres, but it is not an exclusive position and it is interesting to see how people in different areas perceive their accountability.

Within the White Papers published in the UK countries in December 1997, great value has been placed on clinical staff, in its widest sense, and their value systems. That is reflected in other documents including the Human Resources Strategy document in Scotland (NHS in Scotland, 1998) and it is up to us all to make sure that attitudes and behaviours match this faith. This is probably the bit that makes people a little uncomfortable; the 'touchy-feely' things that people don't really want to talk too much about in the macho world of business. Well, we are not in the macho world of business, no matter how business-like we need to be. We are in one of the caring professions, and if we can't think about our own values then we have no business advocating others' values.

From an individual perspective

In terms of leadership, it is both the values of others and of oneself that are manifest in particular attitudes and behaviour that are of interest. Clearly, this is not a treatise on psychology or the humanities and you can get the lists of acceptable behaviour almost anywhere. One of the items on the induction programme we had many years ago was entitled 'Etiquette and behaviour' but I am sure that has been superseded by something a bit more empowering to individuals. So I have no list, but over the years I have come to remind both myself and others of some thoughts on the matter.

> Be nice to people on your way up because you'll meet 'em on your way down.
>
> Wilson Mizner (1953).

Do not go around trying to score points over others. It is usually only a cheap victory anyway and can do immense harm. You don't see successful leaders bothering with that. As a leader, be generous to others – not with money of course, but with time and effort and give them chances to succeed when you have already reached the position. You could always try humility but the problem with that is expressed by one author as follows:

> Humility – a great quality that disappears the moment you think you have it.
>
> E. D. Hulse (1993).

And frankly there is so much change going on it is really important to hold on to your values in the midst of it all.

Tools and measurability

> A leader is best,
> When people are hardly aware of his existence,
> Not so good when people praise his government,
> Less good when people stand in fear,
> Worst, when people are contemptuous,
> Fail to honour people, and they will fail to honour you.
> But of a good leader, who speaks little,
> When his task is accomplished, his work done,
> The people say, 'We did it ourselves!'
>
> Lao Tzu (5th Century BC).

I've seen this quote in more than one book on leadership and it does seem to epitomise rather well the perceptions of leadership. However, it is unlikely that someone will write a poem to you about your leadership capabilities, so how do you know whether or not you have successfully achieved anything? How do you know that you are a leader and that you are leading well? Are there any tools and how can you measure qualities which are so difficult to describe?

I am tempted to say that people will soon tell you if you are not leading well, but the fact of the matter is that they rarely do. Well, rarely in the health care professions, that is. I found several references to business strategies that depend as much upon the macho image of managers as constructive staff development opportunities.

You may have a job that places you in a position of leadership but you may still not be a leader; you may still not have those abilities, skills and behaviours in the appropriate measures that enable you to reach the right decisions at the right time and for the right reasons and you may not possess the qualities that set you apart. It is all very well to look at strong leaders and describe their qualities and it is equally legitimate to encourage, enable and empower emergent leaders as much as it is humanly possible, but there is nothing so depressing as seeing people destroying, or being destroyed, because they are in the wrong job or making the wrong decisions. You are very lucky if people are prepared to tell you that, although it probably won't feel like it at the time. I do say 'lucky' because there is always an opportunity to do something about it, but only if you know. So I reckon that the best way to avoid the disappointment is to work it all out for yourself.

Know yourself

Firstly, know yourself. This is not as easy as it sounds and many people find that too 'touchy-feely' but if you are to have a fighting chance in this rapidly changing organisation, if not world, then you have to develop some insight. I believe that where people have a lack of insight about what they do or what they are, they quickly become out of touch with what is happening all around them. How do you get to know yourself further? Well, you could try a simple SWOT analysis describing your strengths, weaknesses, opportunities and threats, subsequently designing strategies to turn the weaknesses into strengths and threats into opportunities. The trouble with that may be that weaknesses in one context become a strength in another and vice versa. One may believe passionately in something, for example, which is considered a strength but when severely tested that 'passion' results in 'lack of optimum equilibrium or ill-considered words', that is, you lose your temper and say things you regret. But then, if you didn't do that occasionally, people may not know how strongly you felt or you may simply appear bland and without opinion. I suppose the trick is not to do it too often.

If you are carrying out an analysis, don't limit your thinking to just the descriptive part of the exercise but compare it all to the skills required, the experiences that would add value to you or your job and the behaviours that are desired. Then write the action plan and do it.

Some of you may be saying 'But what about appraisal and staff development. Surely, if that's done properly then people will know.' You may even be adding 'My staff do ...' I'm pleased if that is so, but I have often found that appraisal systems too frequently concentrate on what only one individual perceives to be your good and bad points and is of limited value as a result. If the wider range of skills, attributes and behaviours are well-defined, it is relatively easy to see how far along the development continuum you are and as work progresses within a professional competencies framework, the opportunity for valid and reliable measurement will develop rapidly. One way or the other, you can find out what you think about yourself. Now, what do others think?

Know what others think

This is not very easy either and it does depend upon what is meant by 'others'. In this context I mean your team, your boss and the organisation. Other than asking them directly, and that is possible although you might not get very helpful answers, you could always do one of those 360 degree personality tests. That is where your boss, a number of your colleagues and reportees assess you against various qualities and their views are then compared with your perception of yourself. That can be quite an experience and not one to be entered into lightly if you are not able to cope with the results. What struck me as most interesting in the one that I did was that the views from the people with a clinical background differed from those without a clinical background. That is as far as I am prepared to go about divulging any results because, of course, the whole thing is anonymous and only meant to be of value to me. Nevertheless, such an exercise is interesting. In fact, it is also quite expensive as the whole process has to be well coordinated, and feedback properly handled by experts. If you are interested in doing something like that, people involved in staff development in your organisation should be able to advise you further.

Often, one will get feedback from others in a very direct fashion and then we are back to the section on communication and about how it is as important to receive feedback as it is to give out information.

Do you have anything to show for it?

You will probably remember the film 'It's A Wonderful Life' with James Stewart in the lead when a kindly angel showed him what the world would have been like if he had not been born in order to convince him of his worth. I suspect that that particular strategy may be a bit extreme for most of us, but what would have happened or not have happened (in work terms, of course) if you hadn't been around. Just in case you haven't come up with anything very positive yet and are preparing to jump off the bridge even as we speak, here are some questions that might start you off.

1 Do you have any followers? Are there people who would, without question, do what you suggest and do it, not because they have to, but because they choose to?

2 Do people seek you out and ask for advice, ask you to speak, write or contribute to discussions, again, because they choose to and not because they have to?

3 Do you have examples of people who have 'done well' for whom you have acted as role-model, mentor or supporter?

4 Do you have examples of your own achievements?

5 Do you have experience of a wide variety of work situations in which you have achieved successful outcomes?

I was just thinking about the exhortation that if you want something done you should ask a busy person. Well that's not quite correct. You should ask someone who is known to achieve things successfully and so is asked frequently to do things and is, thus, busy. That is not the same as asking the person who works very hard but achieves very little.

Self-audit tools

For those who would like to consider this area further, there is an excellent 'leadership checklist' in Ruth Tappen's book on *Nursing Leadership and Management* where a number of areas are highlighted and degrees of achievement can be measured. Mind you, you then have to do something about the results! At the end of it all, though, it is really only you who can know if you have succeeded.

> Not in the clamour of the crowded street,
> Not in the shouts and plaudits of the throng,
> But in ourselves, are triumph and defeat.
>> Henry Wadsworth Longfellow (1807–82)
>> from *The Poets* (1876).

And finally:

> Ah, but a man's reach should exceed his grasp, or what's a heaven for.
>> Robert Browning (1855)
>> in *Andrea del Sorto*.

Reflective activities

This chapter is densely written and thought provoking, presenting many of the lessons the author has learned from her own experience. It should raise many trains of thought for newly appointed nurse managers as well as encouraging established managers to reflect on their practice.

In reflecting on this section of the book the following comments draw attention to aspects you may wish to follow up. The complexity of health care organisations is recognised and management gurus are now recognising that complexity. This is the starting point of the chapter. Within that framework did you consider the following:

1 How can you make good use of both good and bad role models, remembering that 'the scum also rises'? Who are your positive role models? Who would you not wish to be like at all costs? Why?

2 How far are you able to develop your own self-awareness? Do you implement the lessons from your role models? If not, why not?

3 Did you take on board the message about recognising your hero in yourself?

4 Are you clear about differences between managers and leaders. Do you see yourself as a manager or a leader? How important is it to you to be a good leader or would you be happy to settle for being a competent manager?

5 Learn to live with change. How are you going to learn and change so as to maintain your own credibility and effectiveness?

6 Have you considered how you network with others? Try writing down your different networks.

7 How effective are your communication skills?

- at interpersonal level?
- have you written for publication?
- how well do you speak in public?
- are you a good active listener?

8 On further reflection have you found that you know more than you thought you did on first reflection? Do you prepare yourself in good time – how much homework do you do before putting things into practice?

References

Adair, J. 1989 *Great leaders.* Surrey, Talbot Adair Press.

Adair, J. 1997 *Effective leadership masterclass.* London, Pan Books, Macmillan.

Argyle, M. 1972: *Non-verbal communication in human social interaction.* In: Brown, H. & Steven, R. (eds.) 1975 *Social behaviour and experience.* London, Hodder & Stoughton.

Bennis, E. & Townsend, R. 1995 *Reinventing leadership.* London, Piatkus.

Bok, D. In: Weber, E. 1991 *The Book of Business Quotations.* London, Business Books Ltd.

Bruning, L. 1993 Managing change in a changing environment. *Today's OR Nurse,* 9–11.

Bryson, B. 1997 *Mother tongue.* London, Penguin Books.

Campbell, L. 1987 *Power; personal and professional.* Paper presented to the World Conference of Operating Room Nurses.(Singapore), Published with Papers for delegates, AORN.

Carnegie, D. 1993 *The leader in you.* New York, Simon and Schuster.

Cioffi, J. 1997 Heuristics, servants to intuition, in clinical decision-making. *Journal of Advanced Nursing* **26,** 203–208.

Crainer, S. (ed.) 1996 *Leaders on leadership.* Northants, The Institute of Management.

Elliot, T. S. 1944 *Four quartets.* London, Faber and Faber.

Esar, E. In: Weber, E. 1991 *The Book of Business Quotations.* London, Business Books Ltd.

Fitzgerald, E. 1859 *The Rubaiyat of Omar Khayyam.*

Fulghum, R. 1986 *All I really need to know I learned in kindergarten.* New York, Ivy Books.

Gardner, H. 1996 *Leading minds.* London, Harper Collins.

Giddens, A. 1991 *Modernity and self-identity.* In: Pattison, S. 1998 What are we here for? *Health Services Journal* **12,** March.

Girvan, J. 1998 *Motivation and satisfaction among Nurse Executive Directors in NHS Trusts.* London, Royal College of Nursing.

Goodall, C. 1993 Raging against Bull. *Nursing Standard* **7,** 51.

Handy, C. 1989 *The age of unreason.* London, Hutchinson.

Handy, C. 1994 *The empty raincoat.* London, Hutchinson.

Hewison, A. 1997 The language of management: an enduring challenge. *Journal of Nursing Management* **5**, 133–41.

Hesselbein, F., Goldsmith, M., & Beckhard, R. (eds.) 1996 *The leader of the future.* San Francisco, Jossey-Bass.

Holmes, T. H. & Rahe, R. 1967 The social readjustment rating scale. *Journal of Psychosomatic Research* **2** (213), April 1967.

Josefowitz, N. 1983: *Paths to power.* California, Addison-Wesley.

Kane, J. 1992 *The executive's role in getting everyone aboard.* In: McPhail, G. Management of change: an essential skill for nursing in the 1990s. *Journal of Nursing Management* **5**, 199–205.

King, L. & Appleton, J. 1997 Intuition: a critical review of the research and rhetoric. *Journal of Advanced Nursing* **26**, 203–8.

Klein, M. 1975 *Envy and gratitude.* Collected Writings. London, Hogarth Press.

Larsen, R. S. 1996 *Standards of leadership. Reference guide.* Johnson & Johnson (eds.). Management Education and Development.

Margach, J. 1979 *The anatomy of power.* London, W. H. Allen.

Mant, A. 1983 *Leaders we deserve.* London, Blackwell.

Mehrabian, A. 1971 *Silent messages.* New York, Macmillan.

Mintzberg, H. 1997 Foreword. In: Pitcher, P. *The drama of leadership.* New York, John Wiley and Sons.

National Health Service in Scotland. 1997 *Designed to care – renewing* the NHS in Scotland. The Scottish Office.

National Health Service in Scotland. 1998 *Towards a new way of working.* The Scottish Office.

Neubauer, J. 1997 Editorial. *Journal of Nursing Management* **5**, 65–7.

Pattison, S. 1998 What are we here for? *Health Services Journal* **12**, March.

Paulson, T. 1991 *They shoot managers don't they?.* California, Ten Speed Press.

Pluckhan, M. L. 1978 *Human communication: the matrix of nursing.* New York, McGraw-Hill.

Scottish Office DOH. 1991 *The Patient's Charter. A Charter for Health.* HMSO.

Smith, P. 1992 *The emotional labour of nursing.* London, Macmillan.

Tappen, R. 1989 *Nursing leadership and management: concepts and practice.* Philadelphia, F. A. Davis.

Toffler, A. 1970 *Future shock.* London, Bodley Head.

UKCC. 1992 *Code of Professional Conduct.* London, UKCC.

Watzlawick, P., Beauvin. J. H. & Jackson. D. D. 1967 *Pragmatics of human communication.* New York, W. W. Norton.

Zola, E. 1997 In: Peters T. 1997 *The circle of innovation.* London, Hodder and Stoughton.

Is nursing going too fast for the law?

8

Suzanne Fullbrook

Introduction
Nursing and the law
Nurses and the law
Conclusion
Reflective activities

Suzanne Fullbrook, the author of this chapter, is an ITU nurse who is also a qualified lawyer. She has contributed articles on the law, ethics and nursing to the British Journal of Theatre Nursing for some years and has also spoken at the National Association of Theatre Nurses Congress, and other NATN conferences.

The chapter begins by defining the law. It goes on to look in some detail at the legal and ethical constraints on the nurse as an individual and as a practising member of the nursing profession. The difference between nursing, frequently being pushed ahead of the law by innovations and change and the individual nurse living, as everyone does, within the law of the land is spelled out.

Suzanne Fullbrook then goes on to discuss how the statutory nursing body acts as a conduit of the law and gives nurses a framework for practice, by means of codes of practice and guidelines, in both day-to-day situations as well as in more difficult and unusual situations. She reviews the social and scientific innovations which have far-reaching ethical implications for all those in health care. It is particularly important for perioperative nurses to be able to think through the ethical and legal implications as they are so often involved when operative procedures are required.

It may be that it will be something of a shock for the reader to realise just how many recent events have major ethical and legal implications, not just for health professionals, but for the whole of society. We may have realised that we are living through a period of great change, but not until we stop and think about it do we always realise just how profound some of those changes are. The section of this chapter on how nursing can be pushed ahead of the law is particularly relevant here.

At a time when perioperative nurses are developing new roles and relationships, perioperative nurses will find the latter part of the chapter useful in considering legal aspects of new roles, especially those which involve the sharing of skills formerly limited to the surgeon.

Introduction

Nursing has changed dramatically over the past 20 years. These changes have manifested themselves in three ways: firstly the way in which nurses themselves view their role in health care provision; secondly the way in which they are expected to conduct themselves professionally; and thirdly as a result of the underlying expectations of society as a whole; not only in respect of existing health care provision, but also the demand for all the latest innovations in treatment and cure. It is, therefore, not surprising uncertainty has emanated from nurses as to their place and worth in health care provision. Nor should it be surprising that those provided for feel insecure as to what may be provided and how.

In this uncertain reality, nurses are finding it increasingly difficult to care for, and advocate on behalf of their patients. It is not only a matter of not feeling secure in terms of role, it is often that the nurse does not feel secure with the changes occurring in employment status (hers and others), and the splintering of available literature and information which nurses need in order to maintain a standard consistent with other nurses.

This feeling of isolation can all too often produce stress in a nurse and a loss of confidence which can result in a lowering of competence (Fullbrook 1995). The law is an area where these changes might be producing uncertainty. I propose to address the issue of how the law affects nurses, how it affects nursing as a profession and how it affects nurses as individuals. I believe that, contingent upon which word is used, comes a seemingly contradictory reply.

Nurses are expected to obey the law as much as anyone else, therefore nurses cannot go too fast for the law. However, nursing as an art and science, must necessarily face innovation and change, which will often if not always occur prior to a law to regulate matters. Therefore, in order to address the title and provide an explanation, what is needed is a review of the law, or legal situation, as it is today, followed by a review of how ethics influence our thinking and responses to innovative changes in health care. Only when these backgrounds are understood can a debate begin as to the merits and expectations of nurses and a review of the legal and professional duties of nurses be undertaken.

Nursing and the law

What is the law?

There are many ways to define the word 'law'. For some it is the power of God to dictate our lifestyles, for others nature itself defines our realities. One strand of legal thought that has come down through the ages absorbing the various thoughts of historical perceptions, calls itself 'natural law' and expounds that we can all know the difference between right and wrong in order to lead moral lives (Finnis, 1980; d'Entreves, 1970; Fullbrook, 1996a). Whilst, for some, the subject is to be discussed from a normative approach, for others an historical emphasis is important. Different societies, throughout history, have produced different systems, for example, that of continental law as opposed to the common law as practised in the UK.

Contributors to the debate

Here in this country, during the last century, Jeremy Bentham rejected natural law doctrine and the common law in favour of utilitarianism and positivist theory. For him, this began with realising that justice tied in with and was reducible to utility. This leads to the tying of justice to rules which must be 'right and proper'. The utilitarian account produced for Bentham the assertion that:

> If then it be that the rule thus exhibited in the character of a maxim or dictate of justice is the same which on this occasion would be found to be a dictate or, say, precept emanating from the greatest happiness principle then ... the dictate or precept ... may be said to be a dictate of justice.'
>
> Postema (1986, p.156).

This theoretical basis for defining and practising law has prevailed but the central question 'Which is law?' remains to be discussed. In *The Concept of Law* (1961) Professor Hart sought to define law and concluded that the foundations of a legal system had to have a precept whereby those affected by laws passed, recognised their validity. This is his so called 'rule of recognition', (p.97). Hart recognised that, despite Bentham, the common law, for some defined as the passage of custom and usage, has remained within our system of law:

> In our own system, custom and precedent are subordinate to legislation since customary and common law rules may be deprived of their status as law by statute. Yet they owe their status of law ... not to a 'tacit' exercise of legislative power but to the acceptance of a rule of recognition which accords them this independent though subordinate place.
>
> Hart (1961, p.98).

To the modern commentator, this model might seem obvious. We live under sets of rules which are pronounced by Parliament as Statutes which have the highest binding force as law(s). We recognise this and obey or disobey them accordingly. It, therefore, follows that nurses will recognise and follow law(s) which oversee their nursing practice. This seems simple, but it is too simple. There are two ways in which a law passed by Parliament, or as a legal precedent, can be cause and/or effect: firstly a law, existing and understood, can apply with full force and all can access and know its terms and sanctions for non-compliance. Secondly, where human affairs and behaviours reflect changes in societal thinking, law(s) can take up the debate and produce an answer or reflection on the new realities.

Social reality

Law is not made in a vacuum. There has to be a preceding social reality which provided the impetus for a law to be recited and codified. Our system, involving statutory and common law, seeks to keep abreast of changes. On the one hand, matters affecting persons in a modern setting can be introduced to law by the statutory method which can involve and inform itself by recourse to older examples carried down as common law principles. However, the key realisation must be that it takes a social reality to produce a situation whereby the mechanisms of law will evolve.

Novel situations

A recent example of this is provided by the reality of the disaster which occurred at the Hillsborough stadium in Sheffield. Here, many people lost their lives when unable to escape the crush of a crowd situation. In the ensuing legal case (Alcock v. Chief Constable of South Yorkshire [1991] 2 WLR 814 and [1991] 3 WLR 1057) the courts were faced with a real situation which had never occurred before. In trying to decide issues relating to who can recover damages for suffering nervous shock due to witnessing such a horrible event, the court relied on existing principles as to identity of claimant and proximity of that party to the event. At the first instance, the court produced a judgement which recognised the originality of the event by extending the categories of claimant further than had been ruled permissible before. The Court of Appeal reversed the decision, which the House of Lords judgement upheld, finding that the proximity needed to a victim was to be proved by evidence (Alcock and others, [1991]). But there was a rebuttable presumption where family ties were found, that one could not claim for nervous shock where the shocking events had been witnessed on a television screen as opposed to actually witnessing the event in person.[1]

This event, the actual disaster, thus began a process of fresh evaluation of existing law, necessary because of the novel event. That is the point here. The courts have, in novel situations, to re-evaluate existing law and, where necessary, pronounce fresh principles and rules. There are those who follow this idea to its ultimate conclusion to suggest that only that which is pronounced by a judge is actually law (American Realism). However, it is argued that this is not so as the courts, when making their pronouncements, always look to legislative pronouncements to find the existing law and to previous cases to provide precedent. It is only the novel cases such as the facts of Hillsborough which produce a situation in which the courts must look to external guidance in order to reach a decision which, if accepted, will then bind future cases on similar facts.

The reality, therefore, is that law can be forward looking or retrospective – it all depends whether or not the social reality under examination has occurred before or not. Legal commentators assure us that it is this combination which allows the law an internal consistency which will allow us to know what is expected of us, whilst simultaneously providing the mechanism whereby the rules which bind us can alter to accommodate altering realities which will occur over time.

It is suggested that it is the concept of alteration over time which concerns us in this essay. How do we produce laws which can provide us with guidance and certainty when real events alter these laws? The answer is that we can't always. Any changes which occur in reality might take time to be assimilated into rules which we can use when practising as nurses. This is due to the nature of a legal enactment.

The formal making of a law

STATUTES

In this country, any subject which might become subject to a statutory framework has to go through a set process. The events or ideas which prompted the recourse to law are introduced into the Parliamentary framework by the introduction of a Bill. This is then debated in the House of Commons and then sent through committee stages to the House of Lords. It will be returned to the House of Commons for a final reading. At any stage of the Bill, it can be amended or even rejected if those concerned decide to overturn all or any part contained within it (Smith & Bailey, 1984). Only when all six stages of the Bill have been completed does the Bill receive the Royal Assent and proceed to the Statute books. This process takes time, maybe years. This is accepted as a price to be paid for our democratic process. The highest form of law which is binding on us all is obtained after rigorous scrutiny and debate by those elected to represent us in the debate.

THE COMMON LAW

The other element to our legal system, the common law, runs over time, often centuries, providing authority and guidance as to how matters were decided in the past. However, as was witnessed in the Hillsborough case the authority of the legal rule depends upon the level of the Court making the ruling. In this country, there are three levels of court which can make a new, binding ruling – the puisne courts. The court of first instance can rule authoritatively but, as Alcock and the case of Tony Bland illustrate, such are the new and complex issues to be resolved that these cases will normally be appealed by the losing side (Airedale HA v. Bland, [1993]). They will thus be heard and reviewed in the Court of Appeal and, where matters are very contentious, novel or of the utmost importance to the public as a whole, the case will probably be appealed to and heard by the Lords of Appeal in Ordinary – the judicial members of the House of Lords.

This takes time. A civil case can take many years to reach the House of Lords, although very perplexing cases can be heard expediently, as with the case of Tony Bland. Here, the parents of a young man, who was so injured at Hillsborough as to be left in a persistent vegetative state, wanted his attending doctors to discontinue his treatment to let him die in peace.

Anxious to avoid a charge of attempting to murder Mr Bland, the doctors sought guidance from the courts. This case was expedited to the House of Lords to be settled promptly. The press was involved and all of us could read and be informed of the issues being addressed by the idea of discontinuing the treatment of a young man. Again, this is an illustration of judges looking to statute and precedent to assist them with their deliberations. Those judges involved in the Bland judgement took all available laws available to them but had to address the point that this was another novel situation which had never occurred before. As a result the judges were being asked to give guidance and certainty for those directly affected and others, for example, health care providers. They decided that Parliament was the correct place for such new and socially important matters to be decided and said so in the judgement (Airedale v. Bland [1993] p.880). This is because of the way we organise matters of social innovations under our constitution. It is also why, I suggest, that the proper place for nurses to look for assistance with novel innovations concerning health care and other related social and ethical issues, is actually politics.

Politics

It should now be apparent to the reader that the process whereby innovations in our society become accepted or outlawed is a political one. We vote for a representative to speak on our behalf in Parliament. Our views are meant to be represented there. We can lobby our member of Parliament, or any member, to have our views expressed. Commentators, from the academic world and the media debate the issues involved and we can all access these thoughts. An example of this was the great debate on the proscriptions on homosexuality in which Lord Devlin and Professor H. Hart conducted a lengthy debate which is recorded in several books (Hart, 1963; Mitchell, 1970). In the Warnock Report (1986), mention was made of all the academic and religious contributions to the debate that led to recommendations which, in turn, led to the Human Fertilisation and Embryology Act (1990) (DOH, 1984; Warnock, 1985).

This is how new social ways of living, or ideas, become a reality. Firstly, by an alteration or innovation in our decisions as to how we do live and should live, which converts into a political process which will then, should we deem it sufficiently important, import into the legal process. The point being made here is that an idea must reflect a real event, or innovation actually existing in the mind, prior to its introduction into a political debate. The twists and turns of political debate, the contributions made by us all, comprise the political system. It is in this way that the codified proscriptions that appear as laws, are actually the consequences of our political thoughts and aspirations. What appears before us today as an ancient law was once a societal change, an innovation.

Two recent developments in the law illustrate this. Firstly, the laws which were so innovative in the 1960s in respect of the de-criminalisation of consenting homosexuality stipulated the age of consent had to be 21 years and the sexual relationship had to be in private. Today, in the 1990s, that age seems discriminatory as, for heterosexuals, the age of consent is 16. Political change brought about the ideas that in turn altered the law. Today the age of homosexual consent is 18, with certain lobby groups campaigning for parity with heterosexuals. When it is considered that the idea of homosexuality being socially acceptable in any form would have been unthinkable to the Edwardians, one can measure the magnitude of societal change and the political reflection of this change.[2] Similarly, prior to R.v. R. [1991] a married women could not be raped by her husband, the prevailing social norm being that a women consented to sex during a marriage. However, such has been the change in climate with regards to woman's autonomy over their persons that this idea is now repugnant and wholly unacceptable. That which today is perceived as morally acceptable is very different from previous times, even times within living memory.

Nursing

If this is accepted, it then follows that nursing as a social subject might go too fast for the law. The pace of change currently occurring in many areas of health care dictates that there is insufficient time for the new procedures to be reintegrated and codified. We will naturally look for guidance to existing law(s) but currently find that some innovations facing us today have not been met before. The existing authorities, the statutes and common law principles, might not have covered the new realities because they were not envisaged by previous social groups.

Bioethics

Nowhere is this more apparent than in the field of bioethics. In the past 10 years science has produced many innovations which threaten to completely rearrange the way we view certain important areas of life. Profound examples flow but abortion, *in vitro* fertilisation and surrogate motherhood, euthanasia and assisted suicide, embryology and genetic engineering and genetic manipulation have to be at the top of the list.

In the 1980s, the issue of *in vitro* fertilisation and surrogate motherhood came to the fore when the practises involved became a scientific reality. The ethical and religious objections to such practises were vocalised by disparate strands of society for different reasons of concern. In order to obtain a truly representative picture of public opinion, a committee was set up under the chairmanship of Professor Mary Warnock. Called the Warnock Committee, it reported to Parliament in 1986 and the response of the government became the 1990 Act.

As with the Hillsborough situation, no law existed to settle all concerns surrounding surrogate motherhood and *in vitro* fertilisation, because they had not been social realities before. The task was more difficult as existing ethical and religious constraints were all that was available to try and form an opinion which best suited the issues. The political, not the legal, rubric[3] was used as the issues were so innovative. The 1990 statute was the result of a long and contracted political debate, trying to take on board a novel scientific reality.

Dolly, the cloned sheep, appeared on the pages of our newspapers in 1997. Also in that year, Diane Blood was given permission to take her deceased husband's sperm abroad to enable her to conceive with external assistance. The sperm had been obtained from him without his consent whilst he was actually unconscious (*Times* and *Telegraph* (London), June and July 1997).[4] In Australia, the year also witnessed the continuation of the debate as to the rights and wrongs of assisted suicide, with the legal process being brought to bear on the latest innovations of the doctors concerned. The Australian courts were asked to rule that there was no right to assist a suicide and that the doctors undertaking this action were in fact assisting a murder. The final decision was that doctors could not assist a suicide, that using the computer to assist the person to kill themselves was wrong and that no further attempts were to be made.

Here in the UK, we have faced a protracted dilemma in respect of cross infection from animals to humans, the so called 'mad cow disease' or bovine spongiform encephalitis. Currently, there is an ongoing debate surrounding the ethics and infection risks which relate to the proposed new technique of xenotransplantation; animal to human transplantation (Fullbrook & Wilkinson 1996a,b and 1997; *The Times,* 1997).

These current issues are perceived as being ethical concerns well before there is a call for legal proscription and or regulation. This is because they are topics so new that they must be examined, debated and pronounced upon before they can enter the legal sphere. This is not to address the ways society might choose to interpret data relating to a new topic only to emphasise that the mechanisms which new ideas in society must necessarily go through will end with a legal announcement, not begin with one.

Individual responses to change

It is, therefore, not surprising that those persons and groups which are directly concerned with the consequences of such rapid changes to our perceptions and the realities in our way of living should feel uncertain and insecure as they so often occur before they are accessible in the public domain. As individuals in society, we will feel change and respond as individuals. This can be an enlightening experience or it can produce a feeling of isolation. Many nurses will meet persons whose lifestyles and thoughts on moral and ethical behaviour are vastly different to their own. This can produce feelings of conflict which, it is suggested, the individual must address before being able to deal competently with the needs of others.

A prime example of this is abortion. The needs of a patient undergoing an abortion are paramount to the nurses, but the social debate surrounding abortion is one fraught with passion and divided opinions which must affect a person despite being a nurse. The Abortion Act of 1967 covers all aspects relating to the clinical needs of women, including elements relating to mental health. Safeguards to avoid the performance of illegal abortions were inserted in the Act. However, whilst a nurse must fulfil a duty of care to a client, a personal objection to abortions might be so profound as to prevent the nurse from discharging the duty. The United Kingdom Central Council for Nurses, Midwives and Health

Visitors (UKCC, UKCC), in their guide to professional practice, respond to this fact by specifically referring to the fact that, legally, a conscientious objection is allowed in just two areas: those under the Abortion Act (1967) and those under the Human Fertilisation and Embryology Act (1990). This is in recognition of the highly emotional nature of the issues and the likely impact on individuals regardless of whether or not they are health care providers. The guidelines allow for a nurse to refuse to work in an area where abortions are being performed, but state that the nurse must inform management to allow arrangements for a replacement nurse to be able to perform the necessary role.

However, these two areas are recognised by law. Other areas of concern to individuals such as HIV and AIDS are oppositely proscribed by the UKCC. Nurses are not allowed to refuse to nurse anyone suffering from either of these conditions. This rule might produce fear in those who are unsure of the risks to their health and the health of their children. The risks of infection are minimised by a range of procedures which all health care personnel should observe always – Universal Precautions.[5] However, it is an area, where the risks to staff and others of any infection are subjects which are debated by the professions, but not to the satisfaction of all. It illustrates the idea that some nurses feel that the stresses of the reality of nursing are not being alleviated in their personal terms.

The nursing profession must address the fears and tribulations of those who act in its service. Nurses are real people who do a difficult and demanding job which is underpinned by a need for an immense amount of knowledge and expertise. Health care innovations are fast and furious and all need to be assessed and relayed to all nurses in such a way as to allow them to practise safely and competently.

This, in the opinion of the author, is why nursing must always be in front of the law where innovative and novel social realities are being acted out. Nursing is one profession, maybe the ultimate profession, which is involved where people are cared for because they are vulnerable. Things which render them vulnerable may often be related to such a concern as being undecided as to the propriety of a treatment or operation to self or to one close to self. Women having abortions, infertility treatment, cosmetic surgery have moved into areas where social opinion and, ultimately, the legal status of each treatment will be divisive and changing, an unavoidable consequence as societies alter their consensus over time.

Nursing cannot ignore this reality nor try to evade responsibility. As a discipline, nursing must always be at the forefront of response to social change as it affects the individuals in their real experiences. There has to be a real communication between nurse and patient otherwise the key essence of nursing, the caring face of human assistance coupled with knowledge and experience of people and their needs, must be eroded or even lost completely.

Advocacy

It is this fundamental requirement of nursing, that of addressing the new and the difficult in a proficient and professional manner, which means that nurses must advocate, sometimes if not always, on behalf of their patients. Not only is a person often rendered physically vulnerable when, due to their condition, they cannot attend to their own health care needs but they are often psychologically vulnerable, either because their condition has denied them the capacity to self care or because they do not know or understand the ways in which innovative health care can affect them.

This does not lead to a conclusion that the general public is unintelligent. Not at all. It merely underlines the consequences of changing ethics and technical innovations. The nurses caring for these patients might find new innovations hard to keep up with, despite their personal endeavours relating to professional development. How much more difficult for their patients who, as lay persons, probably do not have access to, or an inclination to learn about, all the latest health care trends.

This is the rationale for nurses to advocate on their patient's behalf. In all probability, this will include informing the patient of the new innovations, talking and, vitally, listening to the patient and their responses to the treatment option being proposed. There is a mistaken belief that to advocate for someone is to talk exclusively to a third party on the patient's behalf, with the patient sitting mutely with no active part to play. This idea is patronising and misses the object of nurse advocacy. A person receiving health care must always have as full and independent a voice as possible. This is known and understood. But herein lies the problem. How can you have a full and informed voice if you are not aware of or do not fully understand the problems facing you, either due to their complexity or because the idea or delivery of them is so new that you could not have gained an insight into them even if you wanted to?

Ethics

This is where the nitty gritty of the difference between law and ethics can be vital to nurses. Where ideas and innovations are vastly different from that which went before, a law might be passed promptly and very publicly, such as in the situation involving Tony Bland. A behaviour so radical as discontinuing treatment which must result in the person's death will attract the media and commentators with an ethical perspective will join in the public debate. Both nurses and patients will have a greater opportunity to read and digest for themselves, the issues involved. Thus, the nurse might find less of a need to advocate on behalf of the person affected by the changed situation. However, most case law is not so readily available to the public or even to nurses.

As most nurses know, the ethics of health care delivery which affect us daily will not hit the headlines. Nevertheless, they remain of critical importance to the individual affected by them. Here, the nurse might not be in as good a position to know if consensus has been reached in a wider social domain. It is in this situation that the need for good advocacy is greatest but most difficult because the person affected by a proposed treatment care option will also, most probably, be unaware of the relevant issues and ethics.

The problem is how to keep up with changes in social acceptability over a wide range of topics. Another debate taking place since 1997 is on the ethical contradictions in raising the legal age of smoking whilst lowering the age of legal consensual homosexual relationships. Both of these topics concern nurses directly. Both will affect persons receiving nursing care and treatment. Both have been the subject of considerable debate prior to any new legislation being proposed and enacted. Indeed, the Minister for Health said in that year on a television programme that any new law would be not be passed at least until 1998.

The thorny question of the age of consent for homosexuals came perilously close to wrecking the entire 1997 Crime and Disorder Bill as the House of Lords rejected the reduction of the age of homosexual consent to 16. The discrepancy in the legal age of consent still remains under discussion. The question of the ethics of smoking and all the health care-related consequences affect people in the present, not the future, and nurses will be expected to address concerns. The issue of whether nurses should smoke will be pertinent and raises once more the issue of nurses, as individuals, knowing their personal positions in advance when relating professionally to those they care for. How can a nurse who smokes assist a person who is trying to stop, or relate to a patient who has fully anti-smoking sentiments if he or she smokes? How do you relate as a nurse to women having abortions and abortion clinics? Where does a professional and personal commitment to this topic begin and end? Where does nursing relate to infertility, xenotransplantation, genetic engineering, or any research which might involve a human being to their detriment?

The answer must be that, currently, nursing as a professional discipline is threatened with being swamped by innovation. Ethics as a subject, drawing as it does from philosophy, theology, religion proper, and politics will take time to peruse and settle, if possible, questions on current issues. Modern ethics is a huge discipline, one which many nurses will not have been exposed to in a rounded manner. This makes things very difficult for the practitioner faced with a real situation. It also makes cohesive writing on ethical matters difficult and seemingly fragmented. By the time this manuscript is published, many of the concerns of significance today may seem old hat. Some might be settled and some legally proscribed. Some may remain live issues.

This combination plus a lack of accessibility to information or a lack of time to assimilate all available literature, can result in nursing presenting a public face of confusion which undermines attempts to provide a standard, coherent level of health care. Whilst ethics is the forum for the dissemination of information in respect to innovative social ideas, nurses might well not be in a position to receive that information in a way which will guide them in their everyday practices.

Thus far, you have been asked to consider ethical issues facing nursing. In order to address some of the problems raised by nursing as a discipline per se, it is now proposed to look at nurses, not nursing, to try and find a few solutions.

Nurses and the law

The law

Nurses are not going too fast for the law. They cannot do so, because laws exist and we are in the world with our profession being held accountable under existing law(s). In the UK, our Constitution is based on statutes, as previously described, and the common law. This splits into distinct areas, for example, family law, contract and commercial law. The area which concerns nurses, is the civil law of tort, and for the purposes of this essay, the tort of negligence.

The common law

NEGLIGENCE

The common law principle underpinning the tort of negligence is that at certain times, we might owe another person a duty of care. This concept was expounded upon in the case of Donaghue v. Stevenson [1932] wherein Lord Atkin stated that:

> There … is, some general conception of relations giving rise to a duty of care … The rule that you are to love your neighbour becomes in law 'You must not injure your neighbour' and the lawyer's question, 'Who is my neighbour?' receives a restricted reply. 'You must take reasonable care to avoid acts or omissions which you can reasonably foresee would be likely to injure your neighbour.' 'Who then, in law is my neighbour?' The answer seems to be '… persons who are so closely and directly affected by my act that I ought reasonably to have them in contemplation as being so affected when I am directing my mind to the acts or omissions which are called in question'.
>
> Donaghue v. Stevenson [1932, p.580].

This principle has decided the duty of care owed by nurses. Persons who are nursed are ultimately vulnerable and directly affected by the actions and omissions of a nurse. Therefore, reasonable care must be taken to avoid harm to persons in such a position. This law exists and binds all who practice – the nurse can never be said to be going too fast for it.

The modern world of nursing incorporates the notion of individual practice, which reflects a personal knowledge and experience basis. The old idea of a uniform workforce, recognisable as such, is gone. This has immediate ramifications when the principles of negligence are examined. The underlying principle informs one that a duty of care exists, it does not specify what, where and how the duty can be complied with.

However, one can determine more closely the duty by examining other common law cases and principles. Firstly, the question is asked, what is the standard of the duty of care, and how does it relate to each profession or trade? This question, was addressed in Bolam v. Friern Hospital Management Committee [1957]. Lord Denning stated that in most instances those engaged in a profession could identify a correct standard.[6] The test was to be objective, in that a group, say of 20 persons so involved, could elicit a standard which all in the profession could agree on. Those who fell below this standard could be found to be negligent. Therefore, nurses can determine standards for all actions seen by nurses as being acceptable. Aligned to this reasoning, the question of what is or is not reasonable in a given situation can be elucidated.

The question, it is suggested becomes more problematic when nurses undertake new or innovative practices. How do you find your group of twenty fellow practitioners to gauge your practice? The answer can be difficult. Certain protocols and procedures exist whereby those seeking to undertake new practices can be taught by those already undertaking them, acquire a training and be adjudged competent in their new role. This allows for the practitioner to learn new skills safely and for those who are managing to know that staff are competent in all they do. The group of 20 is quickly arrived at. In law, it allows for all to know and accept that safe reasonable practice is undertaken. This is not nurses going too fast for the law; it is nurses utilising and recognising existing law, and applying it to new and innovative settings.[7]

The other element to innovative nursing practice is that nurses, or most nurses, are employed. Therefore, the employer has an interest in what their staff members are doing whilst employed. They have a duty of care to those who seek medical assistance within the hospital or surgery setting. Nurses, like all other employees must obey their contractual obligations. Where a staff member acts in such a way as to warrant a finding of negligence, it is the employer, the Trust or Health Authority, who usually faces a law suit for negligence. Therefore, vicariously, the employer is responsible for the actions of an employee in most situations and there is much law to identify and regulate these issues. One such rule is that, to be covered vicariously, a staff member must be acting within the course of their employment and within their terms and conditions of employment.

Where a nurse acts or omits to act in an area which is considered to be outside these confines, they might find themselves deemed to be on a 'frolic of their own' (Oughton & Cooke, 1989). This would have the effect of releasing the employer from any vicarious responsibility and place the nurse in the unenviable position of being held to account alone. Where an innovative practice is being undertaken, it is essential to inform management of this fact and to ensure the employer's permission and support. In addition, where a new practice is being undertaken, the standard by which the practitioner should be adjudged for a level of competence would be that of the person who usually undertook the practice. In other words, a nurse doing what is usually done by a surgeon could find themselves being judged by the standards of a competent surgeon.

These aspects of the duty of care are recognised and settled legal principles. To realign existing principles and redefine them for the purposes of current practice is not to go too fast. It is different from the idea that societal thinking on certain health issues might develop faster than legislation can be produced. The cutting edge might come from the bodies which seek to represent nurses, for example, the Royal College of Nursing or the National Association of Theatre

Nurses, when they lobby and inform ministers in order to influence new legislation. They are in a position to inform of innovations within the nursing profession but they must act or begin from within existing law. In practice, it is not usually the common law in general which is cited and followed by nurses but a specific set of rules which define and regulate all nurses practising within the UK. I have in mind, the UKCC Code of Professional Conduct 1992.

Nurses and the Code of Conduct

A DISCUSSION OF THIS PRACTICE STATEMENT

The United Kingdom Central Council for Nurses, Midwives and Health Visitors (UKCC) exists to regulate all nursing practitioners. It owes its authority to do so to the Nurses Midwives and Health Visitors Act (1979), by way of delegated legislation. The purpose of the UKCC is to protect the interests and safety of the public; those who seek and need to be cared for and nursed. It is a common mistake to believe that the UKCC acts to protect nurses. It does not; it is there to control and regulate nurses to ensure the highest possible standards of care are given to those who need it. The ways in which it does this are:

- To control and monitor entry to the nursing register.
- To maintain the register by checking qualification and training controls.
- By having the authority to remove from the register those whose conduct and practice falls below the acceptable and accepted standards (UKCC, 1992).

The duty of care

The Code of Professional Conduct (UKCC, 1992) itself reflects the concepts and principles of the common law and refines them, to address specifically the requirements and scope of nurses' practice. Within this document, the rules are there for all nurses to follow and it is from here that guidelines for all aspects of practice can be elicited. The notion that nurses cannot go too fast for the law is identified most exactly by understanding this document. It incorporates the existing law of the UK and applies with legal force and with certainty to all who practice.

This is reflected in the opening statement of the Code (1992) which states unequivocally that:

Each registered nurse, midwife and health visitor shall act, at all times, in such a manner as to:

- Safeguard and promote the interests of individual patients and clients.
- Serve the interests of society.
- Justify public trust and confidence and uphold and enhance the good standing and reputation of the professions.

As a registered nurse, midwife or health visitor, you are personally accountable for your practice. (UKCC, 1992).

This command is mandatory; there is no room for non-compliance. In this document, the nursing profession under the authority of the UKCC self-regulates whilst obeying the general law. The Code identifies all the elements of the common law and codifies them in such a way as to spell out the principles under which nurses must behave. All the common law elements mentioned in the above discussion are covered and set out in a language which reflects the explicit needs of nurses.

1 NEGLIGENCE

The aspect of negligence is encapsulated in Clause 2 of the code as set out in 1992, wherein it is stated that:

[A nurse must] ensure that no action or omission on your part, or within your sphere of responsibility, is detrimental to the interests, condition or safety of patients and clients (Clause 2).

The issue of expanding one's practice and ensuring an adequate up to date knowledge of new procedures and aspects of clinical practice is covered in Clauses 3 and 4.

Clause 3 states:

Maintain and improve your professional knowledge and competence.

Clause 4 states:

Acknowledge any limitations in your knowledge and competence and decline any duties or responsibilities unless able to perform them in a safe and skilled manner.

UKCC (1992).

2 ADVOCACY

Advocacy receives attention in more than one clause: Clause 1 says that a nurse must 'act always in such a manner as to promote and safeguard the interests and wellbeing of patients and clients', whilst Clause 11 states that a nurse must 'report to an appropriate person or authority, having regard to the physical, psychological and social effects on patients and clients, any circumstances in the environment of care which could jeopardise standards of practice'. This clause covers, it is suggested, advocating on aspects of care which would involve concerns as to health and safety. Clause 12 is slightly different; it states that a nurse must: 'report to an appropriate person or authority any circumstances in which safe and appropriate care for patients and clients cannot be provided ...'

For many nurses, this clause will provide the authority they need to advocate on behalf of patients in respect of the one concern which currently occupies so many nurses' time; namely that of low staff numbers and poor skill mixes. All over the UK, this issue is relevant and very stressful to all who are concerned. It is an issue which, for perioperative nurses, has particular resonances when managers wish to make changes in the skill mix balances in an operating department. It is no good having a wonderful Code of Conduct which exhorts all to the highest standards of care if little can be accommodated due to a lack of skilled staff, or worse and often, inadequate numbers of any experience at all. Clause 12 should be known and internalised by all nurses. It is the clause which commands you and places a duty upon you to inform; to advocate on behalf of your patients, but also on behalf of yourselves and colleagues. Where staffing is inadequate to provide safe and appropriate care, tell your senior nurse manager. If you are a theatre manager it will be your responsibility to respond appropriately which may be by doing your utmost to prevent decisions which lead to such a situation occurring in the first place. We remain at all times responsible for our practice. The practical resolution of the current staffing crisis within nursing is an issue which will only be resolved by policy and practical decisions by those in a position to do so. Until then, at least ensure that you document your report clearly, so as to illustrate that you have understood and acted upon your professional Code of Conduct.

3 OTHER CLAUSES

Autonomy (Clause 7), working with other health providers (Clause 6), cooperation with patients and their families (Clause 5), trust and honesty (Clause 9), teaching (Clause 14), refusing gifts and favours (Clause 15) and refining to allow the profession status to be manipulated by commercial concerns (Clause 16) all feature but there are two areas which deserve a more in depth elucidation.

4 CONFIDENTIALITY

Clause 10 relates to the issue of confidentiality. It makes clear that nurses must:

> protect all confidential information concerning patients ... obtained in the course of professional practice and make disclosures only with consent, where required by the order of a court or where you can justify disclosure in the wider public interest.

For many nurses, this is an area where, not only are they not going too fast for the law, they are aware that a law exists which can seem complicated and contradictory. When notes are produced, the patient has a right to see them, but a doctor is not under a fiduciary duty to reveal all[8] (Bartlett, 1997).

Information given verbally to another may not be adequately received and a written version may be needed. Families and friends may want information. On the one hand, the duty is to the patient and to the need for confidentiality to be strictly observed, but there is also Clause 5 which dictates that the nurse work openly and cooperatively with families. The conflicts between competing loyalties, and notions of what is or is not confidential can be stressful and complex. Here, competent advocacy is essential, as is a knowledge of the Code of Conduct and the underlying legal rules. Recent statutes in this area underline the rights of persons to have access to records whilst case law illustrates that doctors might own the property of records but not necessarily their contents (Access to Health Records Act (1990); Bartlett, 1997; R. v. Mid-Glamorgan FHSA ex.p Martin [1995]). The advice to nurses is always to err on the side of caution. Where fearful of giving too much information to persons other than the patient or client, desist and refer to senior management. It is better to keep someone waiting for information a little longer than to speak and find that you have breached the duty of care to your patient in respect of their right of confidentiality. (Fullbrook, 1998).

However, the law makes it clear that there are times when nurses and others must reveal information relating to their patients. The relevant clause mentions court orders and the public interest. The document *Guidelines for Professional Practice* produced by the UKCC in 1996 explains this further. In respect of defining the notion of 'public interest' paragraph 56 states that:

> The public interest means the interests of an individual, or groups of individuals or of society as a whole, and would, for example, cover matters such as serious crime, child abuse, drug trafficking, or other activities which place others at serious risk.

This list assists nurses to know when they must reveal information. It is not so helpful at revealing when they should not. Again, advocacy is an essential skill required here, to support and assist the client, whilst not breaching one's duty of care. It underlines the fact that we are all bound by the law of the land and emphasises some areas more than others. Sometimes, the nurse must know elements of the law in order to practice safely whilst in other areas the law is quiet and the Code speaks sufficiently to guide nurses.

5 CONSENT

An area where the law is complex and where the code is not explanatory is around the issue of consent. In English law, consent is necessary before any treatment or procedure can be undertaken. Even the act of touching a person, let alone intrusion into their personages, in the absence of consent, constitutes a trespass and a claim for battery or bodily harm could follow (Offences against the Person Act [1861]).

The Guidelines for Professional Practice dedicates four pages (17–20) to understanding the duties of a nurse. However, the legal principles are ever being refined and there is a large body of case law. Perhaps this is the biggest issue which concerns doctors and patients when it comes to claims alleging negligence. Such an area cannot be covered here, but again it illustrates the importance for the nurse of an understanding and knowledge of the law as well as the Code of Conduct (Sidaway v. Bethlem Royal & Maudsley [1985] and others). The ways in which the rules of consent, for example, will develop and refine themselves over time reflects once more the notion of utilising existing legal principles and evolving them into rules which reflect current situations. It is not the same thing as being faced with a novel, hitherto unknown or envisaged reality, or of a new idea being formed and regulated by social and ethical considerations.

It is imperative that each and every nurse practising in the UK is fully conversant with the Code of Conduct as well as with relevant areas of the law. The Code exists to ensure patient safety and respect. The list intends to be all encompassing and, to that end, principles applicable to each defined area are rehearsed. However, the specifics of each event are not. This is made clear in the UKCC publication *Guidelines for Professional Practice* which states that:

> The Code does not cover the specific circumstances in which you make decisions and judgements. It presents important themes and principles which you must apply to all areas of your work (Para 10).

6 THE CODE – GUIDING STRENGTH OR WEAK INDICATOR?

For many the weakness of the Code of Conduct is that it fails to identify those situations where a nurse needs specific guidance for appropriate actions to avoid being accused of negligence in practice. However, the reverse can equally be said. It is the very ambiguity of the wording of the Code which allows for new circumstances to be accommodated so as to allow each practitioner to expand and develop a practice according to individual need. As with the reality of the Hillsborough tragedy, no one can predict the circumstances which will be met in the future.

We, as nurses, cannot predict our next client's personal needs or situations. Therefore, the code must be flexible other than in the areas proscribed or defined by law. For example, nurses must give information, if ordered by a court of law, or under a specific Act of Parliament. The Code of Conduct, like the law, is the defining line between the certainty of existing legal pronouncements and the uncertainty of the future need for application to real events.

7 ETHICS

This is where ethics is so important. When nurses make innovations to meet patient needs they must comply with the law. Nurses must look to debate and refine existing principles but also to debate and form new ideas as to the morality and efficacy of proposed new ideas. This has been observable in operating departments and other perioperative areas in recent years. Perioperative practice has been changing radically and has thrown up anomalous situations which have been thoroughly debated to establish existing nursing roles before new roles and relationships were explored and developed.[9]

It is also in the arena of ethics that social responses of the individual client and nurse should be debated and rehearsed. Ethics is where the views of nurses should be heard, formulated and passed on to nurse lobbyists and nurse organisations such as the Royal College of Nursing and National Association of Theatre Nursing, so that they can be relayed in a political framework to those who represent us and form our laws.

Conclusion

I would suggest that it is at this point that a resolution of the seeming conflict between my two assertions can be found. Nursing, the social subject, will always go too fast for existing legal pronouncements where there is a need to keep at the forefront of changes in thinking and in real events. Nurses, at all times bound legally and professionally by that which exists by way of principles and rules, will have to understand and utilise those principles and rules in a way which enables them to be able to respond to changes so as to act always in their patient's best interests. There is no conflict. The bridge which provides for the existing and the innovative is the study and application of ethics. Ethics can encompass everything and alter our understanding of our realities.

Nursing

On the one hand, nursing as a social reality will always be in advance of settled law due to the nature and circumstance of the task. As those closest to persons rendered vulnerable by life and natural events, nurses will witness the consequences of societal change. Nursing as a discipline will always have to respond rapidly to these changes, whilst 'we' nurses react as professionals to the consequences, possibly unenvisaged, possibly covered by previous experience. Nurses are members of society and their personal responses to changes in social attitudes to fundamentally important issues will influence them as private individuals. Unless professional training and discourse is undertaken this will colour their individual responses both off and on duty. Nursing, as well as being a discipline within social reality, is also a subject with an academic background and a need to make innovative advances. The way in which the profession moves with the times will reflect upon the way in which nursing practice is seen by those directly and indirectly involved. Actions and behaviours will be influenced in the professional practical scene by the theoretical responses to the social mores of the time.

The law, alerted to societal thinking will reflect novel situations. Legislation arises as a consequence of change. Existing law will be there to answer all inquiries if possible but essential changes in societal thoughts often arise from reality and are then formed by committee and open discussion into formulated codes of acceptance or prohibition. Thus such issues as homosexual consent and age, abortion and its boundaries, the acceptability of allowing persons to die and assisting them in the medical environment or not, the transplantation of animal organs to humans, infertility issues and surrogacy of motherhood, to say nothing of all those other issues yet to arise, will find their way into our law to guide us and influence us in the future. Society as a whole, and health care providers in particular, must debate and decide upon new ways of caring for and treating all who need such assistance. Ethics is not merely a theoretical subject. It is the examination of human behaviour and aspirations, the area where it is pertinent to examine and renew perceptions of acceptable and desirable behaviours and human responses.

Nurses

Conversely, nurses as practitioners can never go too fast for the law. Those who practice in the UK are accountable under the law as it stands. New legislation will identity and codify new ways of behaviour but that which exists binds all. For nurses, this concept is made real by the existence of the nursing Code of

Professional Conduct. The rules and regulations therein spell out the nurse's duty to patients and others affected by our interventions in their lives, to colleagues and to society as a whole. Never can it be said that we as nurses run ahead of the law. We must understand our existing law, utilise and reform it as necessary, act to promote its message of care and ensure that we participate in social and ethical debates so that we, as nurses, are able to influence the way in which we deliver health care of the highest possible standards.

Reflective activities

This chapter has made clear how the law is used to give a legal and ethical framework for the practice of nursing, to maintain standards and to protect the public. At a time when there are many changes in the role of the nurse it behoves individual nurses to make sure that they are quite clear on the limitations of their role. It emphasises the way in which 'nursing' is often being pushed into areas where public awareness and discussion has often not yet enabled society to think out the full ethical situation of innovative procedures or possibilities. On the other hand the chapter makes clear how individual nurses have been given codes of conduct worked out by their statutory bodies to control and delineate their practice.

1 Whatever your specific role in the perioperative period, are you quite clear about the ethical and legal constraints on your practice? Does a knowledge of professional codes and guidelines for practice help you to clarify your role and accountability as a perioperative nurse?

2 Use the section on the separate clauses of the UKCC Code of Practice and reflect on the differences between the RN First Assistant and a non-nursing person in this role.

3 As new nursing and non-nursing roles develop in the operating department, how does the employer play his part in giving legal protection to both staff and patient?

4 You might find it useful to refer to other chapters in this book and reflect on how professional bodies are playing their part in defining the changes which are taking place in perioperative nursing.

Endnotes

1 Late in 1998 a claim for compensation for emotional trauma on these grounds by the local police was rejected in view of the fact that family members who witnessed events on television were not so eligible (Ed.).

2 This continues to be an active subject for discussion with the concept of discrimination being more of an issue than that of sexual orientation, despite the opposing argument of the vulnerability of teenage boys.

3 Rubric: defined by the Oxford dictionary as 'directions' or 'explanatory words', originally for divine service and printed in red alongside text.

4 The baby was born in December 1998, to great family rejoicing.

5 Turn to Chapter 10 for further discussion on 'universal precautions' or 'universal standards' as they are now known in some areas.

6 A new case (Botillero v. Hackney, H.A. [1998]) states that the courts can, if need be, be the final arbitrator of a *reasonable* course of action by professionals: expert witnesses can all state that they would/would not do something but the *Court* will decide on the facts.

7 This is the legal principle underlying the publication of guidelines or standards by perioperative nursing organisations such as AORN, ACORN, EORNA or NATN and why, once written and published, they have such authority.

8 Fiduciary: related to duty of trust.

9 You are referred to the first section of this book, especially Chapter 3, to see how perioperative nurses have acted professionally in attempting to manage these changes.

References

Abortion Act 1967, in *Halsbury's Statutes* (4th edn). London, Butterworths 1997 **12**, 366.

Access to Health Records Act. 1990.

Airedale NHS Trust v. Bland. [1993] AC 789.

Alcock v. Chief Constable of South Yorkshire. [1991] 2 WLR 814, (1991) 3 WLR 1057.

Alcock and others v. Chief Constable of the South Yorkshire Police. [1991] 4 All ER 907.

Bartlett, P. 1997 Doctors as fiduciaries: equitable regulation of the doctor–patient relationship. *Medical Law Review* **5**, (2), Summer.

Bolum v. Friern Hospital Management Committee. [1957] 1 WLR 582.

Crime and Disorder Bill 1997. HMSO, No 52.

Crime and Disorder Act 1998, chapter 37.

d'Entreves, A.P. 1970 *Natural law and DNA.* London, Hutchinson.

Donaghue v. Stevenson. [1932] AC 562, p.580.

DoH. 1984 *Report of the Committee of Enquiry into Fertilisation and Embryology.* Cmnd 9314. London, HMSO.

Finnis, J. 1980 *Natural law and natural rights.* Oxford, Oxford University Press.

Fullbrook, S. 1995 Duty of care, Parts 1, 2, & 3. *British Journal of Theatre Nursing* **5** 5(9,10–11),6(18–19) & 7(33–4).

Fullbrook, S. 1996 M.Phil Thesis. University of Sussex.

Fullbrook, S. & Wilkinson, M. 1996a Animal to human transplants. *British Journal of Theatre Nursing* **6**, 2.

Fullbrook, S. & Wilkinson, M. 1996b Ethics of animal transplantation. *British Journal of Theatre Nursing* **6** (3), 13–15,18.

Fullbrook, S. 1997 Xenotransplantation and the Law. *British Journal of Theatre Nursing* **7** (2), 21–5.

Fullbrook, S. 1998 Legal implications of relatives witnessing resuscitation. *British Journal of Theatre Nursing* **7** (10), 33–5.

Hart, H. 1961 *The concept of law.* Oxford, Oxford University Press.

Hart, H. 1963 *Law liberty and morality.* California, Stanford University Press.

Human Fertilisation and Embryology Act 1990, in *Halsbury's Statutes* (4th edn). London, Butterworths 1997 **28**, 316.

Mitchell, B. 1970 *Law, morality and religion, in a secular society.* Oxford, Oxford University Press.

Morgan, D. & Lee, R. 1991 *Blackstone's guide to the Human Fertilisation and Embryology Act (1990).* London, Blackstone.

Nurses, Midwives and Health Visitors Act 1979, in *Halsbury's Statutes* 1996 **28**, 69.

Offences Against The Person Act. 1861 Section 47 covers actual bodily harm. Assault and battery are common law offences.

Oughton, D. & Cooke, P. 1989 *The common law of obligations.* Edinburgh, Butterworth, p.495.

Postema, G. 1986 *Bentham and the Common Law Trade.* Oxford, Oxford University Press.

R. v. R. [1991] 4 All ER 481.

R. v. Mid-Glamorgan FHSA ex.p. Martin. [1995] 1 WLR 110 at 116.

Sidaway v. Board of Governors of the Bethlem Royal Hospital and Maudsley Hospital. [1985] 1 AC, p.871.

Smith, P. & Bailey, S. 1984 *The modern English legal system.* London, Sweet & Maxwell. Read: Smith & Bailey, or Smith & Brazier 1973 for accounts of the procedure of the formation of an Act of Parliament.

Smith v. Tunbridge Wells Health Authority. [1994] 5 Med LR and Lybert v. Warrington Health Authority, [1996] 7 Med LR and Smith v. Barking, Havering and Brentwood Health Authority, [1994] 5 Med LR.

The Telegraph. 7.3.1997 and 5.6.1997.

The Times. 25.2.1997, 26.2.1997, 28.2.1997 and 7.7.1997.

UKCC. 1992 *Code of Professional Conduct.* London, UKCC.

UKCC. 1996 *Guidelines for professional practice.* London, UKCC.

Warnock, M. 1985 *A question of life.* Oxford, Basil Blackwell.

Further reading

Jones, M. & Morris, A. 1992 *Blackstone's statutes on medical law.* London, Blackstone Press.

Knight, B. 1992 *Legal aspects of medical practice.* Edinburgh, Churchill Livingstone.

Lee, S. 1986 *Law and morals: Warnock Gillick and Beyond.* Oxford, University Press.

Lewis, C. 1992 *Medical negligence. A practice guide.* Croydon, Tolley.

Macintyre, A. 1988 *Whose justice? Which rationality?* London, Duckworth.

McHale, J. 1993 *Medical confidentiality and legal privilege.* London and New York, Routledge.

Marks-Maran, D. & Rose, P. 1997 *Reconstructing nursing.* London, Baillière Tindall.

Skegg, P. 1988 *Law, ethics and medicine.* Oxford, Clarendon Press.

Smith, S. & Brazier, R. 1973 *Constitutional and administrative law.* London, Penguin Books.

Tredennick, H. 1976 *Aristotle: ethics. The Nicomachean ethics.* London, Penguin Books.

Tschudin, V. & Marks-Maran, D. 1992 *Ethics.* London, Baillière Tindall.

Journal articles

Allridge, P. 1996 *Consent to medical and surgical treatment.* The Law Commission's recommendations. *Medical Law Review* **4** (2), 129.

Almond, B. 1988 Philosophy, medicine and its technologies. *Journal of Medical Ethics* **14,** 173–8.

Butler, D. 1994 Europe plans convention on social impacts of biomedical technologies. *Nature* **370** (7).

Carson, D. 1986 How the law affects nursing. *Professional Nurse* July **1** (10), 275–7.

Carson, D. 1987 Negligence: defining responsibility. *Professional Nurse* February **2** (5), 141–3.

Cartwright, W. 1996 The pig, the transplant surgeon and the Nuffield Council. *Medical Law Review* **4** (3).

Chellel, A. 1991 Nursing standards stranded. *Nursing Standard* **3** (41), 52–3.

Crossley, T. 1993 Too scared to care. *Nursing Standard* **7** (40), 48–9.

Dimond, B. 1991 Accident, negligence or crime? *Nursing Standard* **5** (21), 22–3.

Duke, C. 1996 HIV and the paediatrician as the child's advocate. *The Lancet* **348,** 247–9.

Finch, J. 1989 Legal notes; employer's liability. *Nursing Standard* **4** (4), 47.

Finch, J. 1989 Legal notes: vicarious liability. *Nursing Standard* **4** (7), 47.

Gillon, R. 1994 Ethics of genetic screening: the first report of the Nuffield Council on Bioethics. *Journal of Medical Ethics* **20,** 67–8.

Giordano, B. 1995 High-tech health care is great, but our first duty is to do no harm. *AORN Journal* **61** (2), 314–15.

Gray, J. 1990 A conflict in embryo. *Nursing Standard* **6** (4), 23.

Hand, D. 1992 Taking a giant leap towards freedom. *Nursing Standard* **6** (42), 23.

Jones, C. 1991 Confidence trick? UKCC guidelines on confidentiality. *Nursing Standard* **5** (41), 54–5.

Keown, J. 1993 Courting Euthanasia? Tony Bland and the Law Lords. *Ethics and Medicine* **9,** 3.

Richards, J. 1991 Ethical issues in clinical genetics. *Journal of the Royal College of Physicians of London* **25** (4), 284–8.

Rieu, S. 1994 Error and trial: the extended role dilemma. *British Journal of Nursing* **3** (4), 168–9 & 172–3.

Shapiro, R. 1986 Whatever happened to Warnock? *Nursing Times* **29** (82), 31–2.

Tingle, J. 1993 The extended role of the nurse: legal implications. *Care of the Critically Ill* **9** (1), 30–4.

Tingle, J. 1989 The law and the nurse. *Nursing Standard.* **4** (12), 20–2.

Tudor, M. 1993 Persistent vegetative state: some clinical observations. *Ethics and Medicine* **9** (3), 37.

9

New ways for managing change

Marilyn Williams

Introduction
Professional change
Personal change
Critical incident analysis
Organisational change
Reflective activities

Anyone who has read thus far in this book cannot fail to be aware that the book is concerned with perioperative nursing in a period of major change for health care and for nursing. It is one of those times in history when events move rapidly, probably because society has reached one of those critical points when the way things are can no longer hold society together. Historians call this phenomenon discontinuity and a considerable amount of historical research is devoted to analysing the causes of continuity and discontinuity. Using the exact science of hindsight it may seem that some events or developments were inevitable but a well-known historian will tell you that 'nothing in history is inevitable' (Carr, 1987). Carr goes on to point out that 'to have happened differently the antecedent causes would have had to be different.' This is a salutary thought to keep in mind when considering not only change itself but the process of change and how we can have some control over change.

Marilyn Williams has spent considerable time during the last few years in studying change and change management. Her chapter considers how the current time of change is affecting perioperative nursing on a professional, personal and organisational level. After reviewing the changes which have taken place, and continue to take place, during the century both generally and in the nursing profession, she turns to the effects of change on the individual, especially the perioperative nurse. The section on strategies for coping with change will be particularly helpful. Many nurses may find themselves in a working environment very different from that into which they first entered. Rather than feeling threatened and dependent, Marilyn Williams suggests that there are ways in which self-empowerment can help individuals to develop themselves to turn the challenges of today and tomorrow into the opportunities of the day after that. She suggests critical incident analysis as a starting point to gain insights into self and the organisational environment in which the nurse is working.

To design your future, visualise where you want to be, and then build your bridge from your present, to that place.

Your vision becomes your destiny, and your bridge becomes your path.

Blackwolf and Gina Jones (1998).

Introduction

This chapter looks at change and ways of dealing with it from both a personal and organisational point of view. Nurses and other people working in the National Health Service (NHS) will have witnessed and may have been a part of many organisational changes over the 50 years for which the NHS has existed. Ways in which individuals can deal with change and ways in which organisations may manage change, are analysed.

Approaching the new millennium is an appropriate time to reflect on changes during this century. Many of the changes in the world during this time have been brought about by revolution and conflict. Two world wars and other conflicts have engaged man's ingenuity to produce yet more terrible weapons, providing the crucible in which many industrial advances were smelted and forged. Many millions of people have died in wars in the service of their countries, making the ultimate sacrifice for causes they may or may not have believed in. The resultant changes can sometimes be seen in the drawing of new borders, or new political systems, or simply in the freedoms which so many of us take for granted.

Other changes have been brought about by peaceful means and scientific advances. These changes have contributed so much to the increasing well-being and comfort of mankind. New medicines, devices and techniques have enabled the eradication of some diseases, or increased the range of treatments available for others. There are philosophical arguments about when or what has changed during this century (Fulcher, 1997), but the fact that change has occurred is undeniable. Theories are offered to explain change in an historical context, differentiating between planned and unplanned change, offering the rationalisation that change is an inevitable and natural occurrence, the result of changes in the ways in which people think and behave over time (Elias, 1977).

The development of information technology and the communications systems which enable information to be shared all over the planet have enabled change on a massive and rapid scale. This change has contributed significantly to the good of mankind. However, some of these advances have proved to be double-edged; nuclear power for example, with its enormous potential for good in medical diagnosis and treatment, remains a fearful weapon of war, and has, as yet unknown long term consequences for the future of the planet. Similarly, the Internet, where the global sharing of information can be subverted for exploitative and destructive purposes as well as for good. Controlling the use to which new developments are put may not always be possible (as with the Internet) but by being aware of what is available, individuals and groups, such as nurses, are better placed to keep pace with developments and use them for the benefit of patients in their care.

Benjamin & Levinson (1995) describe a framework for change based on the use of information technology. Essential to this process is the empowerment of workers who have to use the technology, or instigate new processes which result from it (Roberts, 1983). This is a pertinent point in dealing with change in any context. Changes imposed by management are so often instigated with no preparation or discussion with those affected. Nurses in operating theatres often feel disempowered to start with, reacting to change by resisting it rather than being a part of it, resulting in a feeling of helplessness (Conway, 1996). A sympathetic and supportive approach to change where all those involved feel a part of the process, produces a shift of power based on possession of information, thus enabling change to progress with less fear (Benjamin & Levinson, 1995).

Lilley (1995) believes that the future must be our own creation, and that we should not expect help to deal with it, but rather be at the forefront of change, prepared and ready by our own efforts to meet the challenges of tomorrow. This dynamic new world is, according to Lilley, an 'arena of opportunity that may be impossible for some to enter and for others to exist in' but, he adds significantly 'there is an overlooked opportunity in the health arena for the nursing profession' (Lilley, 1995). Accepting such profound personal responsibilities would require a fundamental change in thinking for most nurses who tend to rely on regular employment and the salaries that go with it, as well as expecting employers to fund and/or provide continuing education. Employers carry no obligation to provide continuing education (Williams, 1996a), and, these days, NHS Trusts can and do change conditions and contracts of employment with consequent effects on salaries. Such issues as redundancy and major downgrading are painful and very threatening. Nurses have still not fully accepted that there is no longer such a thing as a guaranteed job for life.

Professional change

Many nurses, including this author, were told when they qualified that they had a secure future. This is obviously no longer the case; changes in the structure of health care and the development of support staff mean that many of the tasks which nurses previously undertook are now done by others. An American experience of managing profound changes in nursing structure and function is described by Boynton & Rothman (1995). They admitted, at the outset, that the change process would be 'charged with considerable pain, as well as opportunities for disillusionment, anger, and even a sense of malaise in the organisation'. Johnstone (1993) describes the similar integration of nurses in Australia into general management posts in spite of a heavily prejudiced political and organisational system.

In the UK, a significant change in health care management has been the development of integrated care pathways (ICPs). These are rather like package holidays: 'simple and clear plans of proposed clinical activities developed by multidisciplinary teams, expert in the diagnostic group for which the ICP is written' (Luther, 1997). Unfortunately, there exists the potential for a conflict of nursing ideology in this approach, as it flies in the face of the holistic, individualised care of patients promoted by Henderson (1980) and embraced and developed by Benner (1984) ... 'caring cannot be controlled or coerced; it can only be understood and facilitated'. The task of nursing in dealing with this is to find a halfway house where the diagnostic and curative approach of medicine can be reconciled with the caring and nurturing approach of nursing, in a political climate which supplies the funding. No easy options here!

Nurses, too, have shifted their traditional role towards medicine and medical tasks, discarding duties deemed to be less skilled.[1] Doctors have been happy to discard tasks which they consider to be mundane and routine and not requiring medical skills. These are the tasks which some nurses have embraced. Under the banner of the Scope of Professional Practice (UKCC 1992a)[2], nurses are now encroaching into medical roles. Nurses are undertaking invasive diagnostic and surgical procedures, as well as instituting treatment and monitoring its effects. The arguments about 'mini doctor' or 'maxi nurse' will continue until each profession is satisfied that it is performing in the most appropriate role. There is no way of knowing how long this process may take, but these are significant changes of which nursing and nurses will continue to be a part.

The shifting of practice boundaries is influenced by many things. Politics, markets and money are probably the most influential. The delivery of health care is an endlessly expensive business and the shifting of practice boundaries is one approach to containing or reducing costs. The influence here of both politics and markets is obvious. Consumerism is not a new idea. Regarding patients as clients was once regarded as revolutionary, now our patients are not only clients but also customers.

> Consumerism ... is about customer relations, not patients rights. It is concentrating its efforts on waiting lists, on delays in outpatients.
>
> Winkler (1987).

In the UK internal market, the competition it has brought means that providers are anxious to secure contracts at competitive rates. This means looking at the delivery of health care from many angles.

As wages and salaries are a considerable part of providers' costs, ways of reducing these costs have become imperative. Engaging a cheaper workforce, by whatever means, is tempting.

> The NHS reforms were instrumental in focusing providers' attention onto marketing ... economic survival is a powerful motivation for adopting a marketing strategy.
>
> Neylon (1995).

It is more cost-effective to train and employ nurses to function in expanded roles than to employ more doctors. It is also 'cheaper' to train and employ support staff than to take on more nurses. The potential for conflict between the groups affected by these changes is obvious. At the top of this skills exchange it appears that everyone is a winner, but in exchanging skills and roles there is a danger that such divisions of labour and delegating of tasks will lead to deskilling for some.

An example, here, would be helpful: if a nurse is trained to perform endoscopy procedures, these will be carried out within very strictly defined parameters. This would restrict that nurse's practice to a narrow set of tasks, the nurse would not be a doctor although he or she would be operating in a doctor's role. That nurse would bring other useful and relevant skills to the task, possibly enabling the delivery of more holistic care. However, the restrictions of the role might well outweigh the advantages.

This scenario could be repeated in other situations. The support worker who measures blood pressure and temperatures of patients, may not fully understand the significance of the readings and, therefore, not report potentially important signs. A qualified nurse would bring greater knowledge to the task, and, therefore, be able to act upon the readings, as well as making them. The question of accountability and responsibility is also significant here as the qualified nurse is bound to account for his or her practice to the professional body, whereas the support worker is not.

In terms of ownership and control, nurses have demonstrated, and are continuing to demonstrate, that they are happy to take on semi-medical roles as endoscopists and surgeons' assistants. The same innovations have opened up new avenues and career pathways for nurses and also for Operating Department Assistants (ODAs) and Operating Department Practitioners (ODPs). Such competition for careers is another dimension of change which perioperative nurses have to deal with, and this process is going to continue.

> We have moved into a world where conventional business approaches make very little sense. Technology and invention will make today's products and services redundant. Just as we master the skills we need to survive for today, we will need to learn new ones for tomorrow.
>
> Lilley (1995).

This puts the responsibility for managing change firmly in the hands of each and every individual.

Denying the need to change is futile. Research in all disciplines and walks of life means that knowledge is expanding and crying out to be used. We cannot 'disinvent' computers, lasers, space travel or any of the other significant developments of the century. Sensible people would not wish to do so. Some of these inventions have touched almost everyone and may have required the acquisition of new skills and learning in order for these inventions to be useful to us. Creating the right environment for learning is as important as the learning itself. In order to learn effectively, adults need:

> an ethos of support, encouragement, non-judgmental acceptance, mutual help and individual responsibility.
>
> Meizrow (1981).

If this environment is not provided for you, you may have to create it for yourself.

Learning to use a computer may have been seen as a threat where you work. Maybe your employer had not prepared you properly or given you the opportunity to become properly skilled in the use of computers. In such circumstances it would not be surprising if you believed that the introduction of computers was a threat to your position. The same would apply to theatre nurses who have had to accept a whole new range of surgical procedures and a new and very complex set of instruments with which to perform them. The rapid introduction and expansion of minimal access surgery is a good example.[3] The surgeon is interested in having the appropriate equipment and he will be developing skills in using it. The theatre nurse will have to become intimately familiar with all of the variations in the instruments and the operations they enable. Both of these roles require a considerable amount of new learning, and this learning will need to be mastered whilst working, and in a relatively short time. However much support is provided in such situations, a shadow of threat may persist in the background. Many perioperative nurses will find the preceding description familiar and could justifiably take a great deal of satisfaction from the realisation that they have mastered the skills of a considerable range of procedures and the instrumentation that goes with them.

Those already mentioned are a few of the changes which have contributed so much to the increasing wellbeing and comfort of people. New medicines, new devices, and new techniques have enabled medicine to eradicate some diseases and increase the range of treatment for other ailments. Few would wish to return to the days when many people suffered and died in epidemics.

The advancement of medicine has been accompanied by a corresponding advancement in nursing as well as in the development of other professions allied to medicine. Nursing has responded positively in a variety of ways to the challenges these changes have brought. But in some ways nursing is still struggling to shake off the shackles of the suppression of women during the 19th century. In many ways, nurses display the characteristics of an oppressed group (Roberts, 1983). For all of the feminists' progress in highlighting the inferior and unfair treatment of women worldwide, it remains a fact that gender issues are still influential in determining the progress of women in nursing today and this can often be seen in the microcosm of society created in operating theatres and hospital wards. Female nurses can still be seen acting as handmaidens to doctors and surgeons (Conway, 1996). Nursing, itself, is not always comfortable with this situation. Medicine is now almost equally divided by gender. Nursing is still female-dominated, yet advancement in nursing turns the gender issue on its head by promoting men more rapidly to higher managerial positions and in much greater numbers than women. This situation is ripe for change. Nurses at all levels and regardless of their gender need to accept responsibility and take control of their situation, as ownership and control are fundamental to managing change:

> Freedom … involves rejecting the negative images of one's own culture and replacing them with pride and a sense of ability to function autonomously.
>
> Roberts (1983).

Personal change

Reflection on nursing experience, its processes and consequences, is one way of dealing with the feelings created when change is proposed or introduced. There is no universal agreement about exactly what 'reflection' means (Conway, 1996) but its value as a learning process comes from examining:

> the total response of a person to a situation or event: what he or she thinks, feels, does or concludes at the time and immediately thereafter.
>
> Boud *et al.* (1985).

Those unfamiliar with reflection as an enquiring and learning process may be tempted to relate to its physical manifestation, associated with reflected images in mirrors showing what we can already see (Boud *et al.*, 1985). That is a useful starting point as reflection requires starting with what is and then asking how this came to be and how we might then move on to a new point of knowledge, based on learning from our personal questioning of past experiences and actions.

It is important to note here that reflecting on the past in order to find pathways through the future may require challenging long held beliefs and letting go of scientific certainties which are often the hallmark of practising professionals (Schon, 1983). Benner (1984) makes this point succinctly for nurses, declaring:

> Behaviour can be seen as having potentially multiple rather than single meanings. To understand behaviour, therefore, one must look at its larger context.

Your reflections will, therefore, be influenced by many things from that larger context, including your childhood, upbringing, religion, faith, education and many other life experiences. In order to understand behaviour, you first have to know and understand yourself. This can be an uncomfortable and challenging experience, leaving you dissatisfied or disillusioned and no further forward in dealing with change. Or it could reveal things you need to know in order to move on. One widely accepted method of understanding behaviour is by using the 'critical incident technique' (Flanagan, 1954).

Critical incident analysis

Critical incident analysis involves taking specific incidents in which you were personally involved and analysing the significance of them in terms of your feelings, thoughts and responses at the time and later (Williams, 1996b). As a starting point, write accounts of critical incidents you have been involved in and reflect on them. In order to guide your reflections, the nursing literature provides many useful sources, some of these are listed as recommended reading at the end of this chapter. This exercise would be a useful beginning to your professional portfolio.

Your own unique humanity is based in your personal philosophy and value system, the result of all of the already mentioned influences and many more. Reflection on one particular incident may lead to:

the more general questioning of accepted practices and traditions, whether religious or otherwise.

Hanfling (1987).

The question 'why?' obtrudes itself everywhere, and answers are not always available. Raya (1990) also emphasises the importance of promoting values along with learning, declaring that they:

> ... can increase the student's respect for truth, for the worth and rights of other persons, his appreciation of his own worth, assets and limitations, his love of wisdom and desire to serve humanity, his outlook about man's position in the world and his inquiring mind in order to discover the higher perspectives of life.

Such deep and meaningful explorations of self may create more questions than answers but the process of discovering your true self can reveal 'important insights into ... nurses as individuals and the workplace cultures which they inhabit' (Perry, 1997). This has particular significance for operating theatre nurses as the supportive cultures and social systems created in operating theatres may have a profound effect upon those nurses and the way they practice. Dealing with proposed changes within such systems would require this context to be acknowledged (Whitmeyer, 1997), so that the supportive mechanisms remain in place. The tremendous potency of reflection as a way of managing change is perhaps best summed up by Johns' (1998) declaration:

> The reflective practitioner is the creator of her world.

The presence or absence of socially supportive systems in hospitals and operating theatre suites may be a reflection of the overall culture of the hospital. Organisational culture is a profoundly influential phenomenon acknowledged in the literature on quality assurance (Atkinson, 1990; Stebbing, 1990; Thomas, 1995). Thomas points out the roller coaster of expectation followed by disappointment that can be created by change:

> Staff are often seduced by the promise of autonomy and freedom of action only to be bitterly disappointed when they discover that empowerment means 'empowerment to a point'. Real power commonly remains exactly where it was.

Thomas (1995).

Empowerment means control of your own destiny, and this is frequently denied to nurses facing changes such as the closure of hospitals or the reorganisation of services. In these circumstances, passive acceptance or self determined relocation may be the only options. Either of these courses might have long term consequences, for better or worse in the face of the outright brutality of some decisions made by employers.

Wicker (1998) illustrates all too clearly that loyalty, length of service, and experience can be dismissed out of hand, leaving nurses not only disempowered but unemployed. Berry (1995) explains how empowerment is central to success:

Empowerment is a state of mind ... management creates an empowered state of mind by treating employees as part owners of the business and expecting them to behave like owners. Employees have not only the authority but also the responsibility to use their skills, knowledge, judgement and creativity to serve their customers effectively and contribute to their company's success.

Whilst these sentiments are noble and admirable, it is unlikely that they would be applied in hospitals, even though the employees are in fact 'owners' of the business by virtue of their financial contributions to it. Adopting the principles on a small scale, say within one operating department, would be possible, under the supervision of a suitably motivated manager. Creating a culture in which the skills, knowledge and judgement of individuals are acknowledged and used would be the first step.

Organisational change

Organisational cultures are the result of many factors, and evolve over time, they are:

affected by the events of the past and by the climate of the present, by the technology of the type of work, by their aims and the kind of people who work in them.

Handy (1993).

Creating a supportive culture where individuals are valued, respected and given the opportunity to contribute to change and progress is a long-term process. The will to begin it has to be there from the start, and the success of Japan in rebuilding its economy after the second World War is quoted as an outstanding example (Atkinson, 1990).

Expanding on this Japanese approach, the concept of 'kaizen' has clear lessons for managing change in a health service context.

The essence of kaizen is simple and straightforward: kaizen means improvement. Moreover, kaizen means ongoing improvement involving everyone, including both managers and workers. The kaizen philosophy assumes that our way of life – be it our working social life, our social life, or our home life – deserves to be constantly improved.

Imai (1986).

The underlying philosophy of this approach is sound, making small changes, reviewing their effects, and responding by making more changes in a continual process which becomes a way of life at work and at home. Expecting British health care workers to absorb and incorporate this culture wholesale is probably not feasible, but applying it to the process of change in hospitals may be a practical way forward, if the management support for it is in place.

The message in respect of organisational culture as an effective method of change management is that evolution rather than revolution is the sensible approach. Respecting and empowering individuals, using their skills and knowledge, and listening to their ideas, removes or reduces the threat that proposed change often brings. If the whole organisation cannot or will not create a supportive culture, then small groups of individuals may be able to create a subculture 'pocket' for their own progress or survival. Staff in operating theatres often do this without realising it.

If you are facing, or dealing with, changes in your working life, it is understandable that you may be feeling threatened, insecure and powerless. On the other hand, you may feel stimulated and excited at the prospect of change and gratefully accept the opportunities it brings. Whatever your feelings are, you have choices. If the fear and threat are too great, you have the choice of changing your job, however difficult this might seem when first contemplated. Proposed radical changes affecting contracts, terms and conditions should always be discussed with your professional representative. If you do not have one, you should seriously consider contacting an appropriate organisation. For perioperative nurses, professional organisations exist in all countries. In the UK, the National Association of Theatre Nurses provides advice, both legal and professional, as well as indemnity for practice.

Taking responsibility for your own destiny can be an enlightening experience, even if it is borne out of fear. Change, indeed even total transformation, can be successfully managed in operating departments and hospitals, as illustrated by Davidson's (1998) account of making quality an everyday event. Further evidence of the success of involving people at all levels in decision making comes from Jackson's (1998) description of a shared governance initiative, where she admits that:

> as a member of theatre staff I found that I had become isolated and unaware of what was happening outside my own department.

This has been a common situation for nurses to find themselves in when working in the operating department. Keeping in touch with the wider world of nursing, through reading, attending study days, conferences or similar events and by visiting ward areas can help to keep knowledge up to date.

If you feel your knowledge and skills are out of date and this prohibits a change of job, blaming your employer for not sending you on any courses is futile. Continuing education has always been your own responsibility under the UKCC Code of Professional Conduct (UKCC, 1992b). Decide what it is you need to know and investigate ways of learning it. Review your career to date and compile a professional portfolio. You may be surprised at what you have to offer. Brown (1995) offers a very user-friendly and comprehensive guide to portfolio building.

It is easy to adopt a pessimistic and fatalistic view of change, blaming 'them' or 'the system' or 'the Government' for the situation you find yourself in or faced with. Things which are outside an individual's control have to be accepted and dealt with. Nurses must be prepared to take control of their own destiny, accept those things which cannot be changed and be a positive change agent for those things which have to change. Facing a brave new world of work need not be a daunting or negative experience as long as you keep your feet firmly on the ground and your mind focused on the reality of today. Today's National Health Service is not the one which most of us joined and trained in. As Wicker (1998) realises:

> You must believe that your employers owe you nothing. Then you are free to take personal responsibility for your career instead of relying on what you think are your rights, and you will be able to develop the skills which you need to adapt to an ever-changing workplace.

Reflective activities

Now you have read this chapter, why not sit down and reflect on how far the job you, as a nurse, now carry out has changed from the job you expected to carry out when you first started nursing. It is assumed that you work in some capacity in the operating department but you can still carry out this exercise wherever you are working.

1 Are the factors which have affected your job organisational, professional, economic or political or even personal? Are you still going through the change process or do you feel that the major changes have been completed? Are you sure they have? How much are you involved in or informed of decisions?

2 Now consider your personal reactions. Do you feel disempowered and threatened or can you seize the opportunity for self-development? Perhaps you have already done so.

3 Reflect on the last paragraph of this chapter to identify where you go from here. Change does not stop.

4 This chapter is advocating the use of reflection as a way of managing change and of empowering yourself and has proposed both further reading and the use of critical incident analysis. It is suggested that, if you have not already done so, you should use some of the methods described by the author and which will be found in the further reading to help you to analyse your personal situation or to address some of the organisational problems in your own work situation.

Endnotes

1 The first section of this book concentrates on discussing the developing roles of perioperative nurses. Refer to those chapters to identify how nursing practice is changing in ways discussed here.

2 The scope of professional practice has been discussed in some detail in the preceding chapters most especially in Chapters 3 and 8 to which you are referred.

3 Chapters 13 and 14 discuss the problems facing nurses as they took on minimal access surgery skills and offer an outline of how they were prepared and supported to develop these new skills.

References

Atkinson, P. 1990 *Creating culture change: the key to successful total quality management.* Bedford, IFS Publications.

Benjamin, R. & Levinson, E. 1995 A framework for managing IT enabled change. *Sloan Management Review* Summer, 23–33.

Benner, P. 1984 *From novice to expert: excellence and power in clinical nursing practice.* California, Addison Wesley.

Berry, L. 1995 *On great service.* London, The Free Press.

Boud, D., Keogh, R. & Walker, D. (Eds.) 1985 *Reflection: turning experience into learning.* London, Kogan Page.

Boynton, D. & Rothman, L. 1995 Stage managing change: supporting new patient care models. *Nursing Economics* **13** (3), 166–73.

Brown, R. 1995 *Portfolio development for nurses,* 2nd edition, Central Health Studies. Salisbury, Quay Books, a Division of Mark Allen Publishing.

Carr, E. H. 1987 *What is history? George Macauley Trevelyan Lectures, Cambridge, 1961,* 2nd edition. Davis, R. W. (Ed.) London, Penguin.

Conway, J. 1996 *Nursing expertise and advanced practice.* Key Management Skills in Nursing Series. Salisbury, Quay Books, a Division of Mark Allen Publishing.

Davidson, D. 1998 Quality: an everyday event. *British Journal of Theatre Nursing* **7** (10), 28–32.

Elias, N. 1977 Towards a theory of social processes – English translation by Dunning, E. & van Krieken, R. *British Journal of Sociology* **48** (3), 355–83.

Flanagan, J. 1954 The critical incident technique. *Psychological Bulletin* **5** (4), 327–58.

Fulcher, J. 1997 Did British society change character in the 1920s or the 1980s? *British Journal of Sociology* **8** (3), 514–21.

Handy, C. 1993 *Understanding organisations.* London, Penguin Books.

Hanfling, O. (Ed.) 1987 *Life and meaning, a reader.* Oxford, The Open University.

Henderson, V. 1980 Preserving the essence of nursing in a technological age. *Journal of Advanced Nursing* **5**, 245–60.

Imai, M. 1986 *Kaizen, the key to Japan's competitive success.* London, McGraw-Hill.

Jackson, P. 1998 Shared governance – a personal view. *British Journal of Theatre Nursing* **7** (11), 24.

Johns, C. 1998 Illuminating the transformative potential of guided reflection. In: Johns, C. & Freshwater, D. (Eds.) *Transforming nursing through reflective practice.* Oxford, Blackwell Science.

Johnstone, P. 1993 Why not a nurse as a general health service executive? *Australian Health Review* **16** (4), 430–45.

Lilley, R. 1995 *Futureproofing.* Oxford, The Radcliffe Press.

Luther, T. 1997 Managed care: development of an integrated care pathway in neurosciences. *NT Research* **2** (4), 283–91.

Miezrow, J. 1981 A critical theory of adult learning and education. *Adult Education* **32** (1), 3–24.

Neylon, J. 1995 Put your trust in the future. *Nursing Management* **2** (2), 14–15.

Perry, L. 1997 Critical incidents, crucial issues: insights into the working lives of registered nurses. *Journal of Advanced Nursing* **6,** 131–7.

Raya, A. 1990 Can knowledge be promoted and values ignored? Implications for nursing education. *Journal of Advanced Nursing* **15,** 504–9.

Roberts, S. 1983 Oppressed group behaviour: implications for nursing. *Advances in Nursing Science* **5** (4), 21–30.

Schon, D. 1983 *The reflective practitioner, how professionals think in action.* Basic Books, a Division of Harper Collins.

Stebbing, L. 1990 *Quality management in the service industry.* London, Ellis Horwood.

Thomas, B. 1995 *The human dimension of quality.* London, McGraw-Hill.

UKCC. 1992a *Scope of professional practice.* London, UKCC.

UKCC. 1992b *Code of professional conduct.* London, UKCC.

Whitmeyer, J. 1997 Mann's theory of power: a (sympathetic) critique. *British Journal of Sociology* **48** (2), 211–25.

Wicker, P. 1998 Editorial: A brave new world. *British Journal of Theatre Nursing* **7** (12), 3.

Williams, M. 1996a *Managing continuing education, a consumer's and provider's point of view.* Key Management Skills in Nursing Series. Salisbury, Quay Books, a Division of Mark Allen Publishing.

Williams, M. 1996b Reflection, thinking and learning. *British Journal of Theatre Nursing* **6** (5), 26–7.

Winkler, F. 1987 Consumerism in health care: beyond the supermarket model. *Policy and Politics* **15** (1), 1–8.

Further reading

Andrews, M. 1996 Using reflection to develop clinical expertise. *British Journal of Nursing* **5** (8), 503–13.

Argris, C. & Schon, D. 1974 *Theory in practice: increasing professional effectiveness.* Massachusetts, Addison-Wesley.

Atkins, S. & Murphy, K. 1993 Reflection: a review of the literature. *Journal of Advanced Nursing* **18**, 1188–92.

Campbell, I. 1991 The reflective practitioner. *Nursing Standard* **5** (19), 34–5.

Carr, E. 1996 Reflecting on clinical practice: hectoring talk or reality? *Journal of Clinical Nursing* **5** (5), 289-95.

Clare, J. 1993 A challenge to rhetoric of emancipation: recreating a professional culture. *Journal of Advanced Nursing* **18** (7), 133–8.

Johns, C. 1996 Using a reflective model of nursing and guided reflection. *Nursing Standard* **11** (2), 34–8.

Jones, A. 1995 Reflective process in action: uncovering the ritual of washing in nursing practice. *Journal of Clinical Nursing* **4**, 283–8.

Kolb, D. & Fry, R. 1975 *Towards an applied theory of experiential learning.* In: Cooper, C. (ed.) *Theories of group processes.* London, John Wiley.

Richardson, G. & Maltby, H. 1995 Reflection-on-practice: enhancing student learning. *Journal of Advanced Nursing* **22**, 235–42.

Keeping abreast of issues in infection control

10

Kate Nightingale

In Chapter 2 Doreen Kalideen defines infection control as one of the main areas of expertise of the perioperative nurse. I would agree with this. Perioperative nurses were often regarded as the experts in this field in their own hospital and were often asked for advice or became involved in teaching the subject to others. Nowadays, we have specialist infection control nurses who provide invaluable information to both surgeons and theatre personnel, but students still find that the one placement during which they begin to understand how infection spreads and to value the measures taken to prevent the spread of infection is that which is spent in the operating department. At a time when outpatient surgery is being carried out in general practice procedure rooms and day care units, it is particularly unfortunate that many schools and colleges of nursing see this aspect of nurse education as of little value and no longer include time in the operating department as part of the practical experience of student nurses.

The earlier part of this chapter takes a broad view of infection control issues whilst the later part focuses on the issues of current concern for perioperative nurses. Recent years have seen new threats of infection as well as new challenges from the revolution in surgery. The increased risks from blood-borne viruses and the rapid growth in minimal access surgery have given new opportunities for perioperative nurses to liaise with pathologists, engineers, managers, lawyers and others to develop revolutionary, safe and effective methods of infection control. All of this requires constant vigilance and awareness of current changes and innovations. Risk assessment is of considerable importance in this field. For further information on that you are referred to Chapter 11.

Introduction

The programme of the World Conference of Operating Room Nurses (WCORN) in Vienna in 1989 contained, for the first time, a session on 'universal precautions'. I wonder how many of us realised at the time that this signalled the end of the bright confident morning of infection control as we had known it. Before the 1980s we knew which microorganisms were the main dangers in surgery and we perceived those largely as a small number of well-known bacteria. There were the staphylococci, resident on the skin of all of us, many of which were non-pathogenic. We knew we had streptococci lurking in our nasopharynxes and respiratory tracts. And our theatre technique was largely designed to ensure that bacteria, in particular sporing bacteria, notably tetanus and gas gangrene, stayed where we wanted them to stay, on the floor or outside the operating theatre. We had a battery of techniques, physical methods and chemical agents, to combat those infections which were a threat to the patient. We knew when and how these familiar enemies could gain access to wounds and we knew how both to prevent and treat this. This knowledge provided the foundation of theatre aseptic technique.

Priorities were focused on risks to the patient when the surgeon breached his first line of defence, the skin, and on the risks of nosocomial infection. The major aim was, and remains, the prevention of wound infection. So perioperative nurses took steps to prevent cross-infection from patient to patient, from the operating department environment or from the staff present during surgery. Risks of infection to the surgical team were regarded as minimal unless a cut was sustained from a used scalpel or other instrument. In operating departments, blood was regarded as messy but sterile and, until the recognition of the dangers of the virus responsible for serum hepatitis, treated with scant respect as a possible infection risk to staff and patients alike.

Box 10.1   Theatre technique

1   Theatre design and ventilation designed to reduce airborne particles around wound.

2   All activity preceded by hand washing, cleaning, wearing clean scrub suits and scrubbable shoes. Masks worn during surgery and in sterile areas.

3   Theatre procedures carried out to maintain clean environment.

4   Antiseptic technique used to clean wound site and hands of scrub team.

5   Scrub team don gloves and gowns in aseptic style and practise aseptic technique to maintain sterility of all items and prevent contamination of wound by pathogens.

6   Circulating person (runner, scout) is the link to present sterile materials to scrub team.

7   Following wound closure all items used are either disposed of as clinical waste or are decontaminated before recycling.

(After Brigden, 1988)

These basic principles of aseptic technique, aimed at preventing infection of the surgical site, still apply, but have now been modified to include precautions to protect the operating department staff. National standards or guidelines have been developed which observe universal precautions and allow for the increased use of endoscopes, lasers and other pre-packaged items (see below).

The priorities which formed the basis of theatre technique have not gone away. It is still necessary to protect the patient from bacterial infection during surgery but, also, to recognise the far more complicated nature of the environment in which modern surgery takes place. Surgery itself has become infinitely more complex. The materials and equipment used are far more complex. The numbers of people involved in preparing and undertaking surgical procedures are greater. Sterile materials are prepared far from the operating site and must be transported there. The need for detailed record-keeping is greater – and that means a lot of pens and computers, used by numbers of different pairs of hands. Nor is an operating department a very environmentally friendly place in a world running short of resources and in which man is increasingly polluting his environment. Hand-washing, and scrubbing up remain important and must be carried out correctly (Clarke & Jones, 1998, pp.251–2). Mask wearing, which was beginning to be seen as unnecessary, continues but for self-protection rather than patient-protection (Orr, 1981; Norman, 1995).

There has been a great acceleration in the growing technical nature of instrumentation, bringing with it difficulties of decontaminating and sterilising endoscopes and the complicated electronic equipment which has become increasingly necessary in a modern operating department. Greater awareness was unavoidable for perioperative nurses as such techniques became a regular part of the armamentarium of the surgeon. Yet, much of the increasing technical knowledge and new skills were, at first, confined to those using the newer equipment and comparatively slowly became part of routine infection control techniques in all operating departments.

Today's new infection risks

Perhaps the greatest shock of all was the realisation that the battle against pathogenic microorganisms has not been won and probably never will be won. We had, in fact, very nearly lost it. However quickly scientists have been able to develop new disinfectants and antibiotics, the microorganisms have always had one great advantage in their battle with us. Their reproduction rate is so much faster than ours. They evolve at a far speedier rate, are able to mutate and develop new resistance to whatever weapons we use against them. Their numbers are legion. They have always been able to move into new environmental niches. And how we have offered them new niches into which to move! As a result, perioperative infection control now has to concern itself not only with the prevention of wound infections, but with the prevention of more generalised infections which can affect both patient and staff.

Early principles of infection control in operating departments were aimed largely at those microorganisms resident on the skin. Skin cannot be sterilised and so, even today, we use antiseptic, not aseptic, methods to clean the operation site and the hands of the staff before they put on their surgical gloves. Many modern procedures and operative techniques depend on the ability to enable a sterile field by the use of antibiotics and by good disinfection and sterilisation methods in advance of surgery. Many instruments and much equipment, especially endoscopes, must be decontaminated after use as well as being sterilised before use on the next patient or before being handled in the sterile supplies department.

Box 10.2   Glossary of terms

Antisepsis
usually refers to skin antisepsis. There is no way to sterilise skin, therefore, it is rendered as clean as possible, either mechanically as in 'scrubbing up' or by the use of a germicidal solution as in 'skin preparation' of the wound site(s).

Asepsis
means absence of infection or pathogenic organisms and is achieved by sterilisation. How long sterility persists is variable and depends on a number of factors. Once open to the air sterility begins to be compromised.

Disinfection
is the destruction of all actively reproducing organisms (this excludes spores) and can be achieved by the use of chemicals such as sodium hydrochloride or glutaraldehyde. Soaking in the solution means that the item is potentially de-sterilised as soon as it

emerges from the solution and must be used immediately. More modern methods include the use of such disinfectants in sub-atmospheric autoclaves.

Sterilisation
Strictly speaking the destruction of all life but, in this instance, referring to microorganisms. Because of its nature and intent, sterilisation is inherently destructive. Therefore, a number of methods have to be available to avoid destruction of instruments and equipment. Intricate instruments may have to be single use[1] if the sterilising agent cannot penetrate to all parts. Includes hot air ovens, autoclaving (steam under pressure), ionising radiation, ethylene oxide and low temperature systems. (Irradiation and ethylene oxide gas are more largely used by manufacturers as they need expensive plant, safety precautions and time consuming methods which are not cost-effective in hospitals.)

It is incredible to think that medicine was so complacent as to believe that serious infections had been conquered when we were constantly being given signals that this was not so. The 'hospital staphylococcus', that is a strain of *Staphylococcus aureus* with resistance to penicillin, was recognised at least by the early 1950s. The tubercle bacillus was always difficult to combat other than by multiple medication, and we are now seeing this scourge return as a secondary infection in those with reduced immune defences and/or deprived lifestyles. This time the resistance of the tubercle to antibiotics seems to be even more effective.

Pseudomonas colonies found their way into Winchester bottles of Savlon, into water traps in laboratory sinks and into sucker bottles in intensive care units. How long is it since we first became aware of multiple resistance in *Staphylococcus aureus*? How alarming it has been to watch the progress of the methicillin resistant *Staphylococcus aureus* across the world until it arrived in our own hospital or district. We are running out of antibiotics which are effective against such robust bacteria. Now only vancomycin can be used against some *Staphylococcus aureus* and resistance is being established even against this antibiotic by some strains (Domin, 1998).

We have never been able to control viruses by antibiotics. The nature of viruses, using their host's RNA to replicate themselves, makes sure that they would only be destroyed by methods or substances also harmful to the host. But, did we, and more especially, did doctors become complacent when we thought that the vast majority of infections could be treated by antibiotics? Was there a persistent hope that the 'magic bullet', effective against all infections, would one day be discovered?

The current pandemic of a life-threatening infection, the human immuno-deficiency virus (HIV), focused the minds of many, indeed caused in some degree, the sort of panic reactions not experienced since the days of the great plagues. Reference to old-style epidemics reminds us that the latest figures, as announced on a television programme at the end of 1989, suggest that the death rate for HIV in sub-Saharan Africa may soon reach 30%. This is comparable to the figures now generally agreed for the European death rate during the Black Death of the 14th century, until now the largest percentage of deaths caused by a single epidemic disaster (Porter, 1997, p.123.) There were even suggestions in the early days of the pandemic that those infected should be isolated away from the general population, one of the nastier reactions to such threats not well-understood by the general population.

Reactions in health care varied from total disregard of the possibility of infection to the use of total isolation suits and refusal by some non-professional staff to be involved at all in the care of infected patients. We have had to return to thinking in terms of prevention rather than complacently believing that infections are always controllable. Some of our prevention techniques have thrown up problems of their own. The increased use of latex gloves, for example, has made us all too aware of the dangers of allergic reactions to latex.

I began the literature search for this chapter by turning to Medline and Cinahl on the Internet. Despite limiting the search to English and to the last three years, it was an awesome revelation to realise just how broad are the implications resulting from the emergence of new infections and the developing resistance of old infections. Technical advances, widespread travel and neglect of some old precautions from pre-antibiotic days have also increased the risks. The search also proved a good indicator of the current areas of greatest concern in the field.

By far the largest number of articles listed were about infections due to multiple resistant *Staphylococcus aureus* (MRSA). A second large group were focusing on the traditional areas of operating department infection control: air filtration and circulation in theatres, evaluating impermeable materials for gowns and drapes, hand washing and barriers. (Have new risks made it necessary to check the reliability of our existing infection control procedures? Have new legal controls made it obligatory to know that the processes are meeting statutory requirements?) A considerable amount of ink has been spilt on blood-borne viruses, as one would expect. Most of these items were on HIV, but there are also a number on the multiplying range of hepatitis infections. Serum hepatitis is, of course, the viral infection which presents the highest risk in the operating department. (See discussions below.)

Many new guidelines, some as codes of practice, some as legislation, have been published. A considerable number of organisations are engaged in developing guidelines for infection control, not least the Center for Disease Control in Atlanta which was, of course, the originator of universal precautions (Satcher, 1996). The immunisation of health care workers against hepatitis is also a matter under considerable discussion, a responsibility which has been lodged with occupational health departments in the UK. Another priority is the achievement of cost-effective infection control. Ensuring safety for both staff and patients has considerable cost implications. The World Health Organization has a role in both surveillance and prevention but it faces an enormous task in tackling the new threats from old diseases (Lee, 1996). Perioperative nurses, working in areas of high infection risk, have the support of their professional bodies who monitor the literature and official publications and update their guidelines and standards at regular intervals.

Antibiotic resistance and bacterial virulence

It is interesting to note that areas of nursing and medicine formerly not known for their concern with infection control, such as nursing homes caring for the elderly, have found it necessary to concern themselves with the development of infection control procedures (Brunner & Suddarth, 1992, Chapter 2). Elderly patients have shown themselves to be particularly susceptible to infections by resistant microorganisms (Kerr *et al.*, 1990). Of course, the general public are increasingly aware of the threat of these new 'superbugs', as the media describe them.

The general press quickly got hold of this threat to health, describing necrotising fasciitis in terms more notable for their dramatic effect than their accuracy. The effect on the public of alarmist press reports is difficult to assess. Information which is presented with great elan and drama is often quite old and inaccurate news. How much does this increased awareness influence changes in behaviour? Denial or scapegoating rather than adaptation seems to be the more common responses. We only have to make the comparison with our own experience in the operating department to realise how slowly such change in behaviour is effected.

One of the more measured articles on new infections appeared in the *Sunday Times* of 26 April 1998, following an announcement by the UK Public Health Laboratory that it had found a 'strain of bug resistant to every known antibiotic.' The author, Anthony Daniels, went on to discuss the question of antibiotic resistance in an extremely balanced manner. He pointed out that the 'existence of resistant organisms does not mean that they will ramp ferociously through the population.'

Doctors ready to over-prescribe, farmers feeding their animals antibiotics to encourage growth rates of their stock and greedy pharmaceutical companies have all been blamed for the development of bacterial resistance, to say nothing of patients who do not complete the prescribed course of antibiotics. It is not always possible to assign blame. There are many social and economic reasons why such practices are established. Once established, the same or other reasons may perpetuate them. Have you never left the last few pills in the bottom of the bottle when you felt better, either intentionally or because you forgot to take them? In fact, we have probably been very lucky to keep pathogens under control for as long as we have. Bacterial resistance to antibiotics depends on enzyme production by the bacteria. Not only do the fittest survive by a process of natural selection but, by sharing genetic material, microorganisms are able to transfer resistance to others (Daniels, 1998).

Tuberculosis

Of course, the incidence of disease is not always related to resistance to antibiotics. Take tuberculosis, for example. The disease incidence was already much reduced by the time streptomycin was introduced after the second World War. Despite the fact that medicine now had an effective weapon against the tubercle bacillus, the disease was already in retreat from its highest incidence in the 19th century. Was this due to a change in the organism itself or was the reduced incidence due to better public health, better housing or better diet? Or were there socioeconomic or demographic factors, unnoticed at the time, in operation? The return of the tubercle in a newer resistant format has also been due to social changes. Current predisposing factors include poor standards of living due to demographic and political changes and immunosuppression, including AIDS (Brunner & Suddarth, 1992, p.1186).

Beta-haemolytic streptococcus

Another organism which has changed its presentation enormously over the last 50 years is the beta-haemolytic streptococcus. In the 1940s it was still capable of causing a severe toxic tonsillitis accompanied by a rash and it was known as scarlet fever (Conybeare & Mann, 1954). Children still died of this disease and were nursed in isolation hospitals or sometimes developed long-term heart or kidney conditions. By the 1960s, the disease was much milder, and often did not even entail time off school. Nowadays we talk of 'strep throats'. This is one infection for which the drug of choice is still penicillin (Brunner & Suddarth, 1992, p.1182).

Escherichia coli

Outside the range of pathogens likely to present a significant risk in the operating department we are increasingly becoming aware of new risks. Enteric organisms, such as our old friend *Escherichia coli*, have been presented in the press as lethal monsters following outbreaks of food poisoning in which people died due to infections by a virulent and resistant strain of *E. coli* 0157. Unfortunately, it is just these enteric organisms which are demonstrating resistance to vancomycin (Domin, 1998). There appears to be a strain of the organism which exists in a reservoir in cattle. It can cause bloody diarrhoea, thrombocytopenic purpura and kidney failure. It came into the news after 1989 when a high incidence began to be apparent in Scotland (Sharp, 1998). What happens if we find carriers of this pathogen coming for surgery? At present there do not appear to be sufficient people with immunity to the virulent strain for this to constitute a threat. One thing which is certain is that nature always finds a way to respond, whether it be by developing resistance in microorganisms or immunity in higher animals.

Another interesting case of food poisoning reported in 1998 was an outbreak of botulism caused by potatoes! The significance of this was that the potatoes had been kept for a considerable time wrapped in foil at an ambient temperature. If this can happen with one organism it can occur with others (Angulo, 1998). Temperature control is significant in infection control.

We should remember that before penicillin was discovered many techniques for controlling infection were well established. Once microorganisms were recognised as the cause of infection, basic hygiene, cleaning and the use of antiseptics were able to render our environment cleaner. In operating theatres clean clothes, gloves, first cotton then rubber, and the development of antiseptic and, later, aseptic techniques made surgery safer. Hand-washing, boiling instruments and autoclaving linen drapes and gowns had excluded many pathogens and brought surgical infections under control long before the use of antibiotics. Increasing knowledge of pathogens and their modes of spread enabled us to continuously refine infection control techniques.

> The idea that without antibiotics which work, we should necessarily return to primitive conditions is false. The vast majority of us would be unaffected. The moral of the story of bacterial resistance to antibiotics is that there is no final victory in medicine ... One set of problems is replaced by another, but this is not to deny the reality of progress ...
>
> Daniels (1998).

Transferable spongiform encephalitis

Another phenomenon of which we are now increasingly aware, is the ability of microorganisms to cross from one species to another such as the group of diseases known as transferable spongiform encephalitis (TSE). The classic example of this is bovine spongiform encephalitis (BSE). Known historically as scrapie, a disease of sheep, this disease appears to have crossed the species barrier when man began to grind up unwanted protein material from carcasses to feed to cattle. Eventually, it was recognised that the disease was appearing in man as 'new variant' Creutzfeld–Jakob disease (CJD) and that it had probably been caught from eating low-grade beef, possibly in 'fast food' such as beef-burgers. British beef, reputed to have a particularly high incidence of BSE, became taboo throughout the world with immense economic repercussions for the beef farmers of Great Britain.

CREUTZFELD-JAKOB DISEASE (CJD)

Characteristics of CJD are:

- Long incubation period
- Latent period following infection
- No inflammatory response
- Spongy changes in the brain.

Dyke (1997).

CJD and BSE infections are caused by a protein known as a prion which is still being researched.[2] They have an extremely long incubation period. The problem for perioperative nurses is that it is possible for them to be asked to assist at operations taking place during the latent period without anyone being aware that the patient has the infection. Researchers are now stating that there is no means of knowing whether we shall continue to see a mere handful of cases or whether there will eventually be thousands of sufferers worldwide in the next century (Dyke, 1997).

Do we know what the real incidence of BSE is? Some say there has been massive under-reporting around the world following the effect on the beef industry after the outbreak in Great Britain. How many animals were slaughtered and consumed before the infection was recognised? Many of us continue to eat beef. There is also the risk of iatrogenic transmission. Those who may go on to develop CJD could have been donors of blood or bone for grafting. Were any donors of corneal grafts in the latent period? It has already been shown that those treated with human pituitary growth hormone or gonadotrophin are at risk. Is it possible that the prion may have been transmitted in such reusable medical devices as haemodyalysis equipment, cardiac catheters or pacemakers.

Box 10.3   Effective sterilisation against CJD

The CJD prion is resistant to:

- heat
- glutaraldehyde
- formaldehyde
- ionising radiation
- freezing
- drying
- organic detergents.

Autoclaving at 134–138°C at 30 psi for 18 min is effective as is subatmospheric autoclaving using sodium hypochlorite or sodium hydroxide.

From Dyke (1997).

Helicobacter pylori

One group of operations which has almost disappeared in recent years is that group which was intended to relieve the symptoms of peptic ulceration. We have always believed two simple precepts:

- The stomach secretes acid to keep it sterile.
- Too much acid causes peptic ulcers.

The reduction in surgical treatment was caused by the development of H_2 antagonists which seemed to have a magic effect on gastric and duodenal ulceration from the 1970s. In 1979 an Australian team in Perth published a report on the first culture of *Helicobacter pylori*. They were initially thought to be non-pathogenic but it was noticed that patients with gastritis or ulcers were more frequently infected with these spiral bacteria than healthy controls.

Box 10.4 Helicobacter pylori

Spiral or curved Gram-negative rod with flagellae at one end. Gastric acid kills most bacteria, but gastric helicobacters have evolved features to allow them to cope with gastric acid and the gastric immune response. Under the electron microscope or on video they are seen to be highly mobile and are capable of drilling themselves into the non-acid mucous layer of the stomach wall. It appears that their colonisation of this layer may increase permeability and allow back-diffusion of acid. *H. pylori* also has a mechanism to neutralise the mucosal immune response. There are many strains of this bacteria some of which infect some animals. Some are more likely to cause disease than others.

Researchers sometimes found themselves complaining of vague gastric symptoms when investigating *H. pylorus* – an early sign of helicobacter infection (Calam, 1996).

Patterns of helicobacter infections in developing countries are different from those seen in the West. The one universal factor is that it is more prevalent in groups with lower income and inferior education. The conditions of the childhood home seem to be of some significance. Spread of infection is by direct transmission. This may link with the higher incidence of peptic ulceration seen after the second World War. The poor living conditions of displaced persons, bombed-out populations and armies in the field meant that many more people than normal could have been exposed to the possibility of infection with helicobacter at a time when people were living in poor conditions and in close contact with others. Hence, the high incidence of gastrectomies, vagotomies and pyloroplasties to alleviate peptic ulceration during the 1950s and 1960s. The stereotype of the patient presenting with peptic ulceration in the post-war period was that of the high-powered businessman, always under pressure, not stopping to take proper meals. The cause of this peptic ulceration was related to tension and hyperacidity due to faulty eating habits. This did not fit with the link now established with poor living conditions. It now appears that this may have been a legacy of the war, another infection whose incidence was affected by social factors. It is also an example of opportunist behaviour by a microorganism, unidentified by medical science, replicating itself in ways totally unknown to us and capable of causing disease in man. This was not the first, nor will it be the last example of such a process.

Why is this of relevance to perioperative nurses? It has been established that gastroenterologists are one of the groups infected by helicobacter. This is attributed to the fact that they did not wear gloves and face-masks in the early days of gastroscopy. The lack of face mask was most probably the reason for infection, allowing them to be infected by gastric juices bubbling back through the instrument (Calam, 1997). This is an example of how operating department staff can now be protected from a previously unrecognised infection risk by observing one element of universal precautions, in this instance by using a face shield/visor.

We have moved into a new era of infection which requires new methods of infection control. We do not yet have all the answers. Nor do we have the immunity which we had developed to more familiar infections. We do have universal precautions which, as we shall see, are now an integral part of infection control policies and procedures.

New risks for travellers

The high noon of antibiotics seems to be at an end. In a world which is increasingly politically unstable and increasingly overpopulated, resources are at a premium. Old enemies, like malaria, are also returning as Third World, newly independent countries are economically or politically unable to maintain the controlled environments needed to interrupt their breeding cycle. DDT insecticides can no longer be as widely used after they were found to be entering the food chain. By 1990 three times as many cases of malaria were reported as in 1961 (Porter, 1997). A variety of antimalaria drugs exist but the most effective, mefloquine (larium), has severe side-effects in a minority of subjects and is only recommended for use in high-risk areas such as sub-Saharan Africa and south-east Asia (British National Formulary, 1998). Increased travel continues to spread this and other diseases by a variety of methods. Previously unidentified and rapidly fatal diseases, such as Ebola and other haemorrhagic fevers, occasionally occur far from their original source of infection in returned or evacuated travellers.

Xenotransplantation

This is also the dawn of genetic engineering. One use for this technique has been in the development of genetically changed pigs to provide xenotransplantation material to replace hearts, kidneys and other organs. Two major questions have stopped the implementation of a surgical technique for which we have the technology. One is the ethical question of whether it is right to exploit animals in this way. The second is a realisation that pigs carry viruses which do not cause illness in pigs – but what happens if you introduce these into man? Do we as members of the operating team have an ethical responsibility to ask these questions before we join operating teams who propose to carry out such procedures (Fulbrook & Wilkinson, 1996)?

Perioperative priorities

Once again we are aware that living is dangerous to our health and that we cannot always destroy microorganisms responsible for infections! For perioperative nurses this was brought home, first of all, by the realisation that they were at risk during surgery, not only from some bacteria but more especially from viral infections. Old antiseptic techniques, old disinfectants and some other aspects of theatre technique had to be revised and replaced.

We are not always aware of what is happening in the world of microorganisms, or even in our own world, until a disaster breaks upon us. We, at the grass roots, are not even always aware of what the scientists already know but are not telling us for one very good reason or another. Sometimes, it takes time to assemble all the facts from isolated research findings to draw conclusions on which to make changes. Even as I write I heard an announcement on the radio of a suspected link between Alzheimer's disease and chlamydia, yet another infection which may have more far-reaching effects than we were aware ('Today' programme, Radio Four, 14 August 1998). Where this will lead and when or whether there will be any firm conclusions is to be seen.

Perhaps one of the greatest problems, especially in isolated units and small operating departments, is a tendency to be complacent in relying on established methods of infection control or the technique favoured by the surgeon operating at the time. How far the development of nurse education and an increased research awareness has affected such units is difficult to estimate. This varies across different countries. Despite a considerable accumulation of research evidence, practices such as preoperative skin shaving, wearing of overshoes, use of swab racks persisted long after they were shown to be infection risks (Brigden, 1988, pp.133–69; Nightingale, 1990, pp.49–55). This retrograde tendency was often reinforced by financial stringency or by ignorance on the part of senior medical or nursing staff who had not kept themselves up to date. Is it possible to be out of touch these days when clinical practices are more closely audited and when all members of staff are expected to be accountable to a critical employer and a more informed public and when perioperative nurses are professionally liable?

Many new infection control methods and the purchase of advanced equipment involve considerable expenditure. However, money saved by not spending money on a new infection control measure can be wiped out by an insurance claim from a patient or member of staff who becomes infected due to sub-standard care and practice. In both public and private sectors, and in all countries, perioperative nurses are finding themselves working within a stringent budget which has a number of competing demands made on it. It requires good strategic planning to make sure that infection risks are assessed and controlled. Good infection control can only be achieved if the perioperative environment is clean and well-managed and if the operating department personnel are well trained, aware and meticulous.

> All theatre personnel have an individual responsibility to ensure that all practices within their operating department are based on sound rational research findings and are updated regularly and conscientiously carried out.
>
> NATN (1988).

The approach taken by perioperative nurses in the UK differs from that in some other countries. National standards for practice are not set by professional bodies such as the National Association of Theatre Nurses (NATN), the Royal College of Nursing (RCN) or the United Kingdom Central Council (UKCC). Individual responsibility lies with the practitioners at local level to ensure that their infection control practices meet nationally and internationally accepted standards and guidelines, that they take note of recent research findings and that all equipment is used according to manufacturer's instructions (NATN, 1998). At a personal level perioperative nursing associations have always emphasised the need for a 'good surgical conscience' and awareness of 'margins of safety'.

Staff compliance

Not all infection control measures are expensive. It is vital that all staff understand the basic rules of infection control: why they are expected to wear theatre clothes correctly; why they must respect the basic rules of hygiene by observing such protocols as washing hands before going into theatres; avoiding touching used masks with their hands; or, even worse, putting that used mask into a pocket (Nightingale, 1990). It is these simple aspects of infection control which may make the difference in preventing pathogens from establishing new footholds. It is difficult for untrained staff to appreciate the risks from such an invisible enemy, but it has to be admitted that it is these simple breaks in procedure that can destroy the whole edifice of infection control and allow microorganisms to colonise new areas. You may point out that this does go on all the time without disastrous effects. I would ask, in that case, what happens if you have, among your staff, a carrier of a pathogenic bacteria, a heavy 'skin shedder' (Meers & Yeo, 1978) or someone who is unaware of the virus already circulating in their blood without displaying any clinical symptoms?

Many years ago, as a student nurse, I was taught never to put sterilised packs onto the floor. This never forgotten lesson was backed up by a story, which I have never heard since, of an outbreak of several cases of postoperative tetanus. The outbreak was finally traced back to tetanus spores in a drum of gloves which had been stored on the floor. (Yes, it is a very old story, they still washed, tested, packed and reused gloves in those days!) I never put anything sterile on the floor, but in these days of pre-packed everything, how do your sterile supplies get to you? The floor could be the floor of a van or trolley that was used for something very different before the porters brought the sterile supplies, unless they know that they must use specifically designated transport. And will they all be as individually responsible as you are? The professional responsibilities of a perioperative nurse extend to educating non-professional staff in such a way that they will internalise the principles of infection control so that putting the procedures into practice will become second nature at all times. There are no second chances with multiresistant bacteria.

Blood-borne viruses

From here, the rest of the chapter will be concerned with the really big issues for perioperative nurses, the developments which have had a revolutionary effect on how we approach infection control in operating departments and other places where surgery is carried out. It was HIV and hepatitis B that motivated the changes needed to protect staff as it became clear that an increasing number of operating room staff were known to be infected with hepatitis B. For many, a degree of complacency persisted. Hepatitis was something that happened to other people in other places. As time went on the list of blood-borne viruses grew, but it was the advent of the human immunodeficiency virus in the late 1980s which raised concerns sufficiently to lead to a new approach to infection control. Rather than developing specific precautions the Centers for Disease Control (CDC) in Atlanta, USA, proposed the concept of universal precautions as a baseline for precautions against all infection and, more specifically, to prevent contact with blood and other body fluids (Centers for Disease Control, 1987). This was a rather more sophisticated concept than the old 'barrier nursing' technique. To begin with, our knowledge of how diseases spread was now much more detailed. The recommendations for universal precautions are continuously monitored and updated and provide the bench-mark for other guidelines.[3]

Many nursing, medical and other organisations have now published guidelines for protection specifically against hepatitis B and HIV in a variety of situations. As well as giving guidance on precautions against infection most include information about vaccination, what to do in case of incidents such as needlestick accidents and contact addresses for further information. From these guidelines individual institutions developed their own procedures for both managers and individual care workers.

The original concern has now died down. Even areas of high infection have had to learn to live with the risk of blood-borne viral infection as a fact of life. In some areas it is much easier to do this than others. In politically unstable countries or very poor areas, often identical, the situation is often well out of the control of the health workers. Reports from missionaries and others working in Africa, perhaps in civil war situations, demonstrate how difficult it is to protect oneself and others. It is not so long since the more developed countries were sending unused needles and out-of-date surgical supplies to help out. Even now the response may have to be that 'something is better than nothing' (Rigby, 1997).

Universal precautions

No-one working in health care can fail to be aware of the risk now recognised from 'potentially catastrophic' blood-borne viruses, in particular the human immunodeficiency virus (HIV), hepatitis B (HBV) and now hepatitis C (HCV). The guidelines relating to every area of clinical practice are updated as needed. Research continues and new information is rapidly disseminated, in these days of computers, by the Internet as well as by publication in professional journals. Whatever references are quoted in this article may well be superseded by more recent publications on the subject before the book is available. Different countries will have different local and national guidelines and different institutions for referral. Some of this information is listed in the further reading list to this chapter. Points referred to here are drawn from the most recent publications on universal precautions in the perioperative setting available at the time. The Internet home page address of the CDC has also been included as this will be a useful source for recent information.

Box 10.5   Blood-borne viruses

Human immunodeficiency virus
(Two types: HIV 1 and HIV 2.)

- Infects CD4 lymphocytes.
- Uses the host's own ribonucleic acid (RNA) with its own DNA to produce viral RNA which is then able to replicate new virus particles in other T-cells with disastrous effect.
- Impairs the individual's cell-mediated immune response to pathogens and malignancies. This is AIDS (autoimmune deficiency syndrome).

Hepatitis B

- HBV transmitted by blood.
- Produces inflammation of the liver as the virus replicates there.
- Acute hepatitis may lead on to chronic hepatitis, in turn leading to cirrhosis, liver failure or malignancy.
- Innoculation available; treatment actively sought.

Hepatitis C
(Formerly known as 'non-A, non-B hepatitis'.)

- HCV also transmitted by blood.
- Can cause profound liver damage many years after initial infection.
- No available immunisation or treatment for needlestick.

NATN (1998).

For perioperative nurses it is sometimes all too easy to concentrate on universal precautions as a means of protecting oneself and other health care workers from infection and forget the original underlying concepts. Universal precautions are intended to protect everyone from contact with blood and body fluids. Outside the operating theatres the psychological significance of treating everyone in a similar way is clearer. In the early days of the HIV epidemic, undignified and degrading stigmatisation occurred when potentially or actually infected persons were subjected to 'over the top' precautions. It is no longer good practice to identify patients as belonging to a 'high-risk' group purely on the basis of their social or medical history. The writers of the NATN Guidelines (1998) point out that though universal precautions have now been recommended for a decade, evidence suggests that internalisation of such safe practice has still not occurred in many places.[4]

The theatre nurse of earlier times, in becoming the perioperative nurse of today, is moving out of the operating department. She or he is caring for patients before and after surgery and is establishing more effective caring relationships with patients and their relatives and with other health care workers. As professional nurses, whose speciality includes profound knowledge of infection control procedures, perioperative nurses are in an excellent position to offer good educational support and to act as good role models to ensure, not only awareness, but real understanding on the part of all involved in the care of the surgical patient.

Preventing infection

In the high-risk area of the actual operating room universal precautions must, perforce, focus largely on preventing contact with blood and body fluids and in preventing contamination of the environment. It is important to remember that accidental (intact) skin contact with blood or body fluids is not thought to be implicated in accidental transmission. Far more dangerous is the accidental inoculation by needlestick or sharps injury. However, the principle of universal precautions against infection, including airborne and droplet infections does protect from other pathogens including chicken-pox, tuberculosis, rubella and whooping cough (NATN, 1998, p.11). Exposure of gastrologists to the then unrecognised helicobacter infections could have been prevented by the wearing of protective visors or masks.

Immunisation

Owing to the nature of their work, health care workers are offered inoculation programmes against hepatitis B, perhaps the most aggressive of the blood-borne viruses and certainly the most commonly encountered. All workers in operating departments have a responsibility to follow local policy; their managers' responsibility is to ensure and facilitate that policy and the responsibility of Occupational Health Departments is to carry it out. It should be made clear to staff members that, once vaccinated, they cannot relax their precautions as there are other viruses against which they have no immunity.

> Immunisation is recommended in individuals who are at risk of hepatitis B because of their lifestyle, occupation or other factors ... the Control of Substances Hazardous to Health (COSHH) Regulations (1994) require employers to undertake their own risk assessment and to bring into effect measures necessary to protect workers and others ...
> Recommendations from Immunisation against Infectious Diseases (DOH, 1996, para 18.3, p.98).

Box 10.6 Precautions to minimise risk

NATN recommend that risk assessment be carried out for all procedures. Some precautions are adopted for all patients. From this baseline the risks inherent in each procedure come under the following headings:

1 Skin: cover for cuts/abrasions.

2 Handwashing: use as appropriate and before and after each patient contact.

3 Gloves: use high quality (latex) gloves.

4 Eyes and mouth: protection needed by use of mask, goggles or visor if likelihood of splashing or aerosol.

5 Contact with body fluids: use of impermeable gowns and drapes and/or plastic aprons as appropriate.

6 Sharps: there should be a local policy for sharps use which should include:

- avoid direct hand to hand exchange
- never involve re-sheathing of needles
- early disposal into sharps box.

7 Spillage:

- use disposable towels
- use sodium hypochlorite 1% or sodium dichloroisocyanate granules
- protect self with gloves and plastic apron.

8 Swabs: contained but countable.

9 Sharps injury:

- encourage bleeding immediately
- wash with running water and soap
- take blood sample – and from patient
- advise manager
- report to Occupational Health Department.

Similar procedures are necessary for splashes on eye or mucous membrane.

10 Waste disposal:

- follow the local clinical waste procedure
- contain linen and instruments for recycling according to local procedures.

The fact that the AORN tends to produce 'standards' which are followed universally, i.e. for all patients whilst the NATN publishes 'guidelines' which are used with local policies and risk assessment is an interesting cultural difference. It is suggested that this is due to the different priorities bearing on practice in the two countries, one of which has a private insurance funded health service whilst the other has a (largely) publicly funded national health service with stricter financial constraints. In a private health service costs can be passed on directly to the patient. We are, perhaps, not always sufficiently ready to admit this difference. Patient expectations also enter into the equation. In the more direct contract between the carers and patients in a private health care system the patient can be much more demanding and is certainly ready to be more critical, if not litigious, if standards fall short of the standard which they expect and for which they are paying.

Latex allergy

It is not possible to leave the topic of infection control without some mention of the incidence of latex allergy. There are always new risks in new techniques. This was demonstrated all too clearly by what happened as new infection control guidelines and standards stipulated the regular use of protective clothing, especially latex gloves, to prevent contact with possibly infected material. The demand for gloves increased enormously and new manufacturers appeared. At first, the need to select high quality, low protein gloves was not appreciated, even in theatres. Those team members not part of the scrub team were regarded as sufficiently protected if wearing less expensive gloves to provide a simple barrier. Fay (1996) discusses the choice of gloves to provide appropriate protection in differing situations. She also discusses in some detail the hydration of latex gloves. Latex gloves are capable of absorbing water from the hands of the wearer. It follows that absorption varies over time and depending on the type and quality of the glove. Hydration also plays a part in allergy as it facilitates the transfer of latex proteins and residual chemicals from the manufacturing process. Research continues to show that speed of hydration varies. Criteria for the selection of gloves should not be purely economic, but should ensure that good quality latex gloves from a reputable manufacturer are chosen which form an effective barrier. Gloves are now available with 'early warning' indicators which change colour if the latex is penetrated; others have linings which reduce the porosity to lessen the chance of allergy and to improve ease of putting on. Some synthetic products are on the market which claim to be as good as latex, but whether it will ever be possible to find an effective and total substitute for the latex used in a variety of medical products needs further research.

It is now possible for every member of the surgical team to be wearing latex gloves for a large part of the day. A perioperative nurse who develops latex allergy has come to the end of her career in the operating department. For a patient who relies on latex devices, such as the patient with spina bifida who has been catheterised for most of his or her life, latex sensitisation could be a nightmare, or death. In addition, an increasing number of the general population are finding that they have faulty allergic responses. Establishing whether a patient has a latex allergy or falls into a high-risk group should now be a routine part of preoperative assessment.

Box 10.7   Hypersensitivity to latex

Hypersensitivity to latex falls into two main categories:

- **Type 4   Cell mediated hypersensitivity**
Usually a local reaction which can be delayed for some hours and generally confined to the area of contact . This type presents as dermatitis, erythema, pruritis, skin cracking or, in very severe cases, with vesicle formation. It can present as an eczema affecting also the flexor or extensor surfaces of the forearms.

- **Type 1   Immediate hypersensitivity reaction**
This can be caused by direct exposure to water soluble latex proteins. Direct contact can be percutaneous, parenteral, inhalant or mucosal if occurring in a patient when a latex device is in use. The reaction will be immediate, certainly within 30 minutes and varies from a rhinitis or asthmatic response to systemic urticaria, angioedema or even anaphylactic shock.

At risk groups

Patients with:

- spina bifida
- congenital urinary abnormalities
- myelodysplasia
- long-term bowel or bladder conditions
- repeated surgical interventions.

Others include:

- health care workers
- people with known sensitivities, especially to fruit
- family history of atopy
- latex industry workers.

Thomson (1996).

Glove powder also allows the latex molecules to be carried into the patient's body. At an international symposium focusing on latex reactions and, in particular, the use of glove powder, some surgeons went so far as to blame the latex molecules carried on glove powder for the development of peritoneal adhesions following surgery. An anaesthetist queried the possible effects of the presence of glove powder particles in the epidural space following installation of epidural anaesthesia. A consultant described the effect on her and her practice when she became sensitised to latex. The general consensus was that glove powder should be banned. Others would go so far as to suggest that a complete ban on latex use, or at least the establishment of 'latex free' areas, is essential in health care (Nightingale, 1996). The jury is still out on this, but how far are perioperative nurses accountable for assessing the risk and taking steps to protect both their staff and their patients?

Implications of minimal access surgery

The unbelievably rapid growth of minimal access surgery raised a number of infection control issues whose significance was not at first realised. They were related to two areas, firstly to the differences in the surgical technique and secondly to the complexity and delicacy of the instrumentation.

Once surgeons began to operate using minimal access techniques, rather than using endoscopes for solely diagnostic procedures in body cavities, the issue of sterilisation of endoscopes and the instruments used with them became increasingly urgent. Subsequent patients, the operators and the staff responsible for recycling the equipment could be, and were, put at risk if the instrument was not immediately decontaminated after use and rendered sterile before reuse. In the learning phase surgeons were also more likely to cause more tissue trauma and took much longer to carry out closed procedures than the old open operation, factors which further increased the possibility of infection. Once introduced, in some situations infection takes longer to be recognised whilst having a head start if established in a deep, warm, dark site.

As patients are often discharged much earlier following minimally invasive surgery they are often at home when symptoms appear, leading to even later diagnosis of infection.

Straight endoscopes, in the form of cystoscopes, laparoscopes, laryngoscopes and bronchoscopes, were used for many years without any real recognition that they needed to be treated with radically different decontamination techniques to other surgical instruments. With the arrival of the flexible gastroscope problems were recognised. The new endoscopes were longer, more complicated, narrow tubes within tubes, and often made of materials which did not take kindly to heat sterilisation. There were plenty of lodging places for residual body fluids or cleaning solutions which could be colonised by microorganisms. The instruments used to carry out, in particular, laparoscopic surgery presented a real challenge to ensure safe and certain sterility. It was these instruments which were seriously researched by the manufacturers to establish whether it was safe to reuse them in the face of the new infection risks (Bell, 1998).

A third recognised infection risk from laparoscopic surgery was related to evacuated peritoneal air. A paper by Baggish (1993) demonstrated that HIV particles could be found in evacuated diathermy (or laser) smoke. The paper concluded that staff were at risk of potential infection from 'sprayback' from trochars and that this risk could be reduced by the use of an instrument chamber, as found on some single use laparoscopic instruments.

This resulted in much liaison between users and the manufacturers, the production of sophisticated sterilising trolleys, the use of new chemical agents to decontaminate and jointly produced procedures in an attempt to ensure safe use of endoscopes (Keymed, 1998, which was preceded by earlier editions). Two particularly significant research results showed that existing methods of cleaning and sterilisation of endoscopic instrumentation were not fully effective. In view of what we now know about the spread of infection and the versatility of pathogens we can no longer accept this.

Whitbourne (1994) demonstrated that the core of a laparoscopic instrument often does not reach the required temperature when heat sterilised and that the residual biodebris, some of which could be presumed to be blood, could not always be confirmed as sterile. He also demonstrated the presence of a sporing bacillus. Under the microscope DesCoteaux et al. (1995) showed that cleaned laparoscopic instruments carried a higher burden of debris than open instruments. The Pharma Strategy Group (1996) also suggests that nurses cleaning the instruments in the operating department do not have time to clean instruments to the standard required. Most theatre staff would agree with this in the face of pressure put on them to get on with the operating list!

Single use instruments

As a result of the findings, manufacturers now recommend the use of single use instruments (Bell 1998). Multiple use instruments remain in use. There are economic and other reasons why there cannot always be a sudden and wholesale change to single use instrumentation. There are, on the other hand, very good legal and ethical reasons for moving to single use items as soon as possible. Even those who use multiple use instruments change to disposable single use instrumentation when operating on patients they regard as 'high risk, i.e. those they know to be serum positive for Hb or HIV. This is flying in the face of the principles of universal precautions.

Considerable guidance is available on this topic in Europe. By the terms of the Consumer Protection Act (1987) anyone reprocessing (by sterilising, for example) such a device will become liable for any damage sustained by a future failure in the performance of the device. NATN (1995) published a position statement on the use, misuse and reuse of medical devices and the Medical Devices Agency (DOH, 1995) have issued guidelines on single use. However, reuse of single use items remained a matter of concern as recently as 1997 when Willmer *et al.* (1997) reported on a survey which indicated that 27% of the respondents had resterilised a single use instrument during the previous 12 months. The European Union has become involved in harmonising the presentation of single use items across Europe. From June 1998 all medical devices in the EU will bear the European Union 'mark of conformity' to demonstrate when they are quality assured, as well as other symbols indicating sterility, use-by dates and whether they are for single use only (Medical and Surgical Users Liaison Committee, 1996). The UK Medical Devices Agency guidelines were made compulsory from 1998.

Sterilising and disinfection

Alongside the demand for cost-effective means to decontaminate and resterilise laparoscopic instruments there was another need. It was becoming increasingly necessary to ensure that whatever means were developed should be environmentally friendly and should meet the standards required by the Health and Safety at Work Act (1974). Many disinfectants had been completely phased out leaving glutaraldehyde as the main agent still being used actually in the operating department. Originally regarded as safe in use, glutaraldehyde sensitisation has now been recognised, causing headaches, rhinitis and asthma (Hutt, 1994). Using solutions is, at best, an uncontrolled process with many variations possible during the storage, preparation, use and disposal of the disinfectant (Carrington, 1996). Legislation on the control of substances hazardous to health (COSHH Regulations, 1994) has tightened up some of the more dangerous practices which used to occur as ventilation cabinets, protective masks and use of closed containers reduce staff exposure (Howell, 1998).

A number of new disinfectant agents have been introduced. Paracetic acid was used for years in the food industry before being used for endoscope disinfection. Chlorine dioxide is also effective. Both offer short kill times, but are more expensive. Other properties affect the performance of disinfectants. Are they corrosive? Do they damage plastic? How stable in solution? What conditions are needed for safe storage? Formal tests show that these new disinfectants are effective though more expensive but may be more damaging to the instruments and possibly not effective against all microorganisms (Babb, 1996).

You will increasingly see these symbols on medical devices – do YOU know what they mean?

Recent European Directives harmonize medical device regulation across Europe. These require certain information to be provided. This can be done by means of symbols which minimise the need for text and so multilingual translations – to cover all European Member States. Just as for road signs, however, the meanings of these symbols are not intuitive; they have to be learnt through association.

Does it mean ... ?	Symbols	No, it really means ...
✗ Only one product in the box ✗ Do not use 2 products at a time ✗ Not for use in February ✗ Can be used single handed	②⃠	✓ 'Do not Reuse'
✗ Mine's a half ✗ For keyhole surgery ✗ Cosmetic body shaping product ✗ Short measures ✗ Radical Compression hosiery	⧖	✓ 'Use By'
✗ More than one in a box ✗ Up for auction ✗ You'll like this product, but not a ...	LOT	✓ 'Batch Code'
✗ Staff Nurse only to use ✗ Owned by senior nurse ✗ Sado-Narcissus product ✗ 'Supernatural' product	SN	✓ 'Serial Number'
✗ As used in the House of Commons/Church ✗ Manual prosthesis ✗ Use this way up ✗ Already incinerated	⋀⋀	✓ 'Date of Manufacture'
✗ Infertility device ✗ Sterile field ✗ Do not touch this product during use	STERILE	✓ 'Sterile'
✗ Non-productive senior manager ✗ End of product is sterile	STERILE EO	✓ 'Sterilized using ethylene oxide'
✗ Really sterile (honest!) ✗ Sterile Registrar ✗ Sterile on right side only	STERILE R	✓ 'Sterilized using irradiation'
✗ Thermometers must be sterile ✗ Vasectomy service ✗ Artificial Insemination device	STERILE 🌡	✓ 'Sterilized using steam/ dry heat'
✗ Unfair practice ✗ Whistle blowers beware! ✗ Dyslexic dreamer ✗ If all esle fails, refer to instructions	REF	✓ 'Catalogue Number'
✗ Beware, concealed opening ✗ Dangerous product ✗ Defective Toblerone	⚠	✓ 'Attention, consult instructions for use'
✗ Cavaet Emptor ✗ Chief Executive use ✗ Church of England (see above) ✗ Continuing Education ✗ Clerical Erur	CE xxxx	✓ 'Conformité Européan' In relation to medical devices, the European Union mark of conformity denotes compliance with the European Directive 93/42/EEC which specifies requirements for safety and performance. It provides the purchaser and user an assurance of the quality of the devices. From June 14, 1998, medical devices placed on the EU market must legitimately bear the 'CE' marking.

This document was created by the Medical & Surgical Products Users Liaison Group.

Figure 10.1 European Union symbols for medical devices.

A completely new technological development may offer a system which can be used in the department, allowing instruments to be rapidly resterilised. This low temperature sterilising system uses the lethal effect of free radicals released in a plasma from aqueous hydrogen peroxide subjected to radio frequency energy.[5]

The process uses both chemical and physical means to destroy all microorganisms in a safe, closed container. As long as they are immersible, delicate and sophisticated laparoscopic instruments can be sterilised in time to be ready for use by the surgeon in 30 minutes (Mackay, 1996).

Conclusions

At this time of great social change and ever-increasing mobility, microorganisms of all types have been able to mutate and move into new niches. They have been carried by man over huge distances, sometimes to emerge as new or more resistant diseases. Coincidentally, the range of antibiotics which are not toxic to humans seems to be exhausted whilst the increasing population is polluting the environment to an unprecedented level.

Domin (1998) points out that the arrival of vancomycin-resistant *Staphylococcus aureus* (VRSA) and enteric organisms on a global scale, represents a huge challenge to those committed to the control of nosocomial infection. With the loss of this last effective antibiotic, infection control measures have become imperative. One way to approach the problem is by the development of liaising CDCs (Control of Disease Centres) and the development of codes of practice for:

- the use of antibiotics
- measures for effective infection control
- general guidelines for practice.

The centralisation of this work will ensure speedy development of high quality precautions.

Costly systems will not be supported by administrators; labour intensive or elaborate systems will not be properly observed. It is those procedures, long regarded as essential in operating theatres which will be effective: hand washing, meticulous cleaning and the use of microbial barriers such as masks and gloves. The question of internalising infection control procedures has already been referred to. If, as in Domin's view, this is the greatest challenge since the dawn of the antibiotic era, setting disease control back by 60 years and, if infection control is to depend on simple measures, as suggested, it is vital that all involved in patient care do internalise those procedures so that they become second nature and are rigorously observed.

Perioperative nurses are key players in the fight to control both new and old infections. They are in a unique position to combine human, educational and managerial aspects of infection control with the technical. Their everyday involvement with the control of infection makes them aware of the risks both from pathogens and from the means we use against pathogens.

New sterilisation and disinfection methods appear first in operating departments where surgeons are actively exposing patients and staff to infection risks by the very nature of surgery. In the short term, local finances may force managers into the choice of cheaper methods but only environmentally friendly and effective infection control, utilised with real understanding of the risks and their management, will be economically and socially effective. Perioperative nurses who implement new practices and are exposed to associated risks must be involved in the decision-making process by assessing and evaluating those risks.

Surgeons are committed to the importance of infection control, but achieving it is a team effort and it is the professional perioperative nurse who achieves this by her or his actions before, during and after operative procedures. Easterbrook (1998) also points out the urgent need to set up global and national surveillance systems, adding that these will only be able to function effectively if underpinned by local monitoring to collect relevant information. Perioperative nursing associations are already actively contributing to this through conferences and publications, by education and research and by liaison with other bodies to achieve standardisation of procedures and by promoting the maintenance of scrupulous records and observation of research-based standards.

Reflective activities

This chapter has only skimmed the surface of infection control. Many other aspects of the subject have not been covered due to lack of space and time. The intention has been to make you stop and think about the serious issues now facing us in the field of infection control.

1 Turn to your own operating department and consider how well your staff comply with the basic but vital aspects of infection control:

- Do they, and do you, wear and dispose of masks. Check the next time you go into theatres. How many masks are hanging underneath chins?
- Discuss with colleagues how well you and they wash hands. Do you wash your hands before going into theatres? Do you wash your hands meticulously between patients?
- Has anyone ever considered whether pens, pencils and computer keyboards are contaminated or cleaned? Could this be an infection risk?

2 Had you ever considered that pathogenic bacteria are substances hazardous to health and, as such, are covered by the COSHH regulations (or their equivalent outside the UK)?

3 Review all the decontamination, disinfectant and sterilisation methods used in your department. Can they be improved?

4 What do you consider the greatest infection risk in your working area? Are both staff and patients adequately protected against this risk?

Endnotes

1 The question of 'single use' instruments raises questions of cost which conflict with the demand for foolproof prevention of cross infection. The topic is also discussed in Chapter 14.

2 In early 1999, as this book went to press, the results of research carried out at Imperial Hospital, London, were indicating that the prion has been identified in the tonsils, appendices and spleens of people who are in the latent period of CJD. This raises serious questions for surgical practice and for those handling, using and sterilising instruments after surgery. This may be another situation where it will be necessary to introduce single use instrumentation. (See also Chapter 14 for information on single use instrumentation.) How patients will be screened is to be seen. The Chief Medical Officer is currently reviewing the situation before making recommendations.

3 The term 'universal precautions' may have been changed in general usage to 'universal standards' by the time you read this book.

4 Although references are made here to HIV in relation to universal precautions, the highest risk to perioperative nurses, surgeons and theatre personnel is from serum hepatitis which is a far more virulent virus than the HIV.

5 Plasma: a cloud of positively and negatively charged particles plus neutral atoms and molecules. Occurs naturally in the aurora borealis/australis and in solar flares.

References

Angulo, F. J. 1998 A large outbreak of botulism: the hazardous potato. *Journal of Infectious Diseases* **178** (1), 172–7.

Babb, J. & Bradley, S. 1995 A review of glutaraldehyde alternatives. *British Journal of Theatre Nursing* **5** (7), 20–4.

Baggish, M. 1993 Comparison of smoke and sprayback leakage from two different trocar sleeves during operative laparoscopy. *Journal of Gynaecological Surgery* **9** (2), 62–76.

Bell, S. 1998 Multiple patient use versus single patient use products. *British Journal of Theatre Nursing* **8** (1), Supplement.

Brigden, R. J. 1988 *Operating theatre technique,* 5th edition. Edinburgh, Churchill Livingstone.

British National Formulary. 1998 (March) London, British Medical Association and Royal Pharmaceutical Society of Great Britain.

Brunner, L. S. & Suddarth, D. S. 1992 *The textbook of adult nursing,* Chapter 2. London, Chapman & Hall.

Calam, J. 1996 *Clinician's guide to Helicobacter pylori.* London, Chapman & Hall.

Carrington, A. C. 1996 Reflections – glutaraldehyde glooms. *British Journal of Theatre Nursing* **5** (12), 16–17.

Centers for Disease Control (CDC) 1987 Recommendations for preventing transmission of HIV transmission in health-care settings. *Morbidity and Mortality Weekly Reports* **36** (Supplement No. 2S.), 3S–18S.

Clarke, P. & Jones, J. 1998 *Brigden's operating department practice.* Edinburgh, Churchill Livingstone.

Consumer Protection Act. 1987 London, HMSO.

Control of Substances Hazardous to Health (COSHH) Regulations. 1994 London, HMSO.

Conybeare, J. & Mann, W. N. 1954 *Textbook of medicine,* 11th edition. Edinburgh & London, E & S Livingstone.

Daniels, A. 1998 Why the superbug isn't the end of the world. *Sunday Times* 26 April, 1998.

Department of Health, Welsh Office, Scottish Office, DHSS (NI). 1996. *Immunisation against Infectious Diseases.* Edward Jenner Bicentenary Edition. London, HMSO.

DesCoteaux, et al. 1995 Residual organic debris on processed surgical instruments. *AORN Journal* July, **62**, 1.

DOH Medical Devices Agency. 1995 The re-use of medical devices supplied for single use only. *Safety Action Bulletin* 9501.

Domin, M. 1998 Highly virulent pathogens – a post-antibiotic era. *British Journal of Theatre Nursing* **8** (2), 14–18.

Dyke, M. 1997 Creutzfeld–Jakob Disease. *British Journal of Theatre Nursing* **7** (8), 33–5.

Easterbrook, P. J. 1998 Superbugs: Are we at the threshold of another Dark Age? *Hospital Medicine* **59** (7), 525–6.

Fay, M. 1996 Hand protection against viral pathogens. *British Journal of Theatre Nursing* **6** (5), 5–9.

Fulbrook, S. & Wilkinson, M. 1996 Ethics of animal transplantation. *British Journal of Theatre Nursing* **6** (3), 13–15,18.

Health and Safety at Work Act. 1974. London, HMSO.

Howell, G. 1998 Something in the air. *British Journal of Theatre Nursing* **8** (1), 29–31.

Hutt, G. 1994 Glutaraldehyde revisited. *British Journal of Theatre Nursing* **3** (10), 10–11.

Kerr, S., Kerr, G. E. & Macintosh, C. A. 1990 A Survey of methicillin-resistant *Staphylococcus aureus* affecting patients in England and Wales. *Journal of Hospital Infection* **16**, 35–48.

Keymed Ltd. 1998 *Nurses' and technicians' guide to Olympus endoscopic systems.* Southend, Reynold.

Lee, T. 1996 World Health Organization **18** (4), 8–9.

Mackay, G. 1996 To Sterilise or Disinfect – That is the Question. *British Journal of Theatre Nursing* **5** (12), 13–14.

Medical and Surgical Product Users Liaison Committee. 1996 Symbols on medical devices. *British Journal of Theatre Nursing* **5** (11), 19.

Meers, P. D. & Yeo, G. A. 1978 Shedding of bacteria and skin squames after handwashing. *Journal of Hygiene* **81**, 99.

NATN. 1988 *Principles of safe practice in the operating department.* Harrogate, NATN.

NATN. 1995 *Minimal access surgery guidelines.* Harrogate, NATN.

NATN. 1995 *Use, re-use and misuse of single use items. A position statement.* Harrogate, NATN.

NATN. 1998 *Universal precautions and infection control.* Harrogate, NATN.

Nightingale, K. 1990 *The surgical patient.* In: Worsley, M. *et al. Infection control: guidelines for nursing care.* UK, Infection Control Nurses Association.

Nightingale, K. 1996 Ban glove powder: report on an international symposium. *British Journal of Theatre Nursing* **6** (5), 15–16.

Norman, A. 1995 A comparison of face masks and visors for the scrub team. *British Journal of Theatre Nursing* **5** (2), 10–11.

Orr, N. 1981 Is a mask necessary in the operating theatre? *Annals of the Royal College of Surgeons of England* **63**, 390–92.

Pharma Strategy Group Ltd. 1996 Surgical instrument survey, summary report for the UK.

Porter, R. 1997 *The greatest benefit to mankind.* London, Harper Collins.

Rigby, D. 1997 African diary. *British Journal of Theatre Nursing* **7** (5), 22–4.

Satcher, D. 1996 Centers for Disease Control. *Asepsis* **18** (4), 4–5.

Sharp, J. C. M. 1998 *Escherichia coli* 0157 infections: the Scottish experience. *Hospital Medicine* **59** (2), 98–9.

Thomson, C. M. 1996 The potential risks of latex. *British Journal of Theatre Nursing* **6** (5), 12–14.

Whitbourne, J. 1994 Feasibility study to evaluate the bioburden remaining on reusable laparoscopic instruments following cleaning and sterilisation. STS Test no. M93–1365.

Willmer, S. *et al.* 1997 Re-use of single use items in minimal access surgery. *British Journal of Theatre Nursing* **7** (3), 11–13.

Further reading

Note: This list is not comprehensive and some guidelines have been included in the list of references above.

AORN. 1996 Recommended practises for environmental cleaning in the surgical practice setting. *AORN Journal.* **64** (4), 611–15, 813–16 and **64** (5), 817–21.

AORN Standards and Recommended Practices. 1996 *Recommended Practises for universal precautions.* Association of ORN.

Audit Commission Report. *Getting sorted: the safe and economic management of hospital waste.*

Advisory Committee on Dangerous Pathogens. 1995 *Protection against blood-borne infections in the workplace – HIV and hepatitis.* London.

Editorial. 1996 First of all do no harm. *British Journal of Theatre Nursing* **5** (11), 18.

Klimek, J. J. 1996 Infection prevention update: HIV update from XI International AIDS Conference. *Asepsis* **18** (3), 19–23.

Macluskey, F. 1996 Does wearing a face mask reduce bacterial wound infection? *British Journal of Theatre Nursing* **6** (5), 18–20, 29.

Plowes, D. 1995 Re-using or misusing? *British Journal of Theatre Nursing* **5** (1), 22–3.

RCN. 1997 *Universal precautions.* London, Royal College of Nursing.

Taylor, G. & Chandler, L. 1997 Ultraviolet light in the operating theatre. *British Journal of Theatre Nursing* **6** (10), 10–14.

Internet Homepage address:
US Centers for Disease Control and Prevention (CDC):
http://www.cdc.gov/

Knowing the hazards and managing the risks

11

Gitta Hutt

After working for many years in perioperative nursing, Gitta Hutt took a sideways step into occupational health nursing. In writing about risk assessment in the workplace she has approached the subject as it was primarily intended. That is to say, that she concentrates on the risks to health and safety of staff at work. Nurses are well aware of the more clinical aspects of risks to patients, but in this approach to the concept of risk assessment the focus is, as intended, on staff safety and risks to staff and to any other persons coming into the workplace, in this instance, the operating department. This chapter will give invaluable guidance and food for thought on risk assessment for those perioperative nurses who are moving into management on both a personal and managerial level.

The high rate of illness and accidents to nurses is emphasised. Attention is also drawn to the comment on page 265 on how a healthier workforce gives a better standard of patient care.

This chapter and Chapter 10 are both concerned with risks in the operating department and complement each other in discussion on risks related to infection control, safety and allergic reactions. Both chapters contain considerable information on guidelines for practice and sources of information on these topics.

Risk assessment legislation

For decades nurses of all specialties have been practising risk assessment. If that comes as a surprise to any reader, please consider the following: who has been at the receiving end of nursing care? Of course – the patients. What has been the overriding consideration in all nursing actions? Not to do harm and to prevent anything – including illness or disability – from causing any further upset to the patient's physiological and psychological wellbeing and return him or her to the highest possible state of health. How has this been done? Whether implicitly, as in the past, or explicitly by way of the adopted nursing process, the first step always was and still is assessment of the presenting condition. This leads to the planning and performing of the actions necessary to alleviate or cure this condition and is followed by the monitoring and evaluation of the outcome, reassessing whether it is improving the situation and then beginning the cycle again.

There you have it: the risk assessment cycle. What appears to be so compellingly new to this concept is the requirement, under Health and Safety legislation, for staff to be included in a similar process in order to provide a safe and healthy working environment. Regrettably, this cannot be automatically assumed.

In 1992, following the Government's *Health of the Nation* policy document, the NHS Executive launched the 'Health at Work in the NHS' (HAW) initiative. The Health Education Authority (HEA) was commissioned to take this 10-year project forward. Interim results at the half-way stage do not encourage optimism. A culture ruled by the maxim 'Patients first – don't worry about yourself' is the professional ethos expected and still almost religiously adhered to by tradition. The HEA cited it as one of the conflicts within the NHS, combined with staff perceiving themselves in a sickness rather than health service. It also recognised that most occupational health departments were marginalised and so removed from the management process that they were not involved in management decisions. Understandable, when a further reason given to explain the lack of success of HAW was the lack of management commitment and low priority given to the initiative (Holroyd, 1998).

This culture would also appear to be borne out by Government statistics on occupational illness (HSE, 1998). These showed that highest prevalence of work-related illness, affecting more than 7% of current or recent workers in several groups, included nursing, sharing the company of such groups as coal mining and construction. It also showed that among the top ten work-related illnesses were stress, back injuries, upper limb and neck disorders, skin disease and headache. These are complaints not unfamiliar to many nurses in whatever specialty. Because of work-related illness, nurses were cited as having taken 2.74 days sickness absence in the previous 12 months, nearly four times the all-sector average (Labour Force Survey 1995/96). Add to this the Compendium of Critical Appraisals published by the Health and Safety Executive (HSE) which assesses the ability of substances to be implicated as causes of occupational asthma and includes substances such as latex and glutaraldehyde. Both substances are now known to be sensitisers able to cause long-term debilitating effects on the health of individuals who are regularly in uncontrolled contact with it.

These statistics make clear why RCN Congress resolutions were passed in 1998 calling for a national inquiry into the state of occupational health and safety in the NHS and why articles in the nursing press are concerned with non-compliance by Trusts 6 years after the Management of Health and Safety at Work Regulations (1992) became law (*Nursing Times*, 1998a and b). Why else, after lengthy and costly wrangling in and out of court do nurses still have to settle for financial compensation in exchange for their health and careers? Although managers appear to be obsessed by risk management and quality control, the culture of the organisation combined with the lack of motivation or interest – often referred to as resources – has nurses continuing to care for patients as they should but remaining, themselves, largely unaware of their own and their employer's legal responsibilities for each other.

Legal responsibilities for each other? Where does that come from you may wonder. Section 7 of the Health and Safety at Work Act 1974 (HASWA) states quite clearly that employees must take reasonable care of their own health and safety and that of others who may be affected by their acts or omissions. However, it also states that they must cooperate with their employer, so far as is necessary, to enable the employer to comply with his duties under the Act. Section 8 makes it an offence for anyone to intentionally or recklessly interfere with or misuse anything provided in the interests of health, safety or welfare.

Members of management, who are, of course, also employees, are vulnerable to prosecution under Section 7 if they fail to carry out their health and safety responsibilities as defined in their safety policy statements. How many managers are aware that Section 36 and 37 of the HASWA make provision for personal prosecution of members of management in certain circumstances? Under Section 37 in particular they can be charged as well as, or instead of, the employer if the offence in question was due to their consent, connivance or neglect. And just to make any possible defence for such neglect even more troublesome, the burden of proof is transferred from the prosecution to the defence in prosecutions where it is alleged that the accused person or employer failed to do what was practicable, or reasonably practicable as required, in particular circumstances. From experience, it would seem that most managers are not even aware that health and safety law forms part of criminal law at all. Being found guilty of such neglect of duty would not only end their career but also leave them with a criminal record.

None of this is too far-fetched considering that one NHS Trust's senior hospital management, who failed to take responsibility for health and safety tasks, was found to be in breach of safety regulations and was fined in 1997 without a specific accident having occurred (*HSE News*, 1997). It was found that the Trust did not have adequate arrangements in place to effectively control and monitor health and safety of the employees and others who may be affected by their activities. This was seen as a contravention of Regulation 4 of the Management of Health and Safety at Work Regulations (1992). The trust admitted the charge. Breaches included failing to provide training in Manual Handling (DOH, 1992) which accounts for four in ten accidents reported under the Reporting of Injury, Disease and Dangerous Occurrences Regulations (1995) (RIDDOR). It also involved breaches concerning clinical waste, electrical equipment maintenance and quality of procedures. The HSE at that time did not rule out taking other hospitals to court if similar or other breaches of Health and Safety Regulations should be found.

I hope that this explains better than almost anything why risk assessment is now so important. The general duties of employers are contained in Sections 2, 3, 4, and 9 of the Health and Safety at Work Act (HASWA). These state that employers must, so far as is reasonably practicable, safeguard the health, safety and welfare of employees (Section 2). This extends particularly to the provision and maintenance of:

- Safe plant and safe systems of work.
- Safe handling, storage, maintenance and transport of work articles and substances.
- A safe place of work, with safe access and egress.
- A safe working environment with adequate welfare facilities.

In law, there is an absolute duty on employers with five or more employees to prepare and revise as necessary a written statement of safety policy which details the general policy of the particular organisation and defines the arrangements for carrying it out. Furthermore the policy must be brought to the notice of all employees (Section 2[3]). Risk assessment is implicit in this policy.

Much more explicit and specific requirements are made within The Management of Health and Safety at Work Regulations (1992). These require us:

- to undertake a systematic general examination of our work activity;
- identify the significant risks arising out of work and assess the risks to the health and safety of those in our employment;
- assess the risks to the health and safety of persons not in our employment who are working on our premises or are affected by our business;
- record 'significant' findings of each assessment and details of groups of employees specifically at risk;
- review our assessments if we have reason to suspect that they are no longer valid or there has been a significant change.

What does this legislation mean?

It tells us that we have to carry out 'risk assessments'. It also makes clear that there is no choice. It is a clear legal requirement.

The process of risk assessment offers a proactive approach to enable organisations to avoid incurring losses by attempting to prevent accidents from happening in the first place. It is a careful examination of what in your work could cause harm to people. It must weigh up whether enough precautions have been taken or if more could be done to prevent harm from happening. This would suggest, therefore, that the pattern of waiting for accidents or ill health to happen and then implementing preventive measures for future occasions could and should be broken. That is a reactive version of risk assessment.

An accident is defined as an unexpected event without apparent cause, an unintentional, unfortunate act with possibly harmful consequences. Historically, human error was usually seen as the main contributor to accidents. A survey of human factors estimated that human error affecting accidents in hazardous technologies increased fourfold between the 1960s and 1990s to a maximum of over

90%. It seems unlikely that people have become more prone to error. With the increasing complexity of equipment and improved accident investigations which now take environmental and organisational factors into consideration, people have more opportunity to have accidents. It would, however, be irrational to assume that these are caused deliberately by those who suffer from them.

Lately, recognition has also been given to the fact that organisational accidents based in planning, scheduling, forecasting, designing, policy making, regulating etc. can be created and transmitted along departmental pathways and promote errors at the point of execution. It is people who design, build, operate, maintain, organise and manage in an increasingly challenging environment dominated by technological systems. A combination of latent weaknesses built into the system and active failures can penetrate layers of defence considered 'safe' and which are designed to protect both patients and staff.

Scientists have become interested in the different psychological origins for errors and differentiate between 'slips', 'lapses' and 'mistakes', 'errors' and 'violations'. It has further been recognised that human causes of accidents can often be followed back to organisational factors which have existed over long periods of time. Differentiation between active failures with instant adverse outcomes and delayed action failures which only become apparent when combined with local triggering events has led to classifying human errors either by their consequences or by their presumed causes (Reason, 1995).

A careful assessment of hazards and risks inherent in our daily routine could help to identify problems ahead of the accident waiting to happen and prevent the often cited costs and losses in both human and financial terms. Reason states that 'slips' and 'lapses' occur mainly during the performance of routine tasks performed almost automatically and usually in familiar surroundings. Precisely the environment we should assess for inherent hazards and risks.

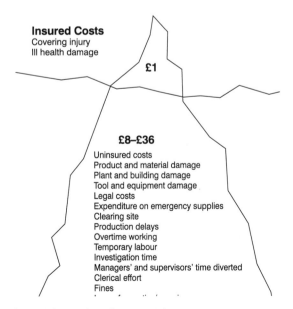

Insured Costs
Covering injury
Ill health damage

£1

£8–£36

Uninsured costs
Product and material damage
Plant and building damage
Tool and equipment damage
Legal costs
Expenditure on emergency supplies
Clearing site
Production delays
Overtime working
Temporary labour
Investigation time
Managers' and supervisors' time diverted
Clerical effort
Fines

Figure 11.1   The Accident Iceberg (source HSE)

The 'iceberg factor' (see Figure 11.1) would seem to concentrate on economic reasons for accident prevention. Mismanagement of health and safety at work is estimated to cost the UK economy between £10 billion and £15 billion per year, or 1.75% to 2.75% of the country's gross domestic product. This translates into 500 people dying in work-related accidents and 30 million working days lost through injury or ill health (McGuinness, 1995). Economically speaking, quite a convincing argument for employers to do something about it. Do not mock profit and loss arguments as a 'hidden agenda' of the employer. Rather, consider who usually carries the burden of the hidden costs. Yes, the remaining work force has to cover absences, carry the extra workload and endure the stresses and strains this automatically brings with it, not to mention the loss of valued friends and colleagues.

It would appear unreasonable to assume that organisations would wish to see their employees injured or killed through their activities. The human suffering involved surely provides enough moral reasons to prevent accidents from happening in the first place, as far as this is ever possible. Managing human fallibility is unlikely to ever be 100% effective. It is understood that, in the final analysis, not all risk can be eliminated. There is no totally risk-free environment. However, that does not stop us from checking for safety before crossing the road in order to prevent the proverbial bus from getting us today.

The legal reasons for risk assessment were explained above. The law is tightening up more and more with increasingly specific requirements and soon more environmental factors will enter the equation. We will all have to learn to consider the consequences of our actions for the environment and for future generations. The presently required risk assessment is only the first step in what one must hope will become a gradual change in attitude and culture.

It is somewhat unfortunate that the risk assessment terminology chosen by the HSE is apt to lead to some confusion. Differentiation between 'risk' and 'hazard' is not necessarily made in common, day-to-day language use. Boyle (1997) also points to some of the inconsistencies between various HSE publications and the possibility of misinterpretation because of them.

- **Assessment** is identifying the hazards present in an activity and estimating the risks involved, taking into account whatever precautions are already being taken. In the dictionary it is defined as 'estimating the magnitude or quality of …'
- **Hazard** means anything that can cause harm, or be a source of danger.

Boyle (1997) argues that we must be able to perceive a hazard, as it can equally well be identified by any of the five senses (with the exception of certain gases and radiation!). We must further have knowledge of the perceived hazard's potential to cause harm, i.e. be able to identify the nature of the harm which could arise and any causal links involved. He divides knowledge into:

- world knowledge – assumed to be possessed by the majority of the adult population;
- domain knowledge – restricted to individuals because of the domain of their activity.

Bringing all of these factors together, we reason and decide whether or not something is a hazard. An HSE definition makes no allowance for the fact that any combinations of hazards can cause harm. Neither does it take into consideration the time and place of the activity, or people's relation to them.

Risk is the chance (great or small) that someone will be harmed by the hazard or, to quote the dictionary again, the 'chance of bad consequences, exposure to mischance or danger'. Considering the large numbers of trivial risks against the decreasing numbers of more severe risks a classification of risk is intended to lead to prioritisation for action. However, there are several elements to risks:

- likelihood
- severity
- number of people possibly affected

which have to be taken on board when assessing the risk.

Since risk assessment is central to any effective health and safety management now and in the future, it is important to be clear about the requirements as set out by present legislation. What exactly does the law require?

The assessment will depend on a number of issues, for example:

- identifying the hazards;
- the circumstances involved in the task/activity that is being looked at;
- evaluating the risk;
- taking into account what controls are already present.

The Approved Code of Practice (ACoP) gives guidance on the regulations and explains further:

- that the purpose of assessment of risks is to determine what measures must be taken to comply with the law;
- that these measures can be identified by looking at the health and safety legislation and any other relevant standards such as Approved Codes of Practice and any manufacturers' instructions which apply.

These should be taken into account when carrying out the risk assessment so that the risk assessment will guide our judgement as to the measures we ought to take to comply with the law.

A guide to risk assessment

In order to explain what knowledge is needed for carrying out risk assessment the following questions are designed to provide a starting point and possible guide through the maze:

WHAT IS RISK ASSESSMENT FOR?

Risk assessment is to encourage safe and effective working practices and to remove or minimise hazards. It is not intended to be a critical assessment of individuals.

TO WHOM DOES RISK ASSESSMENT APPLY?

Risk assessment applies to all staff, and anyone else for whom the organisation has a duty of care where activities on our premises or under our control may cause harm to them. It includes the patient and any possible visitors but should, first and foremost, be considered to be for the benefit of the staff who perform regularly occurring, habitual tasks that have been identified as needing the assessment.

WHAT TYPE OF ACTIVITIES NEED TO BE ASSESSED?

Any work activity where somebody could be injured. The Health and Safety Executive (HSE) points out in its guidelines that one should beware of trivia and should not overcomplicate matters. If the work varies considerably or employees move frequently from site to site any reasonably foreseeable hazards should be selected for risk assessment.

WHO IS RESPONSIBLE FOR CARRYING OUT RISK ASSESSMENTS?

Any manager who has responsibility for an area of work or an activity that could cause harm to staff or anyone else for whom the organisation has a duty of care. Senior management is responsible for directing the programme and must identify appropriately trained individuals to carry out these risk assessments. Details of responsible posts must be reflected in health and safety policies.

SHOULD EMPLOYEES BE INVOLVED IN THE RISK ASSESSMENT?

The people who are most aware of risks are often those actually doing the work/task and they should be involved throughout the risk assessment process. A programme of awareness training in the requirements of the regulations for all staff should be a first step towards gaining staff confidence and to motivate towards active participation.

SHOULD SAFETY REPRESENTATIVES BE INVOLVED IN RISK ASSESSMENT?

Safety representatives, who may have a knowledge of the workplace activities, have been appointed by staff groups and trade unions. It is, therefore, appropriate to involve any appointed safety representatives in the risk assessment.

WHAT COMPETENCE AND TRAINING IS REQUIRED TO UNDERTAKE RISK ASSESSMENT?

To undertake assessments, staff must be competent. This requires information, instruction and training related to risk assessment for managers and sources of assistance from competent health and safety professionals.

WHERE CAN THEY GET THIS TRAINING?

There are numerous software applications on the market. Trade Unions train representatives regularly in order to enable them to fulfil their allocated function. Most large organisations have health and safety experts or an occupational health department who should advise for the organisations particular needs. However, they cannot and should not do it unless familiar with the activities being assessed.

What do you need to do to carry out a risk assessment?

The HSE recommends a 'five steps' approach:

1 Hazard identification

- The first step to consider in your risk assessment is to identify the hazards. This can be done by actively surveying the area where the work activity is being carried out and talking to the people carrying out the tasks, to see how the work is actually done.
- To help you to compile a list of hazards, it is good practice to involve the staff and locally appointed safety representatives.
- Look for the main hazards in your workplace or in specific activities. A decision needs to be made whether a hazard is significant and whether it is covered by satisfactory precautions so that the risk is small. Any unusual hazards spotted at a later date can be added to assessment as they become known.

2 Identifying persons at risk

- Decide who might be harmed and how. This must include cleaners, porters, maintenance personnel etc. who either regularly or occasionally share the workplace with you.

3 Risk evaluation and control measures

- Assess the severity of the risk and whether it is adequately controlled. Taking all precautions into consideration usually leaves some remaining risk. A first check should be concerned as to whether all legal requirements have been met before considering whether generally accepted standards for the profession are in place.
- You cannot necessarily stop there. Think for yourself, if there is anything else you can identify which may be locality specific (inadequate lighting, dangerous stairs, for example). The real aim is to make all risks as small as

possible by adding to your precautions to meet the legal requirement which says you must do what is reasonably practicable to keep your workplace safe.

4   Further action

What more can you do for those risks that are not adequately controlled? If the hazard cannot be removed, controlling and reducing the risk of harm being caused is the next step. Anyone in an operating department should be familiar with the process as it is the same as that applied to the Control of Substances Hazardous to Health Regulations (COSHH) (1998) which should be in force for substances such as glutaraldehyde, for example.

In these days of staff shortages ensure that anyone sharing your workplace on a self-employed or agency basis is aware of any risks identified and what precautions are being taken. In other words, familiarise new staff with your policies, procedures and protocols and do not assume anything.

5   Review your assessment

Activities change, new procedures are introduced, bringing with them new equipment etc. so from time to time you need to consider if a new assessment is required. Amending the assessment for every trivial change is not necessary but, for a new procedure or work activity which introduces significant hazards of its own, assessment in its own right should be considered.

WHAT RECORDS MUST YOU KEEP?

It is not necessary to show how the assessment was done. However, it is expected that it can be shown that:

- a proper check was made
- it was asked who might be affected
- obvious and significant hazards were dealt with
- consideration was given to the number of people who could be involved
- the precautions taken are reasonable, and the remaining risk low.

Written documentation for future reference will be more than helpful if, at any time, an inspector questions your precautions or if any action for civil liability is pending. Most solicitors these days are asking for the relevant risk assessment to be provided.

A written record can also be utilised for keeping an eye on particular matters and detecting possible patterns. It is visible proof that everything the law requires has been done. References to other already existing documents such as hospital policy, local procedure protocols, manufacturers' manuals and instructions can be made in the assessment record. There is no need to repeat all that and it is up to local policy whether all such documents are combined or kept separately.

WHAT IF CONTRACTORS ARE WORKING ON YOUR PREMISES?

Where contractors are working on your premises or on your behalf, they are required by law to undertake risk assessments. These must be available for inspection at any reasonable time if requested. A nominated health and safety contact within the contractor's organisation must be available to advise (via the identified in-house contact) in an emergency situation. All staff should be aware of this and report any observed breaches of local health and safety policy by contractors.

IS HEALTH SURVEILLANCE REQUIRED?

Advice on whether health surveillance is appropriate should be sought from your Occupational Health Department. This will normally be under specific regulations, e.g. Control of Substances Hazardous to Health (COSHH, 1994), Personal Protective Equipment (PPE, 1992), Noise at Work Regulations, etc.

If surveillance is required, the local Occupational Health Department should be able to assist in making the appropriate arrangements. If, for example, glutaraldehyde is still used in the department or there is regular contact with any known hazardous substance for which the COSHH regulations require health surveillance, all new staff should provide base line readings prior to employment. Management should then initiate appropriate surveillance of lung function, skin state, etc. Any identified problems due to latex allergy should be monitored by the Occupational Health Department and appropriate alternative gloves provided for the individuals concerned in line with the PPE Regulations. (These are just examples. There may be more in individual areas.)

Information and instructions to staff

Any briefing given to staff must explain the details of the risk assessment process. This will make staff aware of the aims and benefits of risk assessment so they can take an active part in the assessment. Such briefings can be given during other work related meetings although a record should be kept.

Explain to the staff:

- the reasons for, and benefits of, carrying out risk assessments;
- that they are the people who are most aware of the hazards involved in their work activities;
- they are more likely than anyone else to notice changes in working methods that will require review of the risk assessment;
- they need to take an active part in the process as it is for their own and everyone else's benefit. Staff should be reminded to concentrate on significant hazards.

Compiling a hazard inventory

In order to encourage staff to take part in the assessment and raise general awareness of health and safety matters it might be a good idea if a hazard identification form is given to each member of staff. Ask them to think about any activity needing to be assessed and what they think could reasonably be expected to cause harm. Remind them to ignore the trivial and concentrate on hazards that could cause serious harm. It can be surprising what is discovered that has been a reason for moans for some time but never been brought properly to the attention of management for correction. Explain that the environment in which the activities are performed can also give rise to risk, e.g. lighting, floor condition and so on.

You may wish to agree a return date for the completed form. This will help you to carry out an overall hazard assessment. The returned hazard identification forms will help you to make a list of the hazards and risks identified with a particular activity. Using your own knowledge, add any that you think may have been overlooked. You can then start to compile your Inventory of Hazards. This will also help you to decide what type of assessment is required.

Decide if any identified activities or hazards need to be discussed further with a member of staff or as a group. Most are likely to need to be discussed together or in Health and Safety Committee meetings. This can be picked up during other regular staff meetings arranged with staff to prevent the need for additional distractions.

Under health and safety legislation, you will also need to consider whether existing precautions meet standards set by any Approved Code of Practice, by a British, European or international standard and whether they comply with a recognised industry standard or are included in the latest Department of Health Hazard Notices.

Pointers to help you check all your hazards have been identified:

- Ensure everyone understands the objectives and encourage them to contribute.
- Review every aspect of the work activity, and identify all significant hazards in the workplace/activity which may cause harm. Use feedback from the staff and your own knowledge and experience.
- Actively survey the workplace and talk to staff carrying out the tasks, in order to see how the work is actually carried out.
- Remember that hazards do not only arise from physical conditions but also from working practices. Think about what actually happens in the workplace and during the work activity. Actual practice may differ from policy, procedures, manuals and so on. Hazards can creep in unnoticed.
- Consider non-routine operations including maintenance, loading and unloading, changes in organisation, systems or operations.
- Consider how potential interruptions or irregular work flows may affect the assessment.
- Consider the effectiveness of any controls or preventative measures that are in existence.
- Use past knowledge and experience, both your own and that of your staff and any accredited safety representatives.
- Refer to past accident/incident records and knowledge of near miss occurrences.
- A review of accident records and discussion with staff involved in the activity may help identify any near miss occurrences that are not common knowledge.
- Cross-reference to any specific assessments already undertaken.

- Use any lists or check lists available to help you such as the Risk Assessment Guide (RAG) published by the National Association of Theatre Nurses and any HSE guidance as well as all your procedure books etc.

Specific legal requirements

You will also need to consider and, where possible, identify areas where the law requires you to undertake specific assessments, e.g. under the COSHH Regulations. You should make a list of them and record whether or not they have been carried out. Where outstanding they should be included in the list of hazards discussed above.

Types of risk assessment

There could be three types of risk assessment you may need to carry out:

(a) Specific risk assessments

Specific risk assessments apply to activities for which specific legislation requires an activity to be carried out in a specific way, such as personal protective equipment; manual handling; work equipment; health, safety and welfare; display screen equipment; noise; electricity etc.

For all of these, individual regulations exist and must be adhered to. (This list is in no way complete.) Where other departments are responsible, you must bring the matter to their attention. This should be in writing, and a copy attached to your own records.

(b) General risk assessments

In every operating department there are a number of similar activities or situations which will require risk assessment. To reduce duplication of assessments, in certain circumstances a corporate risk assessment can be created within the organisation and used instead of carrying out a full basic risk assessment. This avoids the duplication of assessments that may to some extent be shared and only need slight adjustments for local requirements. These general assessments should concentrate on key activities which occur on several different sites but within the same Trust or Health Authority. This will save time and standardise assessments across the service. If work activities are the same or very similar, then the assessment should be endorsed, minor amendments being made where necessary and followed through.

Any additional significant hazards that you identify will need full assessment and inclusion in your assessment record. If the circumstances are very different in different areas, the general risk assessment will not apply and a full risk assessment will need to be undertaken, using the general one as a guide.

If your work activities are not covered by specific or corporate risk assessments because the circumstances are very different, or because no previous risk assessment has been carried out, then full risk assessments will have to be undertaken.

(c) Full risk assessments

A 'full' risk assessment is a careful examination of all work activities in order to establish what hazards exist, what risks arise and how these can be removed or controlled to prevent harm. You will now need to carry out a 'full' risk assessment for all the hazards you have identified in your final inventory that are not covered by a corporate general risk assessment or a specific risk assessment. This is covered in more detail below.

The full risk assessment

A full risk assessment means examining the hazards you have identified in order for you to decide whether you have taken enough precautions or could do more to prevent harm occurring. Remembering that a hazard is anything that can cause harm, the risk is the chance that someone will be harmed by the hazard. Therefore, the following must be considered and the assessment carried out in a structured way:

• Check if the law or any recognised standards and practices require you to do anything specific.
• Check if these standards are being met and, if not, identify actions to be taken.
• Check that existing precautions represent best practice.

Prioritising the assessment process

First, where a number of full risk assessments are undertaken, they must be assessed in priority order so that the most serious, or greatest, risk is dealt with first. You should already have identified whether the activity is carried out by an individual or a group.

When carrying out the risk assessment you need to consider both the likelihood of the hazards and risks coming together and the degree of severity. Severity could be determined by the number of people affected.

You need to give a priority ranking to hazards and risks so that, when you assess the level of risk involved, you can prioritise your assessments and the actions that need to be taken. You cannot do everything at once, so it makes sense and is cost-effective to prioritise the health and safety needs and actions that require immediate attention.

Wherever possible remove the risks by:

• stopping the activity; or
• substituting it with a less hazardous one; otherwise
• reduce the risks as far as is reasonably practicable, taking into account what controls are already present.

Remember the risks need to be 'significant' and not trivial unless they have a major impact on the personnel involved. Take care not to obscure the 'major' risks with an excess of information.

Persons at risk

The second step you need to consider in your risk assessment is who might be harmed, how they can be harmed, how badly they may be harmed, and probable or defined length of time exposed to hazard. Do not forget to include people who may not be in the area all the time who will be unfamiliar with the environment (such people are less likely to be aware of fire exits, specific procedures etc.). This will include maintenance staff, contractors, visiting colleagues and representatives from suppliers, medical students, agency staff and members of the public. Also consider vulnerable persons such as staff working regularly in isolated situations, staff with disabilities and new or expectant mothers. Identify such persons on your assessment form.

Risk evaluation and control measures

Third, assess the severity of the hazard, using your experience and common sense to judge the possible outcome. When considering how severe the harm from a hazard could be, it is important to be realistic. Any hazard could result in death. It is possible for someone falling over a trailing lead to be killed, but the most probable result is bruising or, at worst, a fractured bone. However, if the lead is across the top of a staircase, a more severe injury is likely. Similarly, a splinter of wood in the hand could result in tetanus and death but a minor injury is the more realistic outcome.

Risk assessments cover a number of different areas over a wide ranging subject matter. You need to keep the process as simple as possible. The process suggested here uses a high, medium and low estimate for both hazard and risk, as well as for the overall risk assessment. This is explained in the next section.

HAZARD AND RISK CRITERIA

Using the following suggested criteria to decide or assess the severity of each hazard can be a great help in sorting the 'must be done' from the 'should be attended to' and the 'can wait a little longer' actions still outstanding. This is of considerable assistance when allocating scarce budget resources. Make no mistake, any identified high rating risk will need to be controlled immediately and appropriate resources allocated. Hazard levels can be high, medium or low as follows:

HIGH (H)	death or major injury could occur serious illness requiring hospitalisation is almost certain to result.
MEDIUM (M)	serious injury or illness is likely to occur, requiring sick leave for more than 3 days, but not hospitalisation.
LOW (L)	minor injuries or illness could occur, requiring up to 3 days sick leave, or none at all.

When you have decided what you think the level is, enter H, M, or L in your severity column against each hazard. Now consider the likelihood of the hazard actually causing harm, i.e. the risk, using the following criteria:

HIGH (H)   where it is almost certain or very likely that harm will occur.

MEDIUM (M)   where harm is possible or likely to occur.

LOW (L)   where harm is unlikely and will seldom occur.

It is important not to underestimate the likelihood of hazards causing harm, especially if your experience of actual accidents occurring is limited. It is useful to draw on the experience of your safety representatives, staff and colleagues who may be aware of accidents and 'near misses'. These may have actually happened to them or they may have heard of them happening in similar workplaces.

Other factors to consider are:

- the number of times the situation or work activity occurs
- the length of exposure
- the position of the hazard
- possible distractions
- adequacy of lighting
- environmental conditions
- condition of equipment
- competence of people involved
- quantities of materials involved
- maintenance and cleaning.

Now you are ready to assess the level of risk(s) associated with each hazard by using the risk estimator (Figure 11.2).

	LOW HAZARD (slightly harmful)	MEDIUM HAZARD (moderately harmful)	HIGH HAZARD (extremely harmful)
LOW RISK POTENTIAL highly unlikely/unlikely	LOW RISK *(trivial)*	LOW RISK *(acceptable)*	MEDIUM RISK *(moderate)*
MEDIUM RISK POTENTIAL likely/possible	LOW RISK *(acceptable)*	MEDIUM RISK *(moderate)*	HIGH RISK *(substantial)*
HIGH RISK POTENTIAL more likely/near certain	MEDIUM RISK *(moderate)*	HIGH RISK *(substantial)*	HIGH RISK *(intolerable)*

Figure 11.2   Risk estimator

By reading down the vertical hazard column, where it meets the appropriate horizontal risk column, you can calculate the overall level of risk and enter H, M, or L on your risk assessment form . For example:

A HIGH (extremely harmful) hazard
with a LOW risk potential (highly unlikely to occur)
would result in a MEDIUM risk;

A LOW (slightly harmful) hazard
with a MEDIUM risk potential
would result in a LOW (acceptable) risk.

RISK CONTROL MEASURES

You then have to consider whether sufficient precautions have been taken against the risk from the hazards you have identified. Your aim, where possible, is to remove the risks or make them smaller by adding to and improving your precautions.

For example, has the organisation provided:

- Safe systems of work?
- Laid down procedures on how to carry out tasks?
- Ensured adequate training and supervision?
- Provided suitable information and instruction?

Do the precautions:

- Meet the standards set by a legal requirement?
- Comply with a recognised industry standard?
- Represent good practice?
- Reduce risks as far as reasonably practicable?

Enter brief details of control measures on your assessment form. If these adequately control the risk, enter on the assessment; if not or if you are unable to decide and require further advice from some experts make the appropriate entry.

If you have identified the need for further action, move on to the next step.

Further action

The fourth step you need to consider in your risk assessment is what more could the organisation reasonably do for those risks that you found were not adequately controlled.

You will need to give priority to those risks that affect large numbers of people and/or could result in serious harm. Consider the following possibilities when deciding what further action to take:

- remove the hazard completely?
- prevent access to the hazard?
- reorganise work to reduce exposure to the hazard?
- issue personal protective equipment?

> ASSESSMENTS NEED TO BE SUITABLE AND SUFFICIENT, NOT PERFECT

Since it is unlikely that your organisation has unlimited resources, it is probable that all the problems you may have identified are unlikely to be resolved at once. So you will need to list unresolved problems on a priority basis, using a Management Action Plan. List the actions required on a priority basis of High, Medium, or Low. This will provide you with both a record of what is required and a monitoring aid.

You can also list any outstanding specific risk assessments. If a hazard later becomes more or less urgent due to a change of circumstances this can be picked up and the priority altered accordingly.

Review your assessment

The fifth step you need to take in the risk assessment process is to review your findings. The main things that you will have to show are that:

- a proper assessment was made;
- you have considered who might be affected;
- you identified all the obvious and significant hazards;
- you took into account the number of people who may be affected;
- the precautions are reasonable and any remaining risks are considered to be low.

Once you are happy with the risk assessment you have carried out, it should be signed and dated, and be readily available if required for inspection.

WHEN TO REVIEW ASSESSMENTS

Sooner or later activities or personnel change, so it is a good idea to review your risk assessments at regular intervals and if necessary amend or carry out a new one. Changes to be considered include:

- whether any new equipment, substances or processes have been introduced;
- whether any additional persons may be affected, such as new or temporary staff, or where access has been opened up to other people such as contractors or members of the public.

It is not necessary to carry out a re-assessment if the changes are only trivial and have little effect on the risks involved or on the original assessment but a note should be made to the effect that a review has been carried out and signed and dated by the risk assessor line manager. It is good practice to undertake a regular overall review of your risk assessments at least every 3 years, but ideally at more frequent intervals such as annually.

Conclusion

There is no doubt that risk assessment and risk management are central to effective health and safety management and will remain so in the future when environmental aspects will have to be taken into consideration as well. Deployment of limited resources at different levels of the system must include the individual or team, the task, the situation and the organisation as a whole. General improvement of working conditions and ongoing evaluation of work demands and staffing levels in the NHS were included in the recommendations of a report by the Partnership on the Health of the NHS Workforce (Williams *et al.*, 1998). The fact that health care work poses problems of a psychological as well as physiological nature is accepted. The report saw, however, that there is a clear need for urgent and compassionate action by employers to implement recommendations and regulations if the ill health in the NHS workforce is to be dealt with effectively.

As stated at the beginning, the cycle itself is hardly new to nursing. What is new and should be seen as progress, is the application of safety procedures to staff by law and the active involvement of all levels of employees in the assessment cycle. Principled risk management takes into account possible latent failures which may already be embedded in the system long before accidents occur and makes such identified sources of probable failure its prime concern and combines it with the measures described above.

Measures involving sanctions and disciplinary procedures have been shown to have very limited effectiveness, especially when directed at a workforce of highly trained professionals (Reason, 1995). This does not in any way diminish our commitment to excellent nursing care but enhances it as the people giving it should be healthier and better motivated to do so. If we go about claiming that nobody cares for the carers then it would seem appropriate and high time to care sufficiently for ourselves. It has been one of this nurse's maxims that people who cannot care for themselves are hardly the people to entrust with the care of others.

If that means we have to speak up for ourselves, alert management to their responsibilities and cooperate when they accept those responsibilities, even if mainly for economic reasons, so be it. Tackling intrinsic organisational causes subjected to external, political and financial pressures whilst facing ever higher public expectations is not an easy task. It is, however, one task we can and should no longer avoid or hide from, considering that we all have a responsibility in law as well as moral and ethical reasons for caring for ourselves, our colleagues and, last but by no means least, continuing to care for our patients to the highest possible standards in whatever capacity and environment.

Reflective activities

This chapter has gone in some detail into the principles of risk assessment. It could be used as a guide in setting up risk assessment or, more likely, to allow you to explore and understand the difference between the concepts of 'hazard' and 'risk'. At the same time these concepts have been described within the setting of health and safety in the workplace.

1   It is suggested that you reflect on the risk assessment carried out in your department.

2   Is risk management being used as an effective tool on both fronts? That is to say, both to ensure the health and safety of all in the work place and in identifying the clinical risks to patients.

3   Are you identifying and prioritising the risks correctly?

4   Having carried out risk assessment, have the appropriate follow-up actions been carried out?

5   If you have recognised any deficiencies, what actions will you now initiate?

6   Are you aware on a personal basis of the hazards and risks related to your activities in the operating department?

References

Boyle, A. 1997 A fresh look at risk assessment. *The Safety and Health Practitioner* **15** (2).
Control of Substances Hazardous to Health Regulations 1998.
Manual Handling Regulations 1992.
DOH. 1992 *The health of the nation: a strategy for health in England.* Cmmnd.1986. London, HMSO.
Health and Safety Executive Publications.
Free and priced publications can be obtained from:
HSE Books, PO Box 1999, Sudbury, Suffolk, CO10 6FS.
Telephone: 01787 881165; fax: 01787 313995.
Holroyd, K. 1998 Staying healthy in the NHS. *Occupational Health Review,* May/June.
HSE News (Editorial) 1997 Occupational Health Department left to look after safety of staff. *Occupational Health* September 1997 **49** (9), 7.
McGuinness, P. 1995 *Risk assessment. A practical guide.* London, The Industrial Society.
NATN 1995 Risk Assessment Guidelines and Staffing in the Operating Department. *RAG* Harrogate, NATN.
Nursing Times. 1998a **94** (17), April 29, 7. London, Emap Healthcare, Macmillan.
Nursing Times. 1998b **94** (18), May 6, 8. London, Emap Healthcare, Macmillan.
Personal Protective Equipment at Work Regulations 1992.
Reason, J. 1995 Understanding adverse events: human factors. *Quality in Health Care* **4**, 80–8.
The Health and Safety at Work Act 1974.
The Management of Health and Safety at Work Regulations 1992.
Williams, S., Michie, S. & Pattani, S. 1998 *Improving the health of the NHS workforce: report of the partnership on the Health of the NHS workforce.* London, Nuffield Trust.

Further reading

A guide to risk assessment requirements. 1996 IND (G) 218 (L).

Five steps to risk assessment. 1994 IND (G)163 L.

Goldman, L. 1995 *The legal costs of failing to assess risk.* Conference paper.

Health and Safety Commission 1999. *The Management of Health and Safety at Work Approved Code of Practice.*

Health and Safety (Display Screen Equipment) Regulations 1992.

Heimreich, R. L. & Schaefer H. G. 1994 Team performance in the operating room. In: Bogner, M.S. (ed.) *Human errors in medicine.* Hillsdale, New Jersey, Eribaum.

Holt, A. & Andrews, H. 1991 *Principles of health and safety at work.* London, IOSH Publishing.

Manual handling in the health services. ISBN 0 7176 12481.

Manual Handling Operations Regulations 1992.

Provision and Use of Work Equipment Regulations 1992.

The Costs of Accidents at Work. HSE HS(G) 96.

The Management of Health and Safety at Work (Amendment) Regulations 1994.

The Workplace (Health, Safety and Welfare) Regulations 1992.

Acknowledgement

Many thanks are due to Mr Geoff Lloyd, Senior Safety Adviser, Directorate of Occupational Health, Metropolitan Police Service, for his support and advice in all matters of risk assessment principles.

PART FOUR

Change and clinical practice

The value of education **12**

Barbara J Gruendemann

Barbara Gruendemann needs no introduction to perioperative nurses worldwide. She is an educator and author and has been involved in writing and editing many standard publications in the field. In this chapter she reflects on an aspect of perioperative education to which many may have given little thought. As nurse education becomes increasingly expensive and ever more technical, training is required to ensure safe use of complex equipment. Manufacturers are increasingly providing both information and education. A number of questions are asked, and answered, here. Guidance is given to enable perioperative nurses to recognise high quality educational programmes and to become discriminating purchasers of such educational opportunities.

This chapter leads into a section of the book which relates to changes in clinical practice which have transformed much of the actual intraoperative period of perioperative practice. The views expressed in this chapter are very relevant to the descriptions of changes in practice outlined in the next two chapters (13 and 14) and which have followed the introduction of minimal access surgery. Perioperative nurses have sometimes been criticised for their close relationships with industry by those who have not realised how important this training is as new techniques and instrumentation are introduced. The feedback from those using new instruments is also of importance in the research and development of instruments and equipment. It is suggested that it would be appropriate to read this chapter before moving on to Chapters 13 and 14.

Introduction

In 1997, a contractual agreement was forged between the American Medical Association (AMA) and Sunbeam Corporation. The contract stipulated that the AMA would produce valuable health information for consumers, packaging it with Sunbeam's high quality home health care products such as vaporisers and blood pressure monitors. Sunbeam would pay AMA a royalty on sales of products containing the information, with the proceeds supporting the AMA's many educational programmes.

Sunbeam stated that this would be a source of added value to their customers and provide a point of differentiation from competing manufacturers. After all, said Sunbeam, other manufacturers are engaged in similar worthwhile partnering agreements to bring health information and healthy products to consumers. In this agreement, the AMA would benefit from financial rewards as well as an enhanced image as a provider of valuable consumer information and education. The provisions of this contract, however, were never fully realised. Much public and professional criticism and reconsideration by the AMA led to a contract that was voided by the AMA. At the time of this writing, Sunbeam is pursuing its contractual rights in a United States federal court (Dunlap 1997).

This scenario raises several issues that are pertinent to the theme of this chapter:

- What is the value (or 'added value') of education?
- What is the nature of education?
- Is 'information' education?
- Who should provide education? Is education ever pure and without bias?
- How can educational offerings be evaluated?

The value of education

The word 'education' means something different to each learner. Learning is unique to each individual and comes after a perceived or real need. According to Webster's Dictionary (1998), education is the act or process of imparting or acquiring general knowledge and of developing the powers of reasoning and judgement.

Embedded within any definition of education is a process that includes not only the taking in of information and facts, but also doing something with that information. This 'doing something' can be changing a way of thinking, perfecting a new skill or technique, or behaving in a new or different way that furthers one's prowess in a profession.

Education is the key to furthering the goals of perioperative nursing. Perioperative nurses engage in many forms of education: they learn, for example, how to assess patients for potential latex allergies; they become skilled in advanced laparoscopic instrumentation and they come to realise the impact of emerging antibiotic-resistant microbes on their care of patients.

All of these examples may help the perioperative nurse in broadening his or her spheres of thinking and doing. Professional nursing includes both the process of thinking and the actions that ensue. True education is not a frill. It is an absolute necessity for professional growth.

The 'value' of education is determined by the learner who perceives worth and integrates the learning into self, or rejects what has been presented. Learners come with predetermined thoughts, prejudices, and feelings that affect the ability and the willingness to learn. Personal, cultural, and emotional factors also play a role. Value translates into worthiness, appreciation, and usefulness, and is usually subjective and personal. Value is also expressed in the degree of excellence that ensues in the perioperative nurse's practice habits. Education is important to the individual nurse and to the effect it has on group behaviour, policies, and standards of practice.

The nature of education

Education is non-commercial and generic, meaning that it cannot be tainted with biased or one-sided information. (See scenario at beginning of chapter for references to education versus information and where the perception of commercialism may have been present.) Education should be informative in that all views of a topic are presented. In perioperative nursing, education must be current, based on science as much as possible, and taught or brought forward by those who are credentialed, qualified, and considered fit for the subject at hand.

'Inservice education,' on the other hand, is training designed for specific tasks or procedures, is narrow in scope, and is an important part of orientation to a facility, clinical unit, organisation, or a set of workplace practices. Inservice education is usually conducted within a targeted work area or functioning business or clinical unit, and is necessary for a professional's integration into a particular work setting.

For the perioperative nurse, inservice education might include:

- the institution's or organisation's policies and procedures
- safety and emergency procedures
- personnel policies
- dress codes
- job expectations
- evaluation procedures.

Inservice education can also include information about, and instruction in the use of, products that are or will be used in the perioperative setting. These instructional sessions may be taught by a salesperson or another company representative who is very familiar with the product and its application in the operative setting. This chapter does not include a discourse on 'inservice education.'

Methods to further personal and professional growth through generic education can be varied and creative. Some nurses prefer textbooks or self-study programmes; others like on-line, computerised information and many others prefer traditional classroom lectures, discussions, or videotapes where there are opportunities for interaction with the teacher, programme, and other class members. Most want feedback of any variety, and a form of reinforcement when some sort of behavioural change has taken place. All adult learners expect that principles of adult education will be evident in the planning and execution of the educational programme or activity.

Behavioural objectives should be clearly stated, well-defined, and understood by the learners and the teacher(s), at the beginning of any educational endeavour.

Perioperative nurses are usually eager to engage in educational offerings that add to their storehouse of knowledge, increase their technical skills, make them think, and increase their ability to be better persons as well as better nurses.

The nature of education can also be analysed in terms of commitment, for this is integral to the educational process. This commitment can involve time, effort, *and* money. Should sponsors of education charge for their services? Yes, because *value* is often equated with what the learner 'gives' in return for receiving something, and that includes paying for educational programmes. Charges, however, must be perceived as reasonable and fair and must offer returns for the learner, perhaps in the form of education credits or other benefits.

It has been said that what we obtain too cheaply, we esteem too lightly. 'Free' education is often not valued if it has no 'attachments' to which one must commit, even if this means money. To paraphrase a popular cliché, there is no 'free lunch'. Perioperative nurses will place value on education that is relevant, cost-effective, and beneficial in terms of outlay and results.

Is 'information' education?

The imparting and receiving of information is only the beginning of education. Knowledge that is gained or factual information that is received must be used to go to the next level: that of internalising, integrating and making sense of the knowledge so that broader actions and thinking can follow. As an example, the perioperative nurse gains information on several emerging infectious diseases. The nurse then uses the knowledge in several ways:

- to alter Standard Precautions policies for the operating room that include proper disinfection and sterilisation practices which will protect both patient and staff;
- to re-examine clean-up procedures and to assess adequacy of scrubbing and hand-washing techniques.

The nurse may also use new information on infectious diseases to revamp assessment skills for patients who might come to the operating room with one of the diseases.

Whether subtle or obvious, the link from information to actions is a vital component of true education and cannot be ignored. The mere receiving of information can and does lead to education but only if the learner is aware of the process and does not allow it to stop midstream.

Who should provide education?

Providers of education can be organisations, health care facilities, corporations, consulting firms or individuals. Accreditation or endorsement of providers by credible and recognised entities is an absolute 'must'. Accreditation is a 'seal of approval' and a statement of assurance to the learner that the programmes provided are of the highest quality, are accurate and timely, have well-defined goals, and are taught by qualified and experienced persons or groups.

Perioperative nurses should pay as close attention to the qualifications of the instructor as they do to the sponsoring entity. The mere presence of initials or listed degrees after a name may not automatically guarantee competence to teach or competence and knowledge in the topic at hand, although these credentials are important in the total assessment. The teacher should have demonstrated abilities and competencies in the specific subject matter and should be a recognised teacher. Word-of-mouth or networking recommendations on a programme or teacher are often as valuable, if not more so, as written statements in a brochure or programme.

Perioperative nurses often have educational requirements for relicensure, recertification, or other credentialing mechanisms, and will base at least part of their assessment of a programme on the awarding of some type of educational credits or units. This, of course, will be dependent on the requirements of different countries and professional organisations around the world and, therefore, may necessitate different verification procedures. Programmes approved for educational credits must usually undergo vigorous steps to meet requirements. This is another positive sign, assuring that the programme has met at least the minimum requirements for a credible, 'good' course or presentation.

Hospitals and other health care facilities have typically been the primary providers of perioperative nursing education. But in recent years, hospitals around the world have seen budgets for education diminishing and in many cases, disappearing. Therefore, hospitals increasingly are looking to other sources to supply and meet educational needs. Corporations and medical products companies are beginning to fill some of these needs by providing educational videotapes, manuals and other publications, interactive programmes, conferences, and consulting services.

Corporations, worldwide, are understanding the budget restrictions imposed on hospitals and realising that they can help fill some of the gaps. Companies are developing educational resources within 'education departments'; some are sponsoring credible educators who teach in hospitals; and others are restructuring marketing strategies to include 'customer education' in their company's mission. A few large companies that originally provided customer education have now discontinued the practice, citing their own budget restraints and non-measurable 'return on investment'.

Corporations that do provide perioperative nursing (and other) educational programmes cite the following advantages to the company:

- value-added service to customers (real and potential customers);
- good-will and competitive edge;
- development of partnerships with clients;
- establishment of relationships that can lead to 'relationship selling';
- heightened image and credibility;
- inherent part of progressive marketing and sales strategies.

Many of the corporations that provide education are also sources of commercial products for the perioperative area. Although many credible companies have excellent educational activities that are non-commercial and generic, some do not. It is important for perioperative nurses to be able to distinguish the commercial from the non-commercial 'education' programmes (and for the companies to label them as such).

If a corporation-sponsored educational offering has blatant product advertising, it is not truly 'educational'. Sales promotions can be subtle and 'slipped into' education or be slanted towards a certain product or groups of products. If the education teacher is a company salesperson, the presentation will most likely be biased, naturally towards sales and product promotion; this is a commonly expected behaviour for the salesperson, as it should be. It is difficult for a salesperson to 'wear two hats', nor should the company (or the nurse) have that expectation. If there is denigration by the teacher of other products or companies, there is assurance that the programme is commercially oriented and biased. If there is a product display in the same room as the 'education' programme, chances are quite high that there will, subtly or overtly, be a blurring of education and sales goals. Nurses have a responsibility to question the company and its representatives on the programme's objectives, any credits to be awarded, qualifications of the instructor that are directly related to programme content, and the outcomes to be expected.

If the educational programme is inclusive of all aspects of a topic (even if the topic is controversial); free of unnatural aggrandisement of a topic or one aspect of a topic; factual in its content; scientific in its approach; generic, reliable and topical in its treatment of the subject; free of subtle and overt references to products and companies and inclusive of questions, answers, and free discussion of the subject, it most likely is truly educational and will be of great benefit to perioperative nurses.

Can education always be pure and unbiased? Probably not. But becoming aware of possible biases will alert learners to carefully assess the roots of potential influences of programmes in which learners choose to participate. If a generalisation can be made from research to education, the following report on possible conflicts of interest becomes relevant. Citing the fact that very little has been done to examine the influence of corporate funding on scientific opinions, a Canadian study asked if research is influenced by corporate funding. The study focused on researchers who evaluated risks and benefits of calcium channel blockers.

It was found that most of the researchers who publicly supported calcium channel blockers had received financial support from companies that make the drugs, including speaking honorariums, consulting fees, money to attend symposiums, and funding for research.

Published comments on the article itself include the necessity of revealing potential conflicts of interest, understanding the opportunities for problems and abuse, especially in research, but also knowing that there are checks and balances in place, such as disclosure policies of medical journals (Stelfox *et al.*, 1996). Building awareness of a problem, such as cholesterol consciousness, can enable pharmaceutical companies, for example, to market drugs that lower blood cholesterol levels.

As another example, building awareness of the importance of hand-washing in infection prevention can help a university raise funds to further research on increasing compliance with the washing of hands. This in turn can increase the credibility of the researchers and the university, and may lead to findings that benefit both health care professionals and the public.

It is obvious from these examples that the issue of influences (of many types) on education and research can have positive, neutral, or negative outcomes, for the learner and for the researcher (Tanouye 1998).

Evaluation of educational offerings

There are guidelines and criteria for determining the value of an educational offering. Perioperative nurses, familiar with patient assessment skills, can use the same diagnostic techniques for assessing an education programme. It is helpful to couch some salient points as questions. The most valuable criteria are as follows:

Objectives and content
- Thorough description of programme's intent?
- All sides of an issue presented?
- Objectives stated in measurable terms?
- Target audience(s) identified?
- Descriptive, understandable outcomes?
- Adequate evaluation procedures?
- Content not commercial?

Accreditation or sponsorship
- Clear statement of sponsors and promoters?
- Reputable, verifiable accreditation agency (professional associations, universities, or other highly-regarded educational organisations)?
- Offers credits or certificates?
- Offers continuing education credits in reasonable amounts?
- Sponsored/funded by an educationally oriented organisation or institution?

Speakers/faculty/education leaders

- Qualified to speak?
- Appropriate credentials for the topic?
- Qualified regarding the specific content?
- Allow for interaction, discussion, and question and answer times during the programme?
- Sponsored by a reputable school or company that is committed to professional education?

Environment and take-aways

- Pertinent and useful notebooks, handouts?
- Any displays of commercial products outside of the classroom?
- Opportunities for networking?
- Comfortable physical surroundings?
- Come away from programme with new, useful, or novel ideas or practices?
- New perspectives, insights?
- Programme valuable to you, personally, professionally, or both?

Summary

Education is a thread that continually runs through all of perioperative nursing. In this chapter, education is defined, described, and analysed. Examples of the influences that can affect educational programming are discussed. The perioperative nurse must be a sophisticated buyer of programmes, always assessing personal and professional worth of the educational activity and outcomes. Guidelines for evaluating educational programmes are provided. We have not done well in quantifying the beneficial effects of education, let alone described the positive 'fallouts' and changes that do usually occur with a high-quality programme.

Learning is difficult to measure and the true outcome of education can probably only be found in the minds and actions of those who experience it. Regardless, education in its finest form must be carefully preserved, articulately presented, and artistically integrated into one's being.

Reflective activities

Perioperative nurses have, by necessity, always established close relationships with the manufacturers of the instruments and equipment used in the operating room. This has been essential for many years. However, when financial gain by one or both parties is involved there is always the question of bias to be considered.

1 Do you believe that sponsorship of educational programmes is ethical? If so, who would be appropriate sponsors? How much more personally expensive would you find education without sponsorship?

2 How valuable have the contributions of manufacturers been in recent years in ensuring for example, that surgeons and operating department teams have been competent and up to date in the use of equipment needed for minimal access surgery? Has the practical training been backed up by education using the results of current research?

3 Have you ever been uneasy about educational opportunities offered to you? If so, why? Use the criteria offered in the chapter to analyse the situation.

See Chapter 14 for description of inservice education by a company representative.

References

Dunlap, A.J. 1997 Why I'm taking on the arrogant AMA. *Wall Street Journal* 17 November, C:A16.

Stelfox, H.T., Chua, G., O'Rourke, K. & Detsky, A. 1996 Conflict of interest in the debate over calcium-channel antagonists. *The New England Journal of Medicine* **338**,101–8.

Tanouye, E. 1998 Does corporate funding influence research? *Wall Street Journal* 8 January, Cl:B1.

Webster's American Family Dictionary. 1998 New York, Random House, Inc. 300.

Further reading

Anon 1989a Hospitals link education with hard numbers. *Hospitals* 20 May, 64.

Anon 1989b Education centres are subtle marketing tools. *Hospitals* 20 September, 76.

Becker, G.E. 1995 The value of educational meetings. *Infection Control and Sterilisation Technology* **1**, 12.

Crim, B.J. & Hood, A.W. 1995 The educational process. In: Gruendemann, B.J. & Fernsebner, B. *Comprehensive perioperative nursing* Vol. 1. Boston, Jones & Bartlett, pp. 17–48.

Galbraith, M.W. 1991 *Facilitating adult learning: A transactional process.* Malabar, FL, Krieger.

Goldrick, B., Gruendemann, B.J. & Larson, E. 1993 Learning styles and teaching/learning strategy preferences: Implications for educating nurses in critical care, the operating room, and infection control. *Heart and Lung* **22**,176–82.

Hansten, R.l. & Washburn, M.J. 1997 Successful restructuring: Maximising training dollars. *Nursing Economics* March–April **15**, 22–4.

Louden T.L. 1990 Customer education programs show returns. *Health Industry Today* June, 13.

McMurry, P.V. Jr. 1991 Health education: Fulfilling a mission. *Health Systems Review* November/December, 46–7.

Milks, D.A. & Siefert, S.E. 1997 Contracting educational and library services. *Journal of Healthcare Resource Management* **15**, 22–4.

Senge P.M. 1990 *The fifth discipline: The art and practice of the learning organisation.* New York, Doubleday Currency.

13

Introducing minimal access surgery

Inger Lönroth

Introduction
Nurses change to high-tech engineers
Technological understanding – an absolute necessity
Continuous need for education
Accountability

Inger Lönroth is a Swedish nurse who has been heavily involved with the development of minimal access surgery (MAS) in a general surgery theatre. She has chosen to describe the development of MAS surgery from the introduction of diagnostic laparoscopy in surgery to the high technology operations now carried out using TV monitors and the 'three (micro) chip' cameras of today. Her description of the early introduction of minimal access surgery emphasises how difficult it was for operating department staff to cope with a major and rapid surgical revolution without training and support. This chapter and Chapter 14 have a different format from the rest of the book. The two chapters should be read together. The aim was to describe the experience of a perioperative nurse faced with the introduction of new techniques and to follow this with a description of the support provided by the manufacturers.

Introduction

Minimal access surgery (MAS) is designed to reduce the trauma to the abdominal or thoracic wall caused by major surgery. The gains are mainly described as rapid recovery with early return to full activity, accompanied by a short hospital stay. With the introduction of videoscopic surgery, the full development of MAS has been very rapid. The first reported laparoscopy and thoracoscopy in the human was carried out by Hans Christian Jacobaeus at the Karolinska Institute in Stockholm, Sweden in October 1910. It was recognised early that pneumoperitoneum was crucial to the success of laparoscopic examination.

Janos Verres constructed a spring-loaded needle containing a blunt obdurator in 1938. This later became the preferred needle for establishing pneumoperitoneum.

From about 1964, Professor Kurt Semm played the key role in the development of laparoscopy and designed new instruments. Automatic insufflators were introduced in 1966, bipolar high frequency endocoagulation was started in 1971, and endosuture techniques by 1980. Tubal sterilisation by endocoagulation was started in 1972.

The major breakthrough came in 1985 with the introduction of the first computer-chip TV camera which has led to a revolution in surgery. Dr Phillipe Mouret performed the first laparoscopic cholecystectomy in the human in France in 1987. Within one year this procedure was undertaken by a number of centres in the western world. Endosurgery had arrived.

My first encounter with laparoscopy and laparoscopic surgery was within the field of gynaecology. In Sweden, at the beginning of the 1980s, laparoscopy was mainly carried out for diagnostic purposes and occasionally for sterilisation. Videotechnique had not been introduced at that time and only the surgeon could look into the monocular endoscope, so nobody else could obtain an internal view. For a perioperative nurse, this could be unsatisfying because one did not participate in the procedures. Usually, these diagnostic laparoscopies were brief operative procedures. In spite of this, diagnostic laparoscopy occupied a large amount of operating time. Without any statistical documentation, a rough estimate would be up to about 40% of all operative procedures carried out in the gynaecological theatre at that time.

The complete instrumentation was very simple. Apart from the endoscope and the Verres cannula, the gynaecologist used a long probe that was introduced through the abdominal wall without any ports, and used only to manipulate the internal organs to improve the view of the uterus.

The introduction of laparoscopy in general surgery came to Sweden in 1990 with the first laparoscopic cholecystectomies. This new technique was introduced abruptly into our surgical department. The nurses were apprehensive and frustrated. Experienced perioperative nurses became insecure and did not like their new, difficult tasks. In our unit a special nurse had to take care of the maintenance and purchasing of disposable and non-disposable equipment. She had to search through a jungle to find the right laparoscopic equipment. Many questions arose. What kind of instruments were needed? Who were the companies marketing this or that? What was the proper set-up for the patient in the operating room and for the instrumentation?

The majority of staff did not like the new technique, mainly because of fear of something new. It was not like 'the good old days' when you had an open abdomen and you were working in cooperation with the surgeon with scissors and grasping forceps. Now you could only stand passively by his side and watch a television set! You could not participate and help in the wound as before. After the laparoscopic cholecystectomies, newer laparoscopic procedures were successively introduced. These included Nissen fundoplication for oesophageal reflux.

In the beginning this was a struggle. We started with laparoscopy and after a long time, several hours, in fact, the procedure was converted to open surgery. This was very frustrating for the staff with double the work. It was also hard to watch the surgeon more or less 'poking around' without getting anywhere, to say nothing of the effects of long surgery on the patient. This went on until the surgeons overcame the hardships and you found that you no longer had to have extra instrumentation for open surgery ready within the operating room.

At the introduction of a new procedure we always had all the instruments for open surgery unpacked on the trolley as we carried out the laparoscopic procedure. This made the work load very heavy, with many instruments to maintain and a lot of preoperative preparations. Although we had double the work one could not say it was a waste of resources, because this was a necessary learning curve. However, it was tedious for nurses to stand by, waiting, during those initial slow procedures. Once the surgeons had passed the limit where they knew the technique, new procedures were introduced, such as adrenalectomies, which were faster and less cumbersome. These later new procedures were not so demanding for the nurses, although for security reasons, we still had a lot of extra equipment unpacked.

My personal standpoint, as a perioperative nurse, is that I do not feel any apprehension of this surgery today; nor do I find it boring. If you decide to focus your interest on this new surgery, you can follow the new developments and obtain satisfaction in developing a profound knowledge of the instruments and equipment used. The general attitude to minimal access surgery among nurses has become much more positive, thanks to the fact that the process can now be seen. Procedures are accomplished much more rapidly and you experience and understand the 'games' of laparoscopy.

Many nurses would not be prepared to work with laparoscopy every day, but consider it as a complement to other open surgery. One part of the process today, compared with when we started, is that staff can participate by having the right instruments in the operating room, so that they are familiar with all the equipment, stapler machines and so on. To be a good alert nurse during laparoscopic procedures is not actually the same thing as being alert and participating in a large open abdominal procedure. One of the positive things about laparoscopy is that you can also participate by watching the procedure on the TV monitor. The disadvantage is that the surgeons are very concentrated on their work, watching it on the screen. Because of this I feel that the contact with the surgeon is not as good as in open surgery, and this represents a deterioration in our working environment.

Nurses change to high-tech engineers

The new surgical techniques have been accompanied by the introduction of a range of new machines and electronic equipment. These are surgical instruments with a very new look. A whole new vocabulary has accompanied this change. Three-chip cameras with digital videorecorders; TV monitors with carbon dioxide insufflators with flow and pressure meters; cable light sources, straight and angled endoscopes are only some of the new tools to deal with. New applications of monopolar and bipolar electrocoagulation instruments, as well as endoscopic Argon lasercoagulation and endoscopic ultrasound, are other examples.

Very little in the education of perioperative nurses was concerned with dealing with the function of these tools. How electrocautery works with carbon dioxide and other such questions had not been included in our education. Of course we had been taught about electrocautery, but these things can be hard to understand. As a consequence we had to learn a lot of new things by ourselves. When MAS techniques started the surgeons did not seem to know much about this equipment either. Gradually, knowledge has increased in our department. Systematic education for nurses about MAS was only introduced once the new surgery was established. Today, we have company representatives who come to the hospital to introduce new instruments.

It is also necessary to continually inform the staff at internal meetings so that all nurse colleagues understand the instruments, their maintenance and how to use them. A close contact with the product market is necessary as well as meetings where staff can test the equipment and have the opportunity for hands-on training. How does the stapler machine work? How do you connect the video-tower when it does not work? The interest is obvious and the wish to learn. Even though company representatives come into the department to introduce new equipment, it is not unusual to find that you have to assist each other within the operating room to connect the equipment and ensure that all is working correctly.

Another change in the working environment is lack of space. Video-towers for laparoscopy and a large number of other electronic machines, such as ultrasound equipment, monitoring equipment, and mobile X-ray machines occupy a lot of space. This increases the need for large operating theatres and large spaces for pre- and postoperative care. Since it is not easy to adapt the buildings, the working area has a tendency to become more and more crowded, both within and outside the operating room.

In recent years, there has been a reduction in hospital economic resources in Sweden, just as in the rest of the world. As a consequence, the working tempo has increased. At the same time, the introduction of MAS has increased the time occupied by instrument maintenance. Much of this instrument care has to be done manually and is very time consuming. You have to disassemble many of the instruments to be able to clean them. Take-apart instruments can be very complicated to handle and if you do not do it every day you forget how to put them together again.

Today, there are a number of different techniques for cleaning instruments. Ultrasound, dry sterilisation and different types of wet sterilisation with different chemical agents are used. Some of these methods include a number of steps before the instruments are ready to use again. This means that if you only have a limited number of instruments, endoscopes and light source cables, it will need a lot of planning every day to ensure that you do not run out of equipment. During a hectic day, you may not have time to take care of used instruments. This means that maintenance will be done late in the afternoon and by the evening shift. Since the frequency of MAS procedures is increasing all the time, the problem with maintenance is also growing.

Currently, only a limited number of surgeons are doing laparoscopic procedures. The surgeons who mainly perform them know how to handle the instruments and electronic equipment. To a certain extent, they have some understanding of instrument maintenance. This means that they also have to understand that instruments must be easy to take apart for cleaning, and that this is one of the aspects you have to consider when buying non-disposable equipment. The other surgeons know very little about the function of laparoscopic equipment or its maintenance. When new surgeons are starting to do laparoscopic surgery, this is difficult for the nurses, as this means more work for the staff which consumes both time and patience.

Technological understanding – an absolute necessity

The dream situation would be to have medically educated technicians responsible for all equipment who are always present in the operating room. These technicians would assist with all the machines and keep them functioning. There is also a need for a specially trained person for the cleaning, sterilisation and packing of instruments. The alternative is continuous teaching and learning how to handle the instruments and machines in a never-ending round of education. The information has to be continually repeated – a far cry from open surgery when you only cleaned your forceps and packed them for sterilisation.

It is not wise for too many nurses to become involved with MAS. Not only do you have to learn about the instruments you already have, but there are also a tremendous number of new things being introduced into patient care. The need for education is enormous. If you work in the MAS field, you will be able to follow the development of new instruments, but if for some reason you are not involved in this work for a while, it could be hard to catch up on your knowledge when you return. As has been explained, company representatives regularly come to the department with new products, which everyone gets a chance to examine and to handle. In a large department, such as ours, you notice that there are always nurses who are unfamiliar with endoscopic instruments. Perhaps we should have one nurse whose only occupation would be full-time or part-time teaching about these instruments.

Continuous need for education

Today, it has become necessary to have specially trained nurses whose main responsibility is to work with minimal access surgery. These nurses have to learn new things and teach others. In this position you have to have a close contact with the product suppliers, but you also have to attend workshops, courses and other meetings to stay up to date with news. For nurses, it can also be valuable to attend medical conferences such as the Congress of the European Association of Endoscopic Surgeons (EAES) and to visit product exhibitions at other congresses and conferences.

Accountability

It is impossible to have a complete overview of the rules and laws you have to take into account when you start to use new instruments. Today, the European Community has decided that all equipment should have a certain standard (ISO 2000) and a special CE marking. When new electronic equipment is being purchased, the machines are disassembled and completely checked by our hospital engineers before we are allowed to take them into the operating department. They are aware of all the regulations and standards and are able to assist us with our technical problems. This way they guarantee the safety of our equipment in our environment.

We also have contact with a 'hygiene nurse' with whom we discuss the cleaning and sterilisation of laparoscopic instruments so that we can avoid contamination. We have special rules for patients with blood-borne viral infections. Special precautions are used and the operating room is cleaned with disinfectant after the procedures. In laparoscopic surgery there is a new factor about which we are still unsure. The risk from penetrating wounds from suture needles may be reduced and we think that laparoscopic procedures may be a safer approach with these high-risk patients.

On the other hand, there is a new phenomenon, namely aerosol spray from the trocar ports in the abdominal wall. Smoke from electrocautery, fogging and fat drops released by ultrasound cutters may escape from the ports and be inhaled by members of the surgical team. Little is yet known of the risks and consequences of this.

As we learn to prevent certain types of infection, others take their place. Although we apply new standard routines for cleaning after every patient to avoid the risk of contamination, new routes of microbial spread and new risks of infection are encountered, due to changing surgical practice.

As a patient I want a doctor who knows what he is doing. The reputation of minimal access surgery in Sweden has not so far been shattered by any malpractice accidents. Nurses, as well as patients, have a positive view regarding laparoscopic surgery. There are only small scars after this type of surgery and the time in hospital is short. There are people who are sceptical about the benefits of laparoscopic surgery versus open surgery but patients continue to request MAS. On the other hand, patients are hardly able to reflect on who is the most skilled or well-qualified surgeon.

On the question of nurse involvement in the new surgical developments, I think that the surgeons must be responsible for the operative procedure, but nurses have much to contribute to the development of new instruments. How easy is an instrument to take apart? Is it easy to clean and reassemble? How is it to be sterilised? Should it be disposable? Is recycling a cumbersome process? Is it necessary to send it away for maintenance?

Easy handling is a necessity and nurses should participate in this development. Nurses do not usually openly criticise surgeons when they introduce new methods, but there is always a high degree of scepticism until an innovation has shown itself to be successful. The scepticism may then decrease, but you never cease to be critical.

Nurses do not have an influence on operative technique, that is not their profession, but I would like to see nurses having an influence on ergonomics, instrument handling and development. Some surgeons get very upset if nurses try to tell them what to do, but their involvement in the preoperative preparation and postoperative processing of instruments and equipment gives them a right to contribute to the development of those instruments and equipment.

Bibliography

Gordon, A.G. & Magos, A.L. 1989 The development of laparoscopic surgery. *Balliers Clin. Obstet, Gynaecol.* **3**, 429–49.

Edmondson, J. M. 1991 History of the instruments for gastrointestinal endoscopy. *Gastrointest. Endosc* **37**, S27–S56.

Davis, C.J. 1992 A history of endoscopic surgery. *Surg. Laparosc. Endosc.* **2**, 16–23.

Jacobaeus, H.C. 1910 Ueber die Moglichkeit die Zystoscopie bei Untersuchung seroser Hohlunge anzuwenden. *Munch. Med. Wochenschr.* **57**, 2090–92.

Gruendemann, B. J. & Fernsebner, B. 1995 *Comprehensive perioperative nursing.* Volumes I & II. Boston, Jones & Bartlett.

Arregui, M.E., Fitzgibbons, R. J., Katkhouda, N., McKernan, J. B. & Reich, H. 1995 *Principles of laparoscopic surgery: basic and advanced techniques.* Berlin, Springer Verlag.

Supporting a surgical revolution

14

Nicole Nightingale Sinclair

Introduction
Cost is not the only issue
Purchasing
Training
New procedures
Conclusion
Reflective activities

This chapter is a response to the description by Inger Lonroth of the effects of the intro-
duction of minimal access surgery (MAS). Until recently the author, Nicole Sinclair,
worked as a company representative. She has worked for two major companies, one making
and selling endosurgery instrumentation, the other endoscopic equipment.

It is refreshing to have a different viewpoint from this new member of the operative
team who is now increasingly seen inside the operating theatre during operations. The
new viewpoint brings into focus some of the more commercial aspects of choosing and
buying surgical equipment and instruments. At the same time it is obvious that there is
an ethical aspect in choosing equipment which can be respected when buying from a
company which also observes ethical standards. Although the author refers throughout
to the 'company representative' she emphasises the extension of the representative's role
in assisting in the training of the surgical team in the use, maintenance and care of
instruments and equipment used in minimal access surgery.

Introduction

The following are extracts from *Principles and Practice of Surgical Laparoscopy*
(Pateson-Brown & Garden, 1994) and are perhaps best described as the basis on
which the best laparoscopic surgeons work. The principles discussed form the
basis of the current rules and regulations governing the way surgeons are
trained to carry out minimal access surgery (MAS). The good medical
equipment companies are aware of these principles and actively promote and

support training of surgeons based on those principles and assist with the implementation of MAS practice.

It has now certainly become possible to carry out extremely complex procedures on the abdominal and/or thoracic wall. The question that remains to be answered is whether the advantages of this type of approach are sufficient to make them a new standard against which conventional open surgery, with its big exposures and precise Halstedian dissection, should be judged. ... The great plus point for endoscopic surgery in the chest and abdomen is that it avoids the physiological disturbance which is caused by the incision and the distraction of structures required to gain access.

It is reasonably certain that we have underestimated these matters and have tended blindly to ascribe all the diverse features of the response to injury to the operation as a whole rather than to specific aspects such as the extent of the wound required, eventration and the handling of viscera.

The objective biological evidence is not yet fully available ... but it is striking that patients are often so little disturbed by endoscopic procedures that they are able to leave hospital much earlier than convention would expect.

It is reasonable for endoscopic surgeons to assume that they have almost completely removed the 'wound factor' both in relation to its general effects and also, of more importance to the patient, in terms of the subjective disturbance created by pain which is also an important trigger of adaptive events. It is, however, as yet unclear whether endoscopic surgery may not lead to problems of its own.

...as in all forms of laparoscopic surgery, the lessons learnt from years and years of open surgery must not be abandoned just to simplify the laparoscopic approach ... rigorous preoperative and postoperative assessment should be carried out, not just for clinical audit and subsequent publication but as a quality control for the surgeon so that the technique can be monitored constantly, and, if necessary, improved upon.

Pateson-Brown & Garden (1994).

At the risk of 'teaching my grandmother to suck eggs' what follows is my personal view of what ideally constitutes the alliance between theatre personnel and a company representative. A good company representative should be doing much more than just selling a product. They should be providing a wealth of services and information. If they are not doing so, ask yourself two questions:

1 Should I be getting more from my supplier(s)?

2 Do I want or need more from my supplier(s)?

You must then ascertain whether or not there are more services available.

When I was deciding which companies I would like to work for, I made a list of criteria I would expect in a company supplying endoscopic instruments.

available in a number of ways. All training related to the instrumentation should be offered by your supplier and your company representative should be able to advise you of availability and any cost implications.

Initial training

The training requirements may vary slightly for MPU and SPU as you will have cleaning and sterilising issues for MPU instruments as well as becoming adapt at assembling and disassembling the modular instruments. Inservice training is a free of charge service and should be offered as a matter of course. It may be advisable to discuss this with the company representative, the surgeon and anyone else on your team involved with the procedure to arrange a series of operations that will allow continuity of training for all involved. Inservice training periods are a good opportunity to identify any other training needs, such as procedure training. If you feel that you and your team would benefit from a formal training course discuss this with your company representative. Although most companies have training budgets for both medical and nursing staff, many hospitals have strict guidelines about accepting what could be interpreted as 'gifts'.[2]

Study days can be a difficult topic. The time is available but not the money or vice versa. If attending a company organised training course is going to cause problems talk to the company representative about holding a formal training course in your unit.

The importance of good training cannot be over-stressed. In order to ensure your patient receives the best possible care and a good outcome from their operation, the surgeon will have (should have) received the appropriate training, the anaesthetist will be familiar with the possible risks. With the advances in MAS you may be seeing an increasingly elderly population with multiorgan disease who previously were not candidates for any invasive technique. Anaesthetic and recovery nurses should be advised of the possible complications. Again, the company representative may be able to advise on any training courses available. Your training requirements should be discussed at the outset and formalised.

New procedures

A team approach to new procedures is much the best approach. Many of the better companies are adopting this technique when offering training courses. The advantages are many but the fact that nursing staff are included from the beginning of the journey means that the whole procedure will run more smoothly once it moves into your operating theatre. This style of training means that more personnel will be out of the department and could potentially cause unwelcome disruption within the department. Bearing this in mind it is worth getting management involved by supplying them with information they find 'interesting'.

Interesting information to hospital management is generally about cost, and occasionally about kudos. New procedures need to offer more to the hospital than just a better operation for the patient. Usually they require an amount of financial investment. Therefore, new procedures must show:

- A definite benefit in the outcome for the patient.
- An overall cost saving to your hospital.
- An overall cost saving to the NHS.

This goes back to the 'silo mentality' and may need some work. Again the company representative can supply you or the management group with the right information. The other benefits are generally considered to be more global and perhaps of interest to the government and the 'world economy'. If patients are recovering better and getting back to work quicker they are more productive individuals. They do not require as much sick pay and are, therefore, less of a 'burden' on the rest of the population. If patient benefits are good, and it has to be said that on the whole the benefits to MAS patients are numerous, and the rest of the population benefits too, then MAS can only be a beneficial step forward.

Conclusion

These benefits can only be reaped if the whole team feels there will be benefits. The only way that this can be communicated is if there is a team and if the information is readily available. Your company representative is your best resource for much of the information, either directly or as a sounding board. It has been my experience both personally and from observing other successful company representatives that the success for the theatre team and the company representative is when the objectives and goals of both parties are the same. This is only achievable by discussion. It is a fact of life that communication plays a major part in this success and this often comes down to personalities. I hope this has given you some food for thought. For those of you who are already lucky enough to have good working relationships, I hope this may help to reassure you that you are covering all the bases. Noone has all the answers. We can all learn something every day, but by questioning what we do we can be sure we are heading in the right direction.

Reflective activities

A main issue which you may like to reflect on after reading this chapter is the question of multiple or single use products. There is a considerable amount of discussion in the perioperative nursing press on the topic. The *British Journal of Theatre Nursing* Supplement named in the references contains considerable information and is well-referenced (NATN, 1995). It discusses the arguments in some detail. As this is still a new and developing field of surgery with constant implications for operating department practices, you should also refer to recent publications in your own country and language and keep yourself up-to-date with manufacturers' recommendations on the care, use and storage of instruments and equipment.

Useful addresses

The following addresses are useful contact points for information on further training and education on minimal invasive surgery. Minimal access therapy (MAT) is a term which can be used to cover all non-invasive procedures and is preferred by some, as in MATTU – minimal access therapy training unit.

Ms P Dunkley
Surgical Skills Unit
Ninewell Hospital
Dundee
Tayside
DD1 9BY

Miss C Caballero
Laparaoscopic Nurse Practitioner
Milton Keynes General NHS Trust
Standing Way, Eaglestone
Milton Keynes MK6 5LD

Alison Snook
Unit Manager, MATTU
Royal Surrey County Hospital
Guildford
Surrey GU2 5XX

Mr J O'Leary
Training Manager
MASTER Unit
Royal Liverpool Hospital
Prescott St
Liverpool L7 8XP

Brenda Valdez
Laparoscopic Course Convenor
Main Theatres
Royal London Hospital
Whitechapel
London E1 1BB

Endnote

1 The term 'silo mentality' means only considering the financial implication of your part of the patient treatment and ignoring the total picture.
2 Refer back to Chapter 12 for the ethics of company sponsored training and education.

References

Pateson-Brown, S. & Garden, J. 1994 *Principles and practice of surgical laparoscopy.* London, W B Saunders, pp 289.

Bell, S. 1998 Multiple patient use vs single patient use products. *British Journal of Theatre Nursing* **8** (1) Supplement.

NATN. 1995 *Use, re-use and misuse of single use items. A position statement.* Harrogate, NATN.

Further reading

European Directive 1993: Medical Directive 93/42 (CE marking).

Medical Devices Agency. 1995 *The re-use of medical devices supplied for single use only.* MDA. DB 9501.

Plowes, D. 1995 Re-using or misusing? *British Journal of Theatre Nursing* **5** (1), 22–2.

Note: You are also referred to Chapter 10 for further discussion on the question of single use or multiple use instruments.

Preliminary Training School with a statutory 'Preliminary, Part I', examination at the end of this time. 'Prelim Part II' was taken at the end of the first year of training. Allocation to wards or departments was often of nine weeks duration, with rotation to night duty as well.

If you were lucky, theoretical study was by the 'Block' system of 4 or more weeks duration, when full-time education took place, with no ward work involved. Hospital Final examinations were taken at the end of the third year and had to be passed before the student was allowed to sit the State Registration Final examination. In teaching hospitals, a fourth year had to be served in order to receive the hospital badge and certificate. Nurses were paid monthly, in cash, and had to line up on the appropriate day at the specified time in order to receive their salary. A board and lodging deduction, income tax, insurance and superannuation contributions meant that for the first few months the student nurse was unlikely to earn more than the princely sum of £7 per month.

Training usually included 3 months' theatre experience in the second or third year in a very junior capacity. Drapes, mops, dressings, gowns, gloves and other sundries were packed in perforated steel drums by the theatre staff, then autoclaved elsewhere in the hospital, a process which took several hours. Surgical instruments were kept in a cupboard or cabinet in the theatre itself and the scrub nurse would select what she needed for a procedure, sterilising the instruments by immersion in boiling water for 10 minutes minimum. Stainless steel bowls, gallipots and receivers were sterilised in the same way, but in a larger and deeper steriliser. Heavy bowl-grasping forceps were needed for these items, but the instruments could be retrieved with Cheatles forceps (of blessed memory!) Glass syringes were used and had to be prepared in a smaller boiling steriliser. Sterile water was prepared from larger vessels specially for the purpose and stored in sterile stainless steel jugs with lids – for use throughout the list.

Suture materials in use were catgut, linen and silk in the main. Silk and linen thread arrived on large reels, and measured amounts were transferred to steel 'eggs', and boiled as necessary. Catgut was packed in alcohol in waisted glass tubes which had to be either opened with a steel tube 'catgut breaker', or smashed in a gauze swab with a sharp blow in a strategic place using a Spencer-Wells forceps. Either way, the catgut had to be separately rinsed and dried in sterile water by the scrub nurse before the required length could be cut and the needle threaded up.

Sharps, such as suture needles, hypodermic needles, bistouries, blades and fine scissors were kept in a solution of Lysol, a phenolic preparation, in a large lidded 'sharps dish'. The scrub nurse removed the required items aseptically from the dish, and rinsed them in sterile water before use. It was important to know the names of the instruments, recognise the size and nature of needles, plus the variety and gauge of suture material to be used.

Used gloves were rinsed and dried after use, tested for leaks, patched if necessary, paired, then packed in linen envelopes with a talcum powder ball, painstakingly prepared by the night or weekend staff. Large 'chest mops' were often reused after soaking overnight in a hypochlorite solution before being rinsed, dried, folded and repacked. Dressings too, had to be cut from large rolls, folded to the required size and packed into drums for processing. There was usually plenty to do during any quiet moments, for the juniors, anyway! At least in theatres there were no hated sputum pots to be washed after the contents had been measured and recorded!

Nursing working conditions in the 1960s

This was a period of rapid economic growth in the country, leading to expansion of health care services along with increasing technology. The MOH became increasingly concerned to rationalise and control expansion, and to this end the Department of Health and Social Security was formed in 1968, responsible for personal social services, health and social security. 'Planning' was introduced into the NHS, and attempted to improve management in the most capital intensive sector, the hospital service.

During this decade it was increasingly recognised that the workforce in the NHS was increasing in size and complexity. There was greater division of labour and new specialities were developing. According to Allsop, the total number of staff employed in the NHS in England in 1949 was 400 000, but by 1980 there had been a two-fold increase to 822 390. Nurses then comprised 37% of the workforce with a great variety of paramedical professionals appearing as technology advanced. The NHS is probably still the largest civilian employer in the UK.

The response of the authorities to the ever-increasing size of the NHS labour force was to adopt a managerialist approach in the search for control. To this end, in 1966, a Committee was set up to look at the reorganisation of nursing services which was suffering from another manpower crisis. The Report on Senior Nursing Staff Structure recommended a division between managers and practitioners, to provide a basis for organising the work under a scheme of scientific management. The critical shortage of nursing staff prompted the government to undertake a review of the profession under the chairmanship of Brian Salmon, a businessman from Lyons, the food distributors.

The Salmon Report as it was inevitably called, published in 1969, created new management structures for nursing, establishing the local professional head of nursing as an equal to his/her medical and administrative colleagues. Management grades were created under the title of Senior Nursing Officer (Grade 8), Nursing Officer (Grade 7), Sister (Grade 6), with staff nurses, enrolled nurses and auxiliaries forming the lower, non-management grades. This imposed a new management structure which swept away nurse matrons, replacing them with a hierarchy of nurse managers.

CENTRALISATION OF STERILE SUPPLIES

Introduction of the pre-set tray system (modified Edinburgh Tray System) during this decade and the establishment of Theatre Sterile Supply Units (TSSU) locally, or Central Sterile Supply Units (CSSD) supplying several units with sterile goods, partially removed one set of responsibilities from the operating theatre team, that of processing and sterilising surgical instruments. Whereas three sets of instruments (or less) for a particular procedure in a theatre (one set in use, one dirty and one clean in cupboard) would have been sufficient when processed in the department, massive amounts of new instruments had to be purchased to cope with the exigencies of new surgical procedures, centralised laundry facilities, and the turnround time for processing and repacking the trays.

A variety of systems developed locally to meet these demands. Since heat-labile and delicate instrumentation still had to be processed in the department, the general availability of, so-called, cold 'sterilising' solutions began, when the toxic effects of formaldehyde preparations, in general use for heat-labile items, was demonstrated. This particular aspect regarding variables involved in instrument preparation failed to be properly recognised by management so the continuing cost of operating department activities was never accurately quantified.

The careful daily manual maintenance and conservation of the instrumentation in use in theatres diminished when processing was transferred to a central location. Mechanical instrument washers with prewash detergent and postwash lubrication cycles automated the drudgery and the health risks involved, but transport and collection restrictions meant that dirty instruments were often not processed for several days, especially over weekends and public holidays. Used instruments, therefore, had to be processed more than once in order to remove the dried-on debris, creating log-jams in the CSSD, and extending turnround times. Nor is it possible for a person who never sees delicate instruments in use to readily understand the care needed to maintain them, especially if there is constant pressure to process the instruments quickly.

Autoclave breakdowns at a central location could have enormous effects peripherally, as could disruption in laundry and transport, on the collection of used instruments and delivery of sterile sets and supplies. Centralisation of hospital stores and other supplies led to a huge proliferation in paperwork and long delays in transactions, encouraging 'hoarding' of vital consumables.

Balancing projected requirements with actual work performed, consumables utilised and available manpower has always been, and continues to remain, virtually a juggling act of the multitude of variables involved.

During the decade, surgical specialisation began to be developed, requiring additional paramedical personnel and the first report of the Cogwheel Working Party, published by the MOH in 1967, on the organisation of medical work in hospitals was an attempt to create more managerial consciousness within the medical profession (Allsop, 1984, p.59). Cogwheel (so-called because of the design on the cover) recommended the groupings of clinicians into firms and divisions, with a Medical Executive Committee to make decisions concerning the allocation of medical resources over the hospital as a whole.

Lewin Report (1970)

The Hospital Inpatient Inquiry statistics between 1961 and 1963 had shown an increase in surgical work of 28% in England and Wales.

- 1961:   1.8 million operations carried out
- 1963:   2.3 million operations carried out
- 1968/69: 2.5 million operations carried out in major theatres only, although the Report does not specify what constituted a major theatre.

This report, entitled 'The Organisation and Staffing of Operating Departments', chaired by Mr Walpole Lewin, consultant surgeon, was the report of a Joint Sub-Committee of the Standing Medical and Standing Nursing Advisory Committees of the Central Health Services Committee of the Department of Health and Social Security.

The report calculated that there was a major shortage of staff in operating theatres in England and Wales, with probably 7000 nurses and 2000 operating theatre attendants working in 19 000 operating theatres – 78% nurses and 22% operating theatre attendants. This report led to the establishment of the Operating Department Assistant, and a nationally agreed training course for this grade of staff, under the Ancillary Staffs (Whitley Council) terms and conditions of service, and not on the Technical and Scientific Staffs structure as proposed in the Zuckerman Report on the Professions allied to Medicine.

The Lewin Report also made other recommendations:

- Operating Department Orderly grades of staff to carry out portering and cleaning duties within the department.
- Specific training requirements for both State Registered and State Enrolled Nurses.
- Provision for permanent night staff to reduce the long working hours, and the 'on call' and 'standby' commitments.
- Provision for payment for 'on call' and 'standby' duties.
- Setting up of Operating Department Committees for the organisation and management of Operating Departments.
- Integration of operating department services with the total hospital services.
- Staffing, training, education and career structures for operating theatre personnel.
- Development of CSSD and TSSUs on a regional and hospital group basis.

Following this report, payment for on call/standby duties commenced. Nursing staff received a specific sum for an 8-hour on call period, whilst ODAs received a small hourly payment for the same period, as ancillary staff. Prior to this period, any overtime incurred on standby and on call had to recovered on a 'time in lieu' basis, with inevitable problems. The payment for these duties, while some compensation for the inconvenience and long hours involved does nothing to lessen the cumulative fatigue still being experienced by today's theatre staff in yet another crisis of acute staff shortages.

NHS reorganisation in 1974

The reorganisation of the NHS in 1974 was designed to produce a more effi-cient and effective service through a change in structure and by the intro-

Career structures effectively vanished along with permanent contracts as General Management has taken over. The working day has been extended for more flexible working hours and now it seems that even more overtime is necessary to cover ever widening gaps in the service. The resultant demoralisation seems to have been the beginning of the major recruitment and retention crisis which faces the NHS and which is particularly severe in those specialised and more highly qualified branches of the profession such as intensive care and perioperative nursing.

Nurse education

As can be seen from the brief historical notes, the education of nurses has mostly reflected the knowledge base of the period, with emphasis on meeting the physical needs of the patient and the cleanliness and order of his environment. There was, in the past, a distinct emphasis on 'task allocation', with tasks delegated according to the level of seniority of the nursing staff. Thus juniors were entrusted with basic hygiene needs, whilst the seniors undertook more complex tasks like dressings and drug administration (Clifford, 1996). The medical management of care was transmitted by the doctor to the Ward Sister and through her to the nursing staff and ancillaries. There was little multidisciplinary work, and roles were jealously guarded. This attitude could be said to have a parallel with industry, where workers were trained to develop optimal performance in relation to a task in order to increase productivity.

During the decades of the 1960s and 1970s the increasing awareness of the psychological and sociological implications and knowledge began to make an impact on nursing and nurse education, with the emergence of nursing models and philosophies of care (Clifford, 1996).

With the publication of the Salmon Report in 1969, policy management was separated from front-line management. The top management, Chief Nursing Officers created policy; middle management, Nursing Officers programmed policy; and the first line managers, Ward/Department Sisters implemented policy. Increasing bureaucracy distanced middle managers from patient care although first line managers continued to retain authority over clinical practice.

Changes in nurse education evolved over the years and by the early 1980s it was recognised that appropriate skills training for the job was necessary at all levels. Project 2000 was launched as a new way of preparing nurses for the future, providing an appropriate knowledge base for a nurse educated to diploma or degree level who would be a 'knowledgeable doer' (UKCC, 1986). This necessitated moving nurse education into higher education establishments and away from the hospital base. Nursing students, for the first time would become university undergraduates with full-time study programmes and clinical placements, and were to be no longer employees, but given full student status. Entry gates to the profession had been widening over the years and students entered from a wide diversity of backgrounds with equally diverse educational attainments and life experiences.

European legislation has significantly affected nurse training since the first document appeared in 1967. This was 'The European agreement on the Instruction and Education of the Nurse', produced by the Council of Europe. The first European Community (EC) Directives on the training of nurses in General Care were published in 1977, when the Advisory Committee on Training for Nurses (ACTN) was established. The work of this group led to the amendments of the Training Directive regarding balance between theory and practice, leading to the reorganisation of nurse training upon the agreed formula for a common period of training to be recognised throughout Europe. The 'Project 2000' proposals for nurse education in the UK were a direct result of the European legislation in nurse training, and the harmonisation programme. Due to their hard work over a period of 4 years, representatives of the National Association of Theatre Nurses of the UK in conjunction with representatives of perioperative nursing groups in a number of European countries have developed an agreed European Common Core Curriculum for Operating Room Nursing.[5]

Effects of European legislation

Europe has also had an influence on the working environment. A Directive on the minimum health and safety requirements for the manual handling of loads was published in 1990. This led to the Manual Handling Regulations of 1993, with its needs for the assessment of handling and moving of loads, and the annual update of Lifting and Moving and training requirements in all areas, including specialist areas such as the operating theatres which had often been left to organise such training themselves in the past.

Other European legislation affecting the workplace includes the European Medicines Evaluation Agency, January 1995 (Brett 1997), Producer Responsibility Obligations regarding packaging waste, and CE marking for medical devices, among other things.[6] New European legislation (General Medical Device EC42/93) on standards of surgical instrument sterilisation, safe decontamination of medical devices, and care, maintenance and safe processing of such devices is pending at time of writing. This has major implications for all operating departments since current practices will inevitably be brought under scrutiny, and may well be found wanting since most departmental reprocessing procedures have no audit facilities to ensure 'sterility assurance'.

The health care service changes dating from this period have induced ever more turmoil, with a marked increase in the turnover of patients in the hospital and intensive monitoring of hospital activity, outcomes and expenditure. Changes in unit design to smaller ward units has not had the desired effect of reducing labour costs. An open plan 'Nightingale' ward was more easily staffed and supervised than numbers of smaller bed bays although this arrangement could be seen as more patient-friendly. The capital charges arising from new purpose-built units were, strangely, not properly accounted for by Health Authorities and the additional costs of running new units seemed not to have been appreciated either. Greater patient activity and turnover must necessarily result in increased costs at all levels, staffing, consumables, and every kind of service required throughout the day or night.

Day surgery

As a 'value for money' exercise, day surgery units were deemed to be the most cost-effective in treating larger numbers of patients requiring surgery, since the costs of an overnight stay in hospital accommodation with its attendant expenses was absent. However, large numbers of short-stay cases require additional staff to look after them safely and effectively, and more patient throughput inevitably results in increased use of consumables with greater costs implications. It escapes me how this could be otherwise!

Additionally, all the many facilities of the day surgery units now lie fallow and unoccupied for 108 hours out of the 168 hours in a week, which hardly makes too much sense regarding the 90% usage level advocated by the Bevan Report!

The increased use of all operating theatre facilities throughout the UK has inevitably resulted in reduction in available maintenance time since maintenance of whatever description, be it just a thorough clean of the drip-stand or the anaesthetic machine now has to be done outside working hours.

Surgeons are constantly pressured by management dictats to keep up the throughput of patients, and teaching and training of staff may be minimal in this climate. A rise in 'consumerism' would also seem to have led to greater demands for the type of surgery the patient perceives as his need and right as patient awareness and expectations increase in line with increased media attention to health issues.

Urgent and 'fast-track' cases for surgery are required to be dealt with in a specified time scale in the regulations, resulting in even more pressure on surgeons and rearrangement of operating lists. In my experience, the published operating list is practically a thing of the past in day surgery terms, since patients may or may not turn up and may have changed their mind about surgery under local anaesthesia, withdrawn their consent for surgery, be unfit, or the condition requiring surgery may have resolved. (The lump or bump may have disappeared.) In other words, the surgical team may not know what patient they are going to be operating on until they see the whites of the patient's eyes! Today's operating list is only an approximation of what may happen in terms of surgery performed. (If I'm honest, in the past that was not such an unknown occurrence either, although it was not deemed to take place, and had different causal factors.)

'Day surgery' would appear to be a misnomer anyway, and '4-hour surgery' would be a more accurate description of what currently takes place in many units. A number of patients are admitted for surgery on the morning list and are expected to be recovered and discharged in time for the next lot of patients due for operations in the afternoon. These afternoon patients may have an even shorter time for recovery since the unit closes before 20.00 hours and all patients have to be discharged by that time to avoid an overnight stay. More 'efficient' use of the operating department resource would seem to have led to even greater inefficiencies and dubious compromises in attempts to comply with Patient's Charter standards and management demands (Patient's Charter, 1995).

The increased throughput of patients for surgery needs more staff time of whatever grade, medical or non-medical, and more consumption of services at all levels, inevitably increasing ALL costs. Increased use of certain equipment and apparatus such as endoscopes and imaging devices will, without a doubt, result in a shortened life for the item, and revenue consequences for expensive replacements. The tyranny of technology means that if you have the equipment, it must be used regardless, because every operating department wants to be seen to be performing in an innovative manner.

Contracting-out for maintenance services arrangements has led to difficulties, with crisis management being largely the order of the day, in the probably mistaken belief that money will be saved. This may be true in the short term, but the ever-increasing use of all technology has implications for the risk managers, and the proper evaluation of cost-benefit.

Cleaning arrangements for the operating theatre have also been a casualty in the drive to cut costs and the daily scrubbing of floors, regular wall-washing programmes and fabric maintenance, formerly deemed essential hygiene requirements for the department have been pared to the minimum, apart from statutory obligations such as pressure vessels (autoclaves) and lifts. Is it any wonder that methycillin resistant *staphylococcus aureus* (or worse) is present in most operating department suites throughout the country and is, therefore, a threat to any vulnerable individual coming through the door?[7]

Away from the operating department, the consultants' outpatient clinics are also subject to increased pressure, with 'walk-in' and 'fast-track' arrangements for consultations agreed by the local GP practice. Additional consultant appointments do not necessarily mean more work done if there are insufficient beds for admission of patients, and no staff to care for them either, following surgery.

The ever-increasing drive to cut costs has virtually eliminated all the older, experienced, skilled, knowledgeable personnel, these being too expensive in terms of salary. More responsibility is being devolved downwards to staff members who are not only expected to work vast amounts of overtime to cover the shortfalls, but also to undertake degree or diploma courses of postregistration education to maintain their professional profile. No increase in remuneration or additional benefits are offered by the employer, however. The European Directive on Working Time 93/104/EC, seeks to standardise patterns of working hours, with maximum and minimum requirements for daily and weekly work and rest periods. The NHS Management Executive published a document entitled 'The New Deal ' in 1991 reducing the hours worked by junior doctors and delegating to nurses some of the activities previously undertaken by medical staff.

Junior doctors' working hours

The decrease in the permitted working hours of junior doctors within the last few years has led to a variety of role-sectors being taken over by non-medically qualified staff, in order to cover the amount of work required. The erosion of the identified medical and nursing boundaries has possibly developed in a somewhat haphazard fashion, adapting to changing working practices and new skills which were previously the province of other professional groups. Successful multiskilling of the operating theatre workforce requires that roles should be clearly defined and that team members understand how each relates to the other.

Training, education, responsibilities and legal implications associated with the new roles for non-medical staff are admirably dealt with in 'Guidelines for Organisations and Employers Developing New Roles for Non-Medical Staff within Perioperative Care' (1997) published by the National Association of Theatre Nurses.

To what standards should these newly-skilled individuals aspire? Mini-doctor, maxi-nurse, advanced practitioner, nurse consultant or simply Jack-of-all-trades? How will they fit into the existing staffing structure and what tensions is this likely to create ? Will these new practitioners be able to carry out their role full-time or will they be expected to 'muck in' wherever necessary, whenever necessary? How do you keep your new skills bright and shining once you've got them, if you cannot practise them every day? We might also ask who is responsible for the new individual's clinical practise and to whom are they accountable, the nurse in charge, the medical staff, the directorate manager, self, their profession or a higher power? There are considerable legal implications for all existing health care professionals.

There are a host of other issues to consider for the future. The future of nursing is not clear. If a qualified nurse is a valuable resource it is possible that an increasing number of qualified nurses will be expected to justify their costs by operating at an advanced level of practice. The concept of educating all nurses to degree level seems to be flawed. We need many caring pairs of hands but those who finance nursing care seem to be happy to settle for lesser trained carers who are 'doers' but not 'knowledgeable'. The registered nurse could be a thing of the past, once the UKCC 's present term of office expires in 2003? Who creates health policy in the UK anyway – the government of the day, the medical profession, the population at large in the shape of the electorate or even the media, perhaps? It is health policy which will influence the future of the profession. Are our expectations of the NHS unrealistic anyway …?

What of the current Government and their avowed intent to dismantle the internal market for health, which I suppose everyone was just getting used to? Is it possible to go back, and how far back should it go? Employment conditions have changed radically to accommodate the economic climate and the perceived necessities of employers to meet the conditions. Can the relevant adjustments realistically be made? The 1997 White Paper, 'The New NHS: Modern, Dependable' rejects GP fundholding and new groups will bring together community nurses and GPs for primary health care commissioning. The new groups thus formed will (hopefully) work in partnership with local authority social services, and may become Primary Care Trusts eventually. Two new bodies are proposed for England and Wales, the National Institute for Clinical Excellence and a Commission for Health Improvement. The former takes over from Clinical Audit, focusing on clinical effectiveness, cost-effectiveness and producing clinical guidelines, an expanded remit. The latter body is designed to support and oversee the quality of clinical services, with special powers of intervention when problems arise. (Big Brother in disguise?)

A new 'taskforce' to be set up will concentrate on staff issues, and could be a golden opportunity for nurses to take a key role in shaping the NHS of the future. There is already the beginnings of a new nurse-led telephone advice service, 'NHS Direct', to give practical advice to callers who cannot visit their local GP or emergency department. It is aimed at reducing overcrowding in GP surgeries and Accident and Emergency Departments. Pilot helplines will be operating in various areas of England from March 1998, to be extended to cover the whole countryside by 2000, if proven successful.

Conclusion

So here we are again, 50 years after the NHS began, with yet another bout of reorganisation along with demands for unremitting extra work, not only in the clinical area, but to educate ourselves, to carry out research or to apply the results of research as well as feeding the voracious appetite for paper of the bureaucratic monster. But, there are opportunities to be seized. The new White Paper proposals include investment in research to develop the evidence base of nurse-led initiatives, which can identify the effectiveness of nursing practice and the value of nurses and nursing. At last, there is a realistic chance to prove that nurses do make a difference !

Reflective activities

Consider the descriptions of nurse education and of perioperative nursing in the 1950s and 1960s (p.304). How different was the perioperative nurse of that time to the perioperative nurse of today? How do you think nursing aspirations and relationships within the theatre team differed from those of the present?

1 Reflect on how events and changes have resulted in the development of the concept of perioperative practice and new advanced roles for nurses working and caring for patients during the perioperative period.

2 Two major government committees have considered the problems of staffing operating departments during the last 30 years – Lewin Report (1960) and Bevan Report (1989).

- What were the reasons for setting up the investigations?
- What were their findings?
- What were their recommendations?
- Do you agree with the recommendations? Were they implemented and have they been effective?

3 Have the changes, technological, professional, social, political and educational continued at such a rapid pace that the recommendations of Bevan have been superseded?

4 Are we now living and working in an environment of such rapid and continuous change that we have to be able to continually adapt to external change?

Endnotes

1 Comparison with contemporary practices at Guy's Hospital described in Chapter 1, may be of interest to the reader.

2 Refer to Chapter 1 for information on contemporary medical attitudes.

3 Removal of pay-beds from NHS hospitals destroyed an important part of hospital income, which could not be replaced. Hence the growth of private health care facilities, and competition with the NHS for appropriately skilled staff.

4 Many references are made in this chapter to White Papers and other government publications. Not all are included in the references list but the sources for the information are Allsop (1984), Ham (1986), Levitt and Wall (1994) and O'Neill (1989). All of these are included in the references to this chapter.

5 See Chapter 6 for work of EORNA to develop the Common Core Curriculum.

6 Regulations regarding waste disposal are also discussed in Chapter 6.

7 These comments make an interesting comparison with Domin's comments quoted in Chapter 10, p.223 when he emphasises the importance of good basic hygiene practices in the control of resistant miocroorganisms.

References

Abel-Smith, B. 1964 *The hospitals 1800–1948.* London, Heinemann.

Allsop, J. 1984 *Health policy and the National Health Service.* London, Longman.

Brett, M. 1997 Daisy Ayris Memorial Lecture. *British Journal of Theatre Nursing* 6 (11), 11–23.

Clifford, C. 1996 Managing care in nursing. In: Copcutt, L. & Clark, J. *Management for nurses and health care professionals.* London, Chapman and Hall.

Concise Oxford Dictionary, 5th edition. 1964 Oxford, Clarendon Press.

DOH. 1995 *The Patient's Charter.* London, HMSO.

Ham, C. 1986 *Health policy in Britain.* London, Macmillan Press.

Levitt, R., Wall, A. and Appleby, S. 1995 *The reorganised National Health Service*. London, Chapman and Hall.

NATN. 1997 *Guidelines for organisations and employers developing new roles for non-medical staff within perioperative care*. Harrogate, NATN.

O'Neill, C. 1989 *A picture of health*. Oxford, Meadow Books.

Porter, R. 1997 *The greatest benefit to mankind*. London, Harper Collins.

Seymer, L. P. 1956 *A general history of nursing*. 4th edition. London, Faber and Faber.

UKCC. 1986 *Project 2000. A new preparation for practice*. London, UKCC.

Reports

CEPOD Report. Buck, N., Devlin, B. & Lunn, J. N. 1987 *Report of a confidential enquiry into perioperative deaths*. London, Nuffield Provincial Hospitals Trust.

The Organisation and Staffing of Operating Departments. 1970 London, Department of Health and Social Security. HMSO Walpole Lewin (Chairman).

The Management and Utilisation of Operating Departments. 1989 NHS Management Executive Value for Money Unit. Prof P.G. Bevan (Chair)

Efficiency of Theatre Services. 1989 Association of Anaesthetists of Great Britain and Ireland and Association of Surgeons of Great Britain and Ireland.

National Association of Theatre Nurses. 1997 Guidelines for Organisations and Employers Developing New Roles for Non-Medical Staff.

Index

Note: page numbers in *italics* refer to figures and tables